The
DIET
CENTER
Program

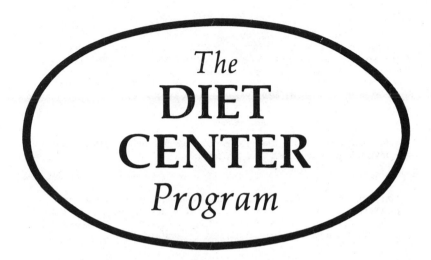

The
DIET
CENTER
Program

Lose Weight Fast
and Keep It Off Forever

SYBIL FERGUSON

Little, Brown and Company — Boston – Toronto

Fourth Printing

Before embarking on any diet or exercise program, including this one, it is advisable to consult with your physician.

"Diet Center" and "How To Win At The Losing Game" are Trademarks and Service Marks owned by Diet Center, Inc. and registered with the United States Patent Office. Rights to the use of such Trademarks are specifically reserved by Diet Center, Inc. — Rexburg, Idaho.

Illustrations by Craig Birch

9 8 7 6 5 4

I know I could never have developed the Diet Center Program alone. I dedicate this book to my husband, family and friends who have helped make all this a reality. And especially to the more than 4,000 Diet Center counselors whose sincere desire to help others is the heart and true spirit of Diet Center.

Contents

The
DIET
CENTER
Program

Foreword

IN 1970, I achieved personal success in conquering my weight problem. It was not based on traditional dieting methods, but on my own beliefs and knowledge gained through research and study. For eighteen years, I had struggled with excess weight, and at last, I had found the answer. I was able to help friends do what I had done; and as I watched them emerge with newfound self-confidence and enthusiasm for life, my own life took on new meaning and direction. It was my dream to help overweight and obese people everywhere who still suffered as I had.

The Diet Center Program represents my belief that you *can* become whatever you desire. This is a book about changing your life, believing in yourself, losing weight and learning to eat correctly so you can be free forever from the physical and emotional problems of being overweight.

Today, I love life! I look forward to getting up each morning and facing the challenges that each new day brings. I can now fully express the love I feel for my husband, Roger, my family, the life that I now have, and Diet Center. I have learned the invaluable lesson that before you can give love to others, you must first learn to love yourself. Each day I count my blessings. Through the concepts of the Diet Center Program, my life has totally changed. I have grown, reached out, and developed my potential. When I was overweight, I could not face people, much less speak in front of a group. Today, I can stand before thousands at an international convention and freely express myself without fear or insecurity. It is a wonderful feeling.

I want to share with you the story of how Diet Center began and how it grew. I want you to understand that I personally know the pain and suffering every overweight person endures. I can only hope that as you read this book, you will come to understand that you are not alone and that you will feel, "She is right! It seems impossible, but if she and millions of others can make such changes in their lives, so can I!" Because I know it is true . . . if you believe you can do it, you can.

I offer *The Diet Center Program* as a promise to every one of the eighty million overweight men, women, and children in this country today that there is a solution — a permanent solution. *The Diet Center Program* can be your guide to better health, a positive self-image, and a slim, new you. Overcoming obesity does not require drastic measures. It can be achieved through simple knowledge and application. *The Diet Center Program* is not just a diet; it is a whole new way of living.

I have included in *The Diet Center Program* a list of criteria by which you can evaluate any weight-loss method, including Diet Center's. I know that overweight people are misled and victimized by fads, gimmicks, and unhealthful diets in their search for a solution that works. I also know that the vast majority of these methods have no chance for long-term success. Overweight people are a tremendous "target market" for profit-oriented big business. Over forty billion dollars was spent last year on books, formal programs, diet foods, exercise equipment, and proposed miracle cures all promising magical results. Tragically, all these efforts result in a nationwide success rate of less than 4 percent! I believe that the only effective program is one that is based on genuine concern for the individual, one that can be expanded to meet your needs for a lifetime . . . a program that places the responsibility and control where it belongs — with you.

Presented in this book are the philosophies of Diet Center. I first learned these insights twelve years ago, and I still stand behind these basic beliefs today, although they have been expanded through continual research and study. Counting nutrients instead of calories, maintaining a stable blood sugar level, and losing the "right" type of fat are examples of philosophies that originated with Diet Center.

Selecting the right foods to eat requires knowledge of how those foods affect your body, both physically and mentally. You must gain control of your life to gain control of your weight. *The Diet Center Program* provides that insight in simple, understandable terms. It is not just a list of foods or a selection of recipes. It is a guide that will provide you with the "why" as well as the "what," a tool that anyone concerned with personal health and sound nutrition can use to make life better.

Also explained are the basic elements that form the foundation of the Diet Center Program: a nutritionally sound and well-balanced diet, our nutrition education and behavior modification series that teaches relaxation and visualization techniques, goal setting, stress management, and the importance of sensible exercise ... and especially, the basis of all Diet Center Diets — the Diet Center Reducing Diet. Again, I have explained not only what, when and how much to eat, but why these foods, in specific combinations, are so important. I have tried, as much as possible, to convey these feelings throughout this book.

At Diet Center, losing weight is only half the battle. Sections IX and X of this book will show you how to remain slim and self-confident forever. They will provide you with practical suggestions for incorporating sound nutrition and self-direction into everyday life. Your grocery shopping list may change forever after reading about food additives and learning how to read labels. Diet Center recipes will show you just how appetizing and satisfying a balanced diet can be, and how easy and inexpensive it is to provide nutritious meals for yourself and your family. The only way to maintain both ideal weight and good health is to develop a nutritional consciousness that you can apply directly to your life.

Diet Center is today, without question, one of the most comprehensive and successful weight-control programs. More important, it can come to be a symbol for you that anything is possible and proof that you can achieve a happier, healthier life and be a slim, self-confident, and self-directed individual.

Introduction

EACH week, I receive hundreds of letters from people across the United States and Canada, describing their success at Diet Center. I try to answer each and every one of these letters. For you see, I know the suffering that comes with being overweight and the wonderful changes that can occur in anyone's life by conquering obesity.

Like millions of other men, women and children, I suffer from the chronic illness of obesity. (Perhaps you've never thought of obesity as an illness; but believe me, it is!) My own memories of how it felt to get up in the morning, dreading another day, are still very real to me. No one can understand what it feels like to be an obese person without having been in that situation.

Twelve years ago, I weighed fifty-eight pounds more than I do today. I used to avoid the sidelong glances at my image in store windows. I used to rush through stores so I could hurry back to the security of my home. I was embarrassed to try on clothes. I was growing out of a size 18, and everything that fit looked like tents, with no style or selection.

Anything and everything seemed to hurt me. I remember overhearing my little daughter say to one of her friends. "Don't say 'fat.' It always makes Mommy cry." Another time a little five-year-old asked me when I was going to have a baby. I was sure that my husband, Roger, could no longer love me. I was so touchy that I took everything he said personally. I was convinced that I was not worthy of being loved. I was very unsure of myself, and I was certain he was ashamed of the way I looked, even though he was always kind and reassuring and careful to avoid words like *overweight, fat,* and *obese.*

I felt so alone — a failure. I kept trying so hard to lose weight. No matter what I did, it seemed the pounds would quickly drop, only to reappear with even a few more added on. My short-lived joy would again revert to feelings of personal failure. I was always depressed, exhausted, and hungry. I knew that I had to lose weight or lose my sanity.

It felt as if I were trapped in a maze, with every new diet or book or pill offering help but turning into a dead end. I felt locked into being obese and unhappy forever. I remember parking in a dark, deserted lot and crying because I hated my body and even myself. I remember thinking, "They are putting men on the moon, with wonderful scientific discoveries. Why can't someone do something for people like me so I can finally lose this ugly fat?"

The turning point came as I lay in a hospital bed, weighing more than I ever had in my entire life. Necessary surgery had to be postponed because it was determined that I was suffering from malnutrition. I could not believe it! The doctor informed me that my body was actually starving! How could this be? How could my body be starving when I weighed 186 pounds? I had to have three blood transfusions before they could operate. While I was recuperating, I had a lot of time to think. I had been dieting most of my adult life. All of my efforts had left me discouraged, depressed, and obese. I remembered pacing the floor and wringing my hands as I struggled between hunger and my desire to lose weight. I was sure that there had to be a better way, and I was determined to find it. I began to realize that obesity is a chronic illness and that permanent control would require a diet that provided my body with the nourishment it needed.

* * *

My realization that obesity was an illness led me to other conclusions. First, I realized that I was placing all the blame for my failures on myself. What if I hadn't failed, but the diets had failed me? Were they lacking an important ingredient that caused my failures? These diets were no more effective in taking off weight and keeping it off than using a sieve to collect water. I also realized that I had literally dieted myself into malnourishment even though I weighed close to 200 pounds! I knew that there were millions of other people, just like me, who were skipping meals, counting calories, and dieting away their good health. I just could not comprehend, however, how someone could be so overweight and yet malnourished.

Perhaps, I reasoned, there was something wrong in the "way" I had previously dieted. I remember counting every single calorie so I wouldn't exceed my quota for the day. I also remember skipping lunch and most of dinner just to make up for the calories in the cake I had eaten that morning. But finally I asked myself, "What good is a calorie-restricted diet when I'm not successful at losing weight and if that diet doesn't provide the essential nutrients I need for good health?"

These ideas sparked my determination to learn more about my body, how foods affected it, and how I could use this knowledge to gain better health and to control my weight. I vowed never again to allow my body to become malnourished.

Many people do not understand how their bodies and minds work, especially regarding the foods they eat. (Most of us take eating for granted — except when we get an upset stomach!) I also realized how hard it is to gain that understanding. When I first began to search for answers, I checked out every library book, magazine, and article that I could find on the subject. I felt like a sponge, absorbing everything I read. I developed an insatiable desire to learn more and study even harder. I was devouring information as fast as I used to devour food!

Unfortunately, I found that many books written on nutrition are far too technical or theoretical to be read easily, much less understood. Many times I skipped over extremely technical sections, only to come back and read them, again and again. I wanted answers and was willing to study. I was so excited, yet so frustrated. Why was basic nutrition so hard to understand? Why did I have to plow through numerous books just to find simple answers? It didn't make sense. I saw the need to restate these principles in nontechnical language so that I could understand them, repeat them to others, and then use these principles in everyday life. Often, when frustrated with a concept, I would turn to my personal physician, Dr. Lester J. Petersen, for his help and understanding, as well as other doctors. As the concepts and principles became clearer to me, I realized that nutrition was largely a matter of common sense!

As everything began to fall into place, I started to formulate a personal diet. I researched every method I could find for losing weight. I also searched for the simplest, most nutritious foods available, being careful to count nutrients instead of calories. I tested each particular food on myself, looking for foods that would help me lose weight, yet keep me feeling satisfied and energetic. At times, I tried a method that did not work. I simply backed up, discarded that idea, and tried again. Each new addition to my list exhilarated me. I was losing weight, and my body was in better health than it had been for eighteen years! I felt as if my mind and body were finally in tune with each other, and I knew I was on the right path.

Every day, I stepped on the scale and weighed myself. Each time the scale showed a pound, half-pound, quarter-pound loss, I was excited. If I registered no loss or even a slight gain, I was not devastated as I had been in the past. I would simply adjust my diet for the day to come. I no longer felt hungry, miserable, literally starving as I had on other diets. I was amazed by the fact that when I ate correctly, I did not need large amounts of food to satisfy me. It was no longer necessary to "live to eat." For the first time, I began to "eat to live."

I also kept careful records of what and how much I ate. I realized how easy it had been for me to grab a handful of candy or a cookie on the way out the door, but never remember eating it. Now, by carefully charting my behavior, I could see the importance of scheduling and maintaining a conscious awareness of what I ate.

Every small success seemed to fuel my determination. I was motivated by each new discovery. I set a goal for my ideal weight based on safe, healthful standards. The greatest day in my life was when I achieved that goal. I felt like a butterfly emerging at long last from the entrapment of a cocoon. I had undergone a complete metamorphosis. I was happy and healthy, loving life. My happiness and pride spread to my husband and family, and I wanted to share this success with everyone else around me.

Soon, friends began to question me about what diet I had used to lose weight and why it seemed to work so well. As I explained my discoveries, my friends asked if I would be willing to help them too.

While I did not yet have a formal system or method, I felt sure that what had worked for me could work for my friends as well. I had kept accurate records throughout the term of my weight loss. I knew success relied on setting a goal and following a plan. But first you must have confidence that the plan will work. My own success provided that confidence for my friends.

I had each new dieter come in separately. To me, dieting was a very private experience, and I felt I could help best when dealing individually with each person's questions and needs. I began to instruct my friends as to why they should do what I recommended. I wanted every one of them to have the fundamental understanding of why certain foods were so important, why eating on time and on a schedule was necessary, and how written food records could help achieve a better weight loss.

My friends soon joined in the "spirit of success." If someone would lose sight of her goal and not come in on a particular day, I would worry and wonder why until I finally called. I began to insist that every single person come in every day. I could better encourage them, check on the foods they ate, and mark their progress. I found that these daily visits were a key to optimum weight loss.

The daily visits also gave me an additional insight into dieting. The communication of each visit was vital to keeping dieters enthusiastic and motivated. Dieting is not, and will never be, simply counting calories. Dieting is an emotional experience. Each one of us has our own personal temptations and challenges to overcome. With each daily visit, I learned more about every dieter and developed a close personal bond — a mutual understanding that went far beyond dieting.

As time went on, I began to see a pattern of slower weight loss when dieters encountered extra pressures or troubles. A family quarrel or personal disappointment can often lead to the refrigerator and the comfort of eating. I knew it is essential that dieters never lose sight of their goals. I learned how important it is that they be able to visualize the end result of a slender, happy, and successful self. I knew personally that these visualizations could become reality. I could guide each dieter by setting goals, and giving positive reinforcement to overcome any problem, no matter how large or small. I also found that some dieters encountered tremendous amounts of stress in their personal lives. I knew that if I could teach dieters the skills of relaxation, visualization, and goal setting, they could stay on the diet and feel good about themselves.

Throughout this period, I continued to study and read. I was in constant contact with Dr. Petersen, referring any dieter with medical problems to him and asking his advice whenever necessary. I would also have weekly group get-togethers to discuss these ideas, share recipes, and practice relaxation and visualization skills. I felt these sessions were an excellent complement to the crucial daily weigh-in and the counseling each dieter received.

*   *   *

As each new friend or neighbor became successful, she would bring another who wanted to learn the secret. All this time, I had been weighing my friends in the front room of my home. With strangers, I kept up the same method that had worked so well for myself, my friends, and my neighbors. However, soon the number of people had grown so large that I felt it was taking most of my free time.

I called Dr. Petersen one day and told him of my growing concerns. I had now been helping people to lose weight for over a year. He said, "Sybil, why don't you open a business? I'm too busy to take the time to help each dieter like you're doing. I'll send overweight patients to you for your help." I responded, "I don't know how to open a business." He said very simply and quietly, "You charge money."

I felt guilty about the prospect of charging for a service that I felt fortunate to be able to give, so I went home to talk to my husband, Roger. Roger had been my right arm and support throughout the develoment of my entire program, for he had seen a great change in my happiness and outlook on life. Yes, he agreed with Dr. Petersen, up to now I had had an idea. If I structured it into a formal program, I would then have a professional service. It is important to realize that in 1970 people were no longer able to receive diet pills from their doctors. There were places for the wealthy to go to lose weight and group organizations were operated, but at this time there were no daily individual counseling services.

It was very interesting! I found that when money was charged, the dieter became very serious and began to lose consistently better weight. It seemed that if they were going to pay money, they weren't going to fool around on this diet! I then began to study even more about the digestion of foods, vitamins, minerals and how to help people become positive thinkers. Each day, as part of the program, I would give dieters a new item of nutritional information or a new way to change their emotional behavior to encourage motivation.

As the number of dieters expanded, so did the Diet Center Program. I was excited to find that the same program that had worked for women also worked for men and children, by making nutritional adjustments using the RDA as a guide. Dieters with special medical problems could also successfully lose weight by adjusting the diet for their health needs.

As dieters lost weight and emerged with newfound confidence, they would hurry to tell their friends. Today, there are over 1,750 Diet Center locations in every corner of the United States and Canada. New centers continue to open almost daily, and millions of men, women, and children have lost weight on Diet Center's program. It is now one of the largest franchised weight-loss programs — where over a million pounds are lost each month and dieters gain good health and a newfound happiness.

*　*　*

Before beginning the Diet Center Reducing Diet, read through the entire book. The Diet Center Program is far more than just a diet. *The Diet Center Program* is organized in a step-by-step format that can make your dieting easier and more successful. Once you have gained a full understanding of the necessary steps for permanent weight control, then turn to "The Total Diet Center Program." Use the preparation techniques in "Before Even Beginning to Diet" prior to starting your diet. Then, while dieting, use the remaining material for additional ways to help change your behavior and attitudes, and to help keep your motivation kindled. Specific dieting tips, creating your own exercise program, and three special recipe sections will prove invaluable to you. To check the nutritional content of the foods you eat, see the nutrition composition tables at the end of this book.

I know that you too can lose weight and achieve permanent weight control. Just take each day, one at a time, and never lose sight of your long-term goal — a slim, healthy you!

I

EXCESS WEIGHT IS THE NUMBER-ONE HEALTH PROBLEM IN AMERICA

1

Obesity Is a Chronic, Incurable Illness

I AM firmly convinced that obesity is an illness, an incurable illness. It is just as serious an illness as diabetes. If left untreated, obesity can ruin entire lives, and even kill.

I call it an illness; in fact, an acute, chronic one. An illness that may not be cured, but one that most definitely can be controlled by eating proper foods, on time and on a schedule. The key to controlling obesity is controlling the concentration of glucose in the blood, which I call the blood sugar level, keeping it stable at all times. In this way, the dieter is in control, not the body. Accepting obesity as an illness is your first step in treating it successfully.

OBESITY IS AN ILLNESS OF EPIDEMIC PROPORTIONS

THERE ARE OVER 80 MILLION OVERWEIGHT MEN, WOMEN, AND CHILDREN IN THE UNITED STATES — ONE OUT OF EVERY THREE PEOPLE IS OVERWEIGHT. Even more alarming is the number of children who are obese. Over 40 million people are struggling to lose 2.3 trillion pounds of unnecessary, harmful fat each year in the United States.

OVERWEIGHT IS COSTLY

Not only is it an extensive problem, but being overweight is also an expensive one as well. Last year, Americans spent an estimated $40 billion in an attempt to burn, sweat, or diet off those extra pounds — not, however, without justification. Being overweight is detrimental to your health, work, and everyday life. Statistically, overweight executives are paid less and receive fewer raises or promotions than their co-workers of normal weight. Heart disease, often traceable to obesity, resulted in an estimated economic cost of $50.7 billion in lost wages, lost productivity, and medical expenses for 1982.

THE EFFECTS ON YOUR BODY OF BEING OVERWEIGHT

Your body can be compared to a supremely complex and magnificent machine. Like any complicated piece of equipment, it needs proper fuel and constant maintenance. For either a machine or your body, neglect in either one of these areas will have destructive results. A machine, however, can always be replaced — your body cannot.

Your skeletal system compensates for extra weight by putting added pressure on joints — arthritis appears, especially in knees, hips and lower spine. Muscles supporting the stomach lose their elasticity and may give way to abdominal hernias. Fat begins to accumulate along leg muscles, preventing proper circulation. Blood collects in the leg veins, swells and hardens — varicose veins may develop. More fat collects in the chest area. Breathing is more difficult — resulting in respiratory problems.

Within the body, the digestive system begins to have trouble assimilating and metabolizing glucose (your body's fuel). Carbohydrate intolerance develops, resulting in high blood sugar — diabetes. A person who is 20 percent overweight is more than twice as likely to develop diabetes as a person of normal weight. Diabetes is a serious, crippling disease that can happen to anyone.

Additional digestive problems produce gout, causing painful swelling in feet and hands. Menstrual abnormalities, cancer, gallbladder disease and gallstones, and severe back problems have also been linked to obesity.

THE MOST DANGEROUS OVERLOAD ON YOUR HEART

Being overweight taxes your cardiovascular system dangerously. Each day, your heart is required to pump over 4,300 gallons of blood through over 70,000 miles of arteries, veins, and capillaries. Every extra pound adds *more miles* of blood vessels through which your heart must pump the needed blood supply. Even worse, fatty tissue requires more blood than lean tissue. Consequently, your heart must pump *faster* as well as harder!

It is no wonder that obesity and being overweight have been directly linked to high blood pressure, stroke, and heart

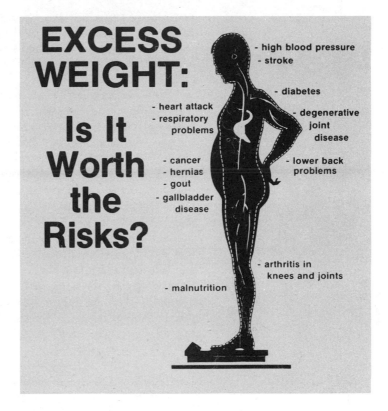

attack. These diseases result in more than forty million deaths each year!

BEING OVERWEIGHT CAN REDUCE YOUR LIFE SPAN

Since the turn of the century, insurance studies have shown consistently that weight affects one's life span. In fact, ONLY 10 PERCENT OF ALL OBESE PERSONS REACH THE AGE OF 80 as compared to 30 percent of slim people — a ratio of one to three.

BEING OVERWEIGHT AFFECTS THE MIND AS WELL AS THE BODY

In a weight-conscience society that sets high values on qualities such as youth, beauty, and slimness, a fat person is often stigmatized. We all grow up with our own stereotype of what a "fat person" is. Positive qualities, such as "happy" and "jolly," and negative descriptions such as "gluttonous," "lazy," and "sloppy" are used to describe whomever we perceive as overweight. Fat people are seen as weak-willed because they just can't stick with a diet and lose that excess weight. The irony is that when someone tries to diet he or she is sabotaged by everything and everyone. Friends, relatives, and even husbands and wives often discourage an obese person from dieting even before they begin.

It is interesting that when a diabetic comes to a dinner party, the hostess caters to specific needs and never questions the necessity of a "special" diet. Yet, when overweight people mention they are dieting, everyone seems to want to undermine their efforts: "For goodness sake, you're not going to diet tonight. You will ruin my party!" "You don't like my cooking?" "But I made this just for you," or "A taste won't hurt you!"

I know the feelings that constant dieting can generate: feelings of depression, listlessness, weepiness, discouragement and self-degradation. This unhappiness with yourself causes unhappiness in relationships with others as well. Marriages can suffer. Families fight more often. In fact, some overweight people have never even had a serious relationship.

RECOGNIZE OBESITY AS AN ILLNESS

First, the key to overcoming obesity is to treat it as a chronic illness. It will never go away, but you can control it by eating the correct nutrients on a schedule and by changing your behavior and attitudes. Left unchecked, this illness can progress through classic stages from a minor weight problem to morbid obesity.

WHAT STAGE ARE YOU IN?

You do not become overweight or obese overnight. There is a point of realization which triggers the painful awareness that those few extra pounds have multiplied to quite a few more. Why and how each of us gains weight is just as individual as dieting. There are, however, general stages advancing toward morbid obesity.

The age at which you become overweight or obese has a direct effect on the severity of the consequences and the difficulty of control. Obesity in very young children and teenagers is potentially more dangerous than obesity in middle-aged or elderly adults. However, regardless of age at the onset, the longer someone is obese, the more serious the physical effects.

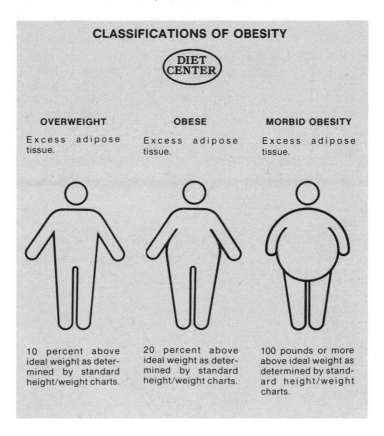

Because of the tremendous long-term effects upon your health, both mental and physical, it is essential that each person recognize the importance of becoming responsible for his or her own health. Each and every one of us must learn how to select nutritious foods. I cannot emphasize this enough. As you read on, I hope you will see the importance of taking on this responsibility for your own good health.

DETERMINING YOUR IDEAL WEIGHT

1. Measure your height (without shoes).
2. Measure your wrist to determine frame size.
3. Consult the following chart to determine your desirable weight.

The ideal weight for a 5′4″ woman, medium frame, would be 119 pounds. If she weighed 131 pounds she would be considered "overweight." If she weighed 143 pounds she would

Desirable Weight Chart

DESIRABLE WEIGHTS FOR MEN AND WOMEN - According to Height, Weight and Frame. Measurements taken with indoor clothing, no shoes. (Subtract 1 pound for each year under 30)

WEIGHTS FOR WOMEN

HEIGHT	SMALL FRAME	IDEAL WEIGHT	MEDIUM FRAME	IDEAL WEIGHT	LARGE FRAME	IDEAL WEIGHT
4'10"	92-98	95	96-107	100	104-119	111
4'11"	94-101	98	98-110	102	106-122	114
5'0"	96-104	101	101-113	107	109-125	117
5'1"	99-107	104	104-116	110	112-128	120
5'2"	102-110	106	107-119	113	115-131	124
5'3"	105-113	109	110-122	115	118-134	126
5'4"	108-116	112	113-126	119	121-138	129
5'5"	111-119	115	116-130	122	125-142	134
5'6"	114-123	118	120-135	127	129-146	137
5'7"	118-127	122	124-139	131	133-150	141
5'8"	122-131	126	128-143	135	137-154	145
5'9"	126-135	130	132-147	139	141-158	149
5'10"	130-140	135	136-151	143	145-163	154
5'11"	134-144	139	140-155	147	149-168	159
6'0"	138-148	143	144-159	151	153-173	163

WRIST MEASUREMENT FOR WOMEN:
Small - 5" to 5½"; Medium - 5½" to 6"; Large 6" to 6½"

WEIGHTS FOR MEN

HEIGHT	SMALL FRAME	IDEAL WEIGHT	MEDIUM FRAME	IDEAL WEIGHT	LARGE FRAME	IDEAL WEIGHT
5'2"	122-130	126	128-139	134	136-151	144
5'3"	125-133	129	131-143	137	139-154	147
5'4"	128-136	132	134-146	140	142-158	150
5'5"	131-139	135	137-149	143	145-162	154
5'6"	134-143	139	140-153	147	148-166	157
5'7"	138-147	143	144-157	152	152-171	162
5'8"	142-151	147	148-162	156	157-176	167
5'9"	146-155	151	152-166	159	161-180	171
5'10"	150-160	155	156-170	163	165-184	175
5'11"	154-164	159	160-175	168	169-189	180
6'0"	158-168	163	164-180	172	174-194	185
6'1"	162-172	167	168-185	177	178-199	190
6'2"	166-177	173	172-190	181	183-204	195
6'3"	170-181	176	177-195	186	188-205	196
6'4"	174-185	180	182-200	191	192-214	205

WRIST MEASUREMENT FOR MEN:
Small - 6½" to 7"; Medium - 7" to 7½"; Large 7½" to 8"

WEIGHT IN POUNDS ACCORDING TO FRAME (In Indoor Clothing)

be "obese." And at 220 pounds she would be "morbidly obese"!

How do you compare? Were you surprised by your own results? If so, you are not alone. Recent health surveys stated an average American woman is 5'3½" tall and weighs 143 pounds. The figures place her as OBESE.

2

The "Yo-Yo" Syndrome

As people gain weight, they seem to reach plateaus. Initial weight gains are slow and steady, but easily dismissed with excuses. The first panic point is reached by most women at 130–140 pounds (ten to fifteen pounds overweight). This "panic point" triggers the feeling of "If I don't do something now I'll be fat!" They crash diet to get rid of those few extra pounds, but unless permanent changes in eating habits are made, a "yo-yo" pattern begins to become a way of life: gaining weight, losing weight, feast or famine while robbing the body of nutrients. Dieters may try to stay below the 150-pound mark and may be able to for a long period of time, but inevitably the weight begins to creep steadily higher: 150, 160 . . . 170. Another panic point seems to occur at each ten-pound increment. Each panic point results in another crash diet and weight is lost, quickly regained, and soon the dieter is resigned just to maintaining her "new" weight of 175 pounds. She is constantly fighting to maintain even that weight, and again panic sets in. A starvation diet takes off twenty pounds, but soon the same twenty (plus five more) reappear. Desperation dieting takes over, and the "yo-yo" pattern now becomes a regular way of life — continually losing twenty pounds and regaining twenty-five — always counting calories, skipping meals, feeling persecuted or even noble while losing weight and then gaining, thinking you have failed and going out of control. You hate what is happening and become desperate, not caring about what you really do to your body, just wanting to be thin.

THE HARMFUL EFFECTS OF "YO-YO-ING"

The yo-yo syndrome is nothing new. Dr. Jean Mayer has labeled it the "rhythm method of girth control." People have been "dieting" for years, using every method and device imaginable to "magically burn off those extra pounds." American consumers are spending approximately $5 billion annually on health foods and vitamins, $6 billion for diet drinks, $54 million on diet pills, and $50 million on diet and exercise literature.

The yo-yo syndrome has harmful effects, both physically and mentally. Picture a rubber band that is constantly stretched taut and relaxed. Eventually, the elasticity of the rubber band reaches its breaking point and it snaps. Now, replace the rubber band with your body and consider the harmful effects of a fluctuating weight on your muscles, skin, heart, stomach, etc. Doctors are alarmed by the effects of losing weight on fad diets only to regain the weight quickly again. These changes exert serious stress and strain on the body. The heart, for example, has to pump harder with every additional pound; and over a period of time, these demands on the heart will cause it to weaken.

Perhaps even more importantly, the yo-yo syndrome can be psychologically devastating, especially to those dieters who have more than just a quick five or ten pounds to lose. The "false encouragement" offered by an initially rapid fluid loss is quickly replaced by discouragement and frustration when those pounds reappear. And when the "battle of the bulge" appears hopeless, it is easy to resort to food for comfort.

The yo-yo syndrome is the most dangerous cycle in which a dieter can become entrapped. You can, however, break this cycle forever.

One dieter, with the help of Diet Center, did just that. Coming from a "thin" family, she was the exception. As a child, she had always been ten to fifteen pounds overweight. At the age of thirteen, she began what was to become her career for the next twenty-nine years — professional dieting. By crash dieting and using diet pills, she was able to control her weight during high school. On her wedding day, her petite frame carried only 118 pounds. That didn't last long. During her two-week honeymoon, she gained fifteen pounds. Married life was great, but she had little time to adjust before finding out she was pregnant. Prior to delivery, she weighed 170 pounds — only one year after her marriage. Just after the

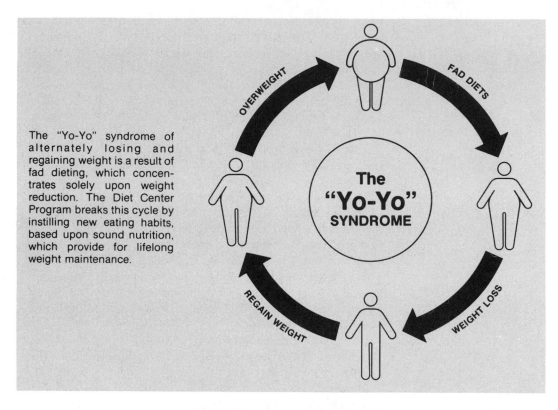

The "Yo-Yo" syndrome of alternately losing and regaining weight is a result of fad dieting, which concentrates solely upon weight reduction. The Diet Center Program breaks this cycle by instilling new eating habits, based upon sound nutrition, which provide for lifelong weight maintenance.

birth of another son, she was able to diet down to 129 pounds before starting to gain again. A third pregnancy found her weighing 211 pounds, and she realized she was trapped in the yo-yo syndrome. Regardless of what new diet she tried, she always weighed more after the diet than when she had started. A determined person by nature, when it came to weight control she considered herself a failure. Having tried almost every program, she had little confidence that anything could succeed. Out of desperation, she enrolled with Diet Center, being careful not to get her hopes up — she couldn't take another failure. After five months, it was no longer a question of whether she could make it, but WHEN! Now, even smaller than on her wedding day at 114 pounds, she couldn't be happier.

FAD DIETING IS HARMFUL

The yo-yo syndrome usually results from nutritionally unsound diets. Whether someone wants to lose five or one hundred pounds, people are desperate for immediate results.

Thus, unusual diets with claims of quick weight losses are far more appealing than well-balanced reducing diets that appear boring. What few people realize, however, is that these "fad" diets work at the expense of good health and have little or no chance for permanent results.

Fad diets are easy to spot. They are characterized by very limited choices of foods and promises of rapid weight losses. However, they often lack essential nutrients. For example, ten days of eating nothing but fruit deprives the body of some fifty essential elements and food nutrients needed to maintain a healthy body. It simply is not good sense.

One group of fad diets involves fasting, starvation, and drastic caloric reduction. Starvation diets drain the body of essential fats used for cushioning and protection, rather than the adipose tissue (the layers of fat that we want to lose), which is the cause of obesity. On a starvation diet, weight is lost rapidly at first; but the dieter feels tired, weak, starved, and is gaunt looking. The person is not alert and cannot concentrate or think clearly. This weight is quickly regained because the body needs these essential fats to survive. Research has shown that weight loss in a starvation diet is only 33 percent fatty tissue, while weight loss from a diet that is nutritionally balanced is 99 percent fatty tissue.

Another group of fad diets are often referred to as "ketosis diets" or low-carbohydrate, high-fat, or high-protein diets and are offered through many widely publicized "book" diets and a number of commercial weight-loss programs. These diets are based on a nutritional fallacy that only fatty tissue is burned in a diet consisting of an excess of proteins or fats and a restricted level of carbohydrates. Eating less than a minimum of 60 grams of carbohydrates daily can result in a condition called ketosis. Over an extended period of time, ketosis can be extremely hazardous to your health. Other complications can also arise from these diets, including dizziness, fatigue, dehydration, hypercholesterolemia (excess of cholesterol in the blood), severe kidney problems, and even death. When weight is lost on this diet, it is not just fat, but also a loss in muscle and other vital tissue. This unnecessary loss of essential tissue and skin elasticity causes rolls of skin to hang on the body, and the dieter may need plastic surgery to remove it.

While large initial weight losses may result on these fad diets, they are also primarily a result of fluid depletion, not the loss of fatty tissue. These diets may also result in loss of lean muscle tissue.

Fad diets invariably cause a dieter to feel deprived, both mentally and physically. Any diet that differs radically from nutritionally balanced eating habits (in amounts or types of food) will be hard to follow on a long-term basis.

WHAT IS KETOSIS?

When, over a period of time, you drastically reduce your intake of carbohydrates (less than 60 grams of "digestible" carbohydrates per day), your body is deprived of its number-one energy source, glucose. One of the major roles of glucose is to supply energy to the brain. Without a supply of glucose, a person would die. Because the body cannot store large amounts of carbohydrates, they must be constantly replenished. If the body needs to find another way to give itself needed energy, it turns to its backup source, stored fats.

When less than 60 grams of digestible carbohydrates per day are eaten over a period of time, the body relies on reserve fuel sources through the emergency process of ketosis. This process obtains energy from two different sources: proteins and fats.

Unfortunately, the body is not capable of burning fats to completion without the presence of carbohydrates; so when the body is forced to rely on fat metabolism (burning of fats) for its energy, a buildup of partially burned fats called ketone bodies occurs.

Ketone bodies are always present, but they appear in a low and tolerable quantity, and are released through breathing and urination. Fat metabolism causes an overabundance of these ketone bodies in the bloodstream; and because they are produced faster than they are removed, they start building up. The result is ketosis. The body then calls for extra water from its cells to flush the ketone bodies from the bloodstream. In this way, ketosis actually increases urination. Consequently, as the kidneys flush out these excessive ketone bodies, vitamins, minerals and necessary body fluids are also lost in the process.

Ketosis is a serious and stressful condition characterized by a peculiar odor of the breath or increased ketone bodies in the urine and bloodstream. Symptoms may also include light-headedness, dizziness, or incoherence. A person may even experience such side effects as calcium depletion, dehydration, fatigue and sleeplessness, loss of hair, sluggishness, and emotional problems.

NORMAL ENERGY

Fruits–Vegetables–Whole Grains–Milk

|

Carbohydrates

|

Glucose (needed daily)

|

Brain

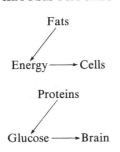

KETOSIS PROCESS

Fats

Energy ⟶ Cells

Proteins

Glucose ⟶ Brain

After a prolonged period of time under this condition, the body's chemistry is also upset. The blood volume is reduced, and the thyroid doesn't produce as much of its essential hormone. Immunity to disease is decreased, and an increase in the uric-acid level of the blood can lead to a gout attack.

Sound serious? It is. If a person's body is allowed to deteriorate further, the kidneys, as well as the heart, may begin to suffer. At the extreme end of the scale, ketosis can induce coma, or even death. So why intentionally put your body into such a potentially dangerous situation? Especially, when you realize that the weight loss it promotes will be short-lived!

On the Diet Center Program, you will not be in ketosis. You will receive 90 to 130 grams of carbohydrates daily.

Losing the "Right" Type of Fat

ONE of the first steps to conquering the yo-yo syndrome is to ensure that your diet results in the "correct" type of weight loss. Fad diets lack essential nutrients and sufficient caloric level needed to keep your body functioning properly.

When I was at my heaviest, I hated my "fat." I wanted to lose every inch of ugly fat from my body. I was determined that "fat" was my worst enemy. Through study, however, I found to my amazement that some fat on my body was ESSENTIAL for good health.

TWO TYPES OF FAT

Essential Fats

The body of primitive man was designed to meet specific needs. Primitive man was a scavenger and hunter and very seldom overweight. Food was not always plentiful, so when it was available, he ate as much as possible. The body stored any excess energy — in the form of fat — in two separate ways. The first was short-term storage that could be used up in case of short emergencies (one or two days without food). Another long-term supply was stored for use during longer periods of famine, such as winter.

The body of modern man has retained these storage capacities, though the need for them has been largely eliminated because of a more constant availability of food. Short-term storage takes place as the essential fat of the body. Essential fat surrounds organs and glands for protection. It also cushions joints. Essential fat creates the soft, feminine curves for women and a more angular look for men.

Each one of us has approximately seventeen to twenty-five pounds of essential fat. This is also the body's short-term emergency supply to be used when the body's nutrient intake falls drastically lower than it should be. Besides being the first used, essential fats are also the first to be replaced!

Essential fat is one of the first places your body turns to in case of starvation or other crisis, to be used as an emergency source of energy. Have you ever gone through surgery or been extremely ill for an extended period of time? Your face begins to look gaunt and haggard; your skin "hangs" on your bones. This is a result of the body using up its store of essential fat for energy. This same situation occurs when you go on a starvation diet (extremely low in calories and nutrients). Your body attacks its store of essential fat for an immediate supply of nutrients. Consequently, you may drop a quick fifteen pounds. However, while the scale drops, your measurements do not. You do not lose those extra rolls around your ribs, hips, or thighs. Your breasts and chest have lost inches, but they sag. The starvation diet has robbed the body of the essential nutrients needed to maintain tissue, skin, and muscle tone. THIS IS A TEMPORARY LOSS ONLY! The lost essential fats are soon replaced as you begin "normal" eating again. Fad dieting results in little more than constantly losing and then regaining the essential fat, while never really losing that outside layer of fat responsible for the bulges.

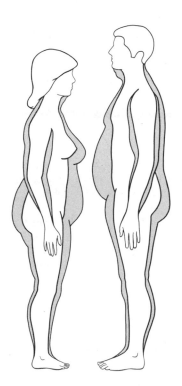

Nonessential Fats (Adipose Tissue)

This type of fat was originally intended as a stored energy supply for prolonged periods of famine or starvation during a prolonged emergency situation. Primitive man built up his supply of nonessential fat to survive long winters or droughts. Unlike essential fats, there is almost no limit to the amount your body can store. Consequently, excess, nonessential fat results in the rolls and bulges most people label as "fat." In the illustration above, excess, nonessential fat is the shaded layer that appears to cover the entire body!

THE DIET CENTER DIFFERENCE

In designing the Diet Center Program, I was determined to create a nutritionally sound, well-balanced diet that would nourish and replenish essential fat, while eliminating nonessential fat. The results from millions of successful Diet Center dieters show that our program does exactly that. Dieters lose approximately one measured inch per pound of weight loss. If a dieter loses twenty-five pounds, he or she will also lose about twenty-five inches. If a dieter loses one hundred pounds, he or she will also lose approximately one hundred inches. This inch loss occurs ALL OVER THE BODY — not just from the face, neck, and chest. Neither tissue nor muscle is lost. If fat is on the back of a woman, she will lose it and decrease in bra size from a 36 to a 32. Unless the fat is on the breast, dieters rarely change actual cup size while on the Diet Center Diet. As one Diet Center dieter relates:

I have now lost 59¾ pounds on the Diet Center Program. I feel great and Diet Center has opened up a whole new world to me. In fact, my whole life is exciting . . . not the least is the joy of buying a whole new wardrobe. I just bought a new suit and it is a size 9/10 Jr.

I can't believe the change in me . . . and no saggy skin either! The fat comes off where it should and I feel just absolutely terrific! My blood pressure is down to normal and I am no longer on medication. It is marvelous to wear clothes that look good on me and feel so comfortable. I can't begin to tell you the confidence it has given me.

Wanda Pitman
Coral Gables, Florida

Men on the Reducing Diet lose only excess adipose tissue, not muscle tone.

Just as important as inch loss is the fact that the body does not starve while on the Diet Center Program. Even dieters who have successfully lost hundreds of pounds do not require plastic surgery. The apron of fat that envelops an obese person literally draws up and disappears. No matter how large a weight loss, dieters remain healthy, and the skin retains its elasticity.

This diet is a "self-eliminating" one. As dieters attain their own individual ideal weight, weight loss ceases. As only the nonessential fats are lost, when the body reaches leanness, weight loss stops. Loss of essential fats only occurs if a dieter does not eat the required foods on the Total Diet Center Program. If you try to eat even less than the program requires, you are inadvertantly turning this into a fad diet. EAT THE QUANTITIES REQUIRED.

Many people are looking for a miracle to lose the so-called cellulite fat. Authorities in the medical world will agree with me that when you lose weight by eating correct nutrients and drinking eight glasses of water a day, you will lose needed inches and the "harder" fat will also leave the body. Neither expensive body wraps nor cellulite gimmicks are effective treatments.

In order to reach your ideal weight, the Total Diet Center Program consists of a Conditioning Phase, Reducing Phase, Stabilization Phase, and Maintenance Phase. These stages will be explained later in the book.

DO NOT GO LOWER THAN YOUR IDEAL WEIGHT! You could go into anorexia. But do not quit dieting before you reach your ideal goal weight, because it is your healthy weight. When dieters quit ten or twenty pounds shy of their goals, they constantly battle to maintain their weight. When weight goal is achieved, dieters find they can follow the Maintenance Diet and easily maintain their weight.

4

Count Nutrients, Not Calories

Too many dieters get so caught up in counting calories that they ignore the importance of nutritious eating. As dieters, we are taught that 3,500 calories equals one pound. To lose one pound, we must reduce our total caloric intake for that week or day and/or increase the amount of calories we burn up. Unfortunately, a reduction in calories often means a reduction in the nutrients needed to maintain energy. Dieters who unconsciously ignore nutrients become weak, tired, depressed, hungry, and . . . unsuccessful!

When I quit counting calories and began paying careful attention to nutrients, I successfully lost weight and kept it off. I realized the importance of maintaining a specific daily calorie level; but for the first time in my life, I began eating foods because of their nutritional content and "staying power" (see the next chapter). No longer did I feel persecuted with that starved, hungry feeling. I was no longer nervous and, amazingly, I quit constantly thinking about food.

I studied to find natural foods high in nutrition and fiber, yet low in fats, refined sugars, and flours. I still looked up information; but instead of searching for a calorie count, I systematically looked up food values to find which were highest in nutrients, vitamins, and minerals, yet lowest in cholesterol and fats.

I was amazed at some of the differences I found. Take meats as an example. An average serving of meat (about 3½ ounces, cooked) contains approximately 22 grams of protein. However, the amount of fat varies drastically among types of meats. A 3½-ounce serving of halibut, for example, has 25 grams of protein and only 7 grams of fat, while a 3½-ounce serving of prime rib has 21 grams of protein and an unbelievable 43 grams of fat. The same serving of prime rib is over two-thirds fat! To lose weight, yet maintain a high level of protein, I chose lean meats, such as fish and chicken.

5

"Staying Power"

As I studied each food group, I gained additional insight into the interaction between foods and the body. I learned that certain foods seemed to "stay longer" in my system. I felt more energetic and satisfied after eating these foods. The hunger that used to plague me between meals was gone. It seemed unbelievable! I labeled these foods with the phrase "staying power."

There are many foods low in calories. Many of these, however, are digested quickly. They lack the "staying power" you need to sustain you, without hunger, between meals, which is so necessary to successfully stay on the diet.

When dieters try to control weight by counting calories, they often rely on prepackaged convenience foods. These foods are easy to prepare. But because they are already pre-processed, they often substitute the goodness of natural foods with highly refined, highly digestible products, high in additives and preservatives. These foods are so quickly digested that they cannot provide the "staying power" needed by every dieter. Craving for more food often results, with the dieter then resorting to even more refined foods, such as candies and pastries.

Instead, dieters need to concentrate on natural foods, and return to basic foods, especially complex carbohyrates, which provide the body with "staying power." The fiber and bulk found in fresh vegetables and fruits help the body to feel full longer and satisfied. The body cannot digest fiber. Therefore, it creates a "full" feeling in your stomach during digestion and improves the body's elimination of waste products.

Foods high in fiber and bulk also require more chewing. They take longer to eat and, therefore, give the body time to signal the brain that it can stop sending out hunger signals while you are still eating. Highly refined foods, those with white sugar and flour as chief ingredients, need little chewing or digestion. It is not long after a meal of these foods that the body is signaling that it needs more nourishment. Selecting foods with "staying power" is essential to every dieter's success.

6

Blood Sugar Level — The Key to Weight Loss and Control

THIS chapter is about a simple remarkable phenomenon that I came across when I was just counting calories or enduring another fad diet. My moods would go up and down like a roller coaster. One minute I would feel energetic and productive, the next I would feel nervous, moody, depressed, indecisive, and, worst of all, HUNGRY! I seemed to crave sweets and constantly think of forbidden foods. Every Monday was "diet day," but I would give in to eating a sliver of that leftover piece of chocolate cake from Sunday's delicious dinner. To make up for all the calories in that piece of cake, I would skip lunch. Inevitably, by late afternoon I would be craving sweets. Again, I'd eat another piece of cake and then, to make up for all those extra calories, I would skip dinner. Within just two days of dieting, I was too exhausted and famished to continue. Finally, I would give up until "next" Monday morning. Each time I felt more like a failure. I kept blaming myself for not having the willpower to stay on a diet. I wanted to lose weight more than anything, and I had every intention to do just that. "Why am I so weak-willed?" I asked myself. But I found that failing to stay on a diet had nothing to do with me or my willpower. The problem was the starvation diet I was on.

While on the Diet Center Program, I noticed a striking difference in the way I felt. I had a sustained energy level, the ability to think clearly and decisively, an overall feeling of well-being, and, most important, *no excessive hunger or craving for sweets*. The difference between the previous diets I had been on and the Diet Center Program is the way in which these foods affect blood sugar level when they are eaten on time and on a schedule. BLOOD SUGAR LEVEL IS THE KEY TO DIETING SUCCESS!

The primary source of energy for the human body is glucose. Every cell in the body relies to some degree upon this most valuable fuel. The brain and central nervous system depend exclusively upon glucose to fuel their various processes. The concentration of glucose in your bloodstream is called your blood sugar level. When that level drops below a certain point, the brain demands an increased supply and signals for more fuel. When the body needs energy, the brain knows that a piece of cake or candy will supply quick energy. It sends out the message, and the body craves sweets.

The body specifically developed to handle the diet of primitive man. Again, primitive man ate large quantities of fresh berries, vegetables, and meats. During digestion, nutrients were slowly unlocked from the fiber and bulk of these foods. These nutrients were then slowly converted to glucose and gradually released into the bloodstream. This gradual release of nutrients also results in a gradual increase in blood sugar level. When the level reaches a point that is adequate for current needs, the excess is stored.

The human body was not designed to utilize the type of food most of us eat today. How many whole grains, fresh fruits and vegetables do you eat each day? If you are like most people, your diet consists of prepackaged breakfast cereals, fast-food meals, sugary treats, TV dinners, spaghetti, pizza, and macaroni. This latter group of foods has one thing in common — a process that strips away the natural fiber and bulk in foods and replaces it with refined sugars, white flours, additives and preservatives. These foods are already "preprocessed" and require little digestion. Instead of a gradual process of digestion, these foods are broken down quickly. Available sugar is converted to glucose and shot into the bloodstream. A skyrocket increase in blood sugar level occurs. The body cannot cope with all this excess sugar, so it sends out a signal to store. The body is fighting to maintain a stable blood sugar level. (Biologically, this signal triggers a release of insulin into the bloodstream and a new series of processes that convert glucose to glycogen and fat.) Once all available glucose is stored, the blood sugar level drops; and you crave more sweets.

Consider this example illustrating the different effects on the blood sugar level of natural foods and of refined foods. A medium-sized apple contains about 100 calories; so does a

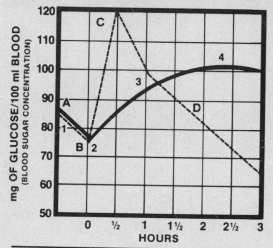

WHAT HAPPENS TO BLOOD SUGAR CONCENTRATION WHEN YOU ATTEMPT TO SATISFY YOUR HUNGER WITH SWEETS (REFINED SUGAR)

Consumption of foods high in refined sugar results in a fluctuation of the blood sugar concentration. When such foods are eaten, they are quickly digested and absorbed into the bloodstream. The blood sugar (glucose) concentration rises quickly, and your hunger is temporarily satisfied. But soon, your blood sugar concentration drops, resulting in feelings of hunger, depression and irritability. You may lack energy and the ability to think clearly. Often, in response to these feelings, sweets are eaten once again and the cycle repeats itself. Maintaining your blood sugar concentration within normal limits is essential to effective dieting.

This chart shows the dramatic rise and fall of blood sugar concentration when you eat refined sugar compared to the effect experienced when you eat an apple.

DOTTED LINE

A BLOOD SUGAR CONCENTRATION DROPS—You become hungry
B You eat a candy bar
C Blood sugar concentration rises quickly
D Blood sugar concentration drops quickly

SOLID LINE

1 BLOOD SUGAR CONCENTRATION DROPS—You become hungry
2 You eat an apple
3 Blood sugar concentration rises gradually
4 Blood sugar concentration remains within normal range for an extended period of time

Note that after sweets are eaten, the blood sugar concentration drops to a point even lower than it was when you first became hungry. You must stabilize the blood sugar concentration in order to maintain a good energy level, control hunger and depression. Be aware that consumption of alcohol, caffeine, most diet pills, amphetamines, etc., can have a similar effect on blood sugar concentration.

Rev. 1/83

scoop of ice cream. If you elect to satisfy your hunger with the ice cream, your system reacts almost immediately. The refined sugar is readily available. It requires very little digestion before all the sugar is converted to glucose and introduced into the bloodstream, causing the blood sugar level to be erratic, rising very high and then dropping extremely low. Only a small percentage of the glucose can be utilized for immediate needs before the rest is gathered and stored. The brain once again signals hunger, and you are right back where you started from, craving more sweets.

If you had selected the apple to satisfy your hunger instead, it would have taken much longer to chew and digest. The blood sugar level would not have risen so quickly or to as high a level. The signal would not have gone out to store, and a continual supply of glucose would have been introduced into the bloodstream over an extended period of time. This supply would be adequate for immediate energy needs, and you would not have experienced hunger. Additionally, your system would be allowed to function properly, working right down to digestion and proper elimination. You would not be nervous or uptight. Your brain would receive adequate fuel to allow you to think clearly; and because your system was in balance, you would experience an overall feeling of well-being. With the apple, you would not be hungry, and because you wouldn't immediately crave more food, you would experience better weight loss.

Many dieters are unconscious victims of their own blood sugar level. Suppose you are ready to begin one "last" diet on Monday morning. Unknowingly, you may be sabotaging your Monday diet by what you eat on Sunday!

In anticipation of dieting, we often go "all out" just before we begin. Vowing that "this time I am going to stick with it all the way," we allow one more day of real eating enjoyment before the deprivation of dieting. Sunday afternoon and evening are filled with "the last feast." And this applies especially to those wonderful chocolates, cookies, cakes, and pastries that will be forbidden tomorrow. When you awake on Monday morning, your blood sugar level (as a result of the process just described) is extremely low . . . perhaps to the point that you have a splitting headache, which makes the task no easier. Most dieters skip breakfast, and by 11 A.M., their bodies are crying out for energy. The brain knows that the leftover cake or pie could supply the body with quick energy. Just one little slice couldn't hurt, could it? Besides, the dieter is counting calories, and therefore will exchange cake for a good lunch. Then, the roller-coaster effect on the blood sugar level begins;

and one piece of pie leads to another and another until the leftovers are gone, along with your good intentions! And another diet has failed.

Now, what if this same dieter had eaten a regular, well-balanced meal on Sunday evening and begun a sound nutritional diet on Monday morning? An early morning dip in blood sugar levels would occur, but not the dramatic decrease from a previous meal high in refined sugars. This time, the dieter can maintain control in choosing a nutritious food — fresh fruits! The fruit provides a natural fruit sugar called fructose, which is "locked" into fiber. The slow digestion of the fruit allows an even, gradual rate of absorption of nutrients from the apple into the bloodstream. The dieter feels satisfied and full, and can easily continue working until lunch.

BLOOD SUGAR LEVEL IS THE KEY TO WEIGHT CONTROL. When the blood sugar level is stable, you won't crave sweets. Maintaining a stable blood sugar level is possible only when basic natural foods are eaten on a schedule that allows this level to remain within a normal, constant range.

Dieters are not weak-willed or gluttonous. They are not failures. Without an understanding of the important role of basic nutritious foods in their own natural state, eaten on a correct schedule, they have no chance for success. One dieter describes her battle with sugar this way:

I was addicted to sugar. My life was like that of an alcoholic. I was living on chocolate with a chaser of Maalox. No wonder my stomach was giving me trouble. My weight bothered me some, but all of my family were short, overweight ladies and I had accepted the fact that this was to be my destiny.

Then, through a neighbor, I found out about the Diet Center Program. Within the first week of the program, I knew my life was about to change. With all the sugar out of my system and a change in my eating habits, I knew I had found something I never dreamed was possible.

No longer did I have to feel uncomfortable around so-called thin people, because now I was one of them. Losing forty pounds and fifty-six inches in 12 weeks is bound to make some changes in a person's life!

Jan Bright
Annapolis, Maryland

If you cannot stay with a diet, you have not failed, but the diet has failed you! Controlling your blood sugar level puts you in full control of your diet and provides the ability to make intelligent decisions about eating.

II

PREPARE YOURSELF FOR DIETING!

Now that I've given you some general background about how your body works and how different diets affect you, we will specifically discuss the Diet Center diet phases. First, let's start with some preparation tips and ideas to help you begin on the right track.

How many times have you lost weight by following a rigid diet just to regain everything you lost (plus even more) only a few months later? The reason for this failure is not because you can't follow a diet (you adhered to every instruction), but because you didn't alter your underlying eating attitudes and behaviors toward food in general. The diet made no provision for maintaining your ideal weight once you reached it.

A diet can teach you what foods to eat, in what amounts and at what times of the day. It can satisfy you physically if nutritionally balanced, but a diet alone cannot teach you "why" you eat. The Diet Center Program includes the crucial importance of learning to diet mentally as well as physically. Maintaining ideal weight often relies on total restructuring of the way you act, think, and feel about food.

How many times have you eaten, not because you were hungry, but because you were tired, angry, depressed, or upset? Food often becomes an object of comfort in our lives, rather than the simple sustenance it should be. Does a quarrel with your children or husband or wife trigger a trip to the refrigerator? One successful dieter correlated her past binges on pizza and ice cream to the monthly arrival of bills and her subsequent money troubles. Another told of how, following a bad day at work, she used to sneak downstairs to raid the refrigerator after everyone fell asleep. Sound familiar?

Few of us realize just how much importance we attach to food, yet how unaware we are of our own eating habits. Can you remember everything that you had to eat yesterday? Start with the main meals: breakfast, lunch, and dinner. Make a mental list of exactly what you ate. Now, try to remember all those snacks during the day. How about that cookie you grabbed on the way out the door or that candy bar you ate while riding home on the bus? Did you "taste-test" the sauce while making dinner or pick at the leftovers while doing the dishes? What about that snack while watching television last night? It is surprising how often and how much each of us can eat without even realizing it.

Try a simple exercise. For the next two days, write down everything you eat. You should also note how much of each food is eaten. At the same time, jot down the reason why you ate each food. Did you have a sweet roll during the morning work break just because everyone else ate one? Was that candy bar eaten because you were hungry or just because you wanted something sweet? Carry a small notebook with you for easy recording and write down every single bite of food you put into your mouth. At the end of two days, you may be astonished by the results.

1

Daily Motivation

PICTURE your dieting efforts as a long climb up a mountain. You need to advance from the bottom to the top, one step at a time. There may be temporary setbacks where you have to retreat to avoid a ravine, but that doesn't mean you have to start all over. Just concentrate on gradually moving upward, a few pounds at a time, until you reach your goal at the top.

The Diet Center Program was designed to assist you in your climb to the top. Each chapter provides another advance. Each advance, motivation to move even farther. You will learn to first prepare for dieting, mentally and physically. You will learn how to choose the correct foods while shopping and the best methods of preparation when you arrive home. You prepare your own personalized weight chart and set goals.

Next come all four phases in full detail, exercising, and other necessary nutrition education and behavior modification tips.

Success can be yours by following each of the steps carefully. Remember, however, to always concentrate on the positive! Refer to the book often. Daily motivation will go a long way in helping you to progress.

As you step on the scale, what do you say to yourself? "One down, ten more to go," or "Great! I lost another pound today!" Your overall attitude will influence not only how fast you lose, but your chance of permanent success.

Realize that every day may not be a "losing" one for you. Some days, you may experience water retention from stress, fatigue, or illness. Don't let these days get you down. Instead, concentrate on keeping positive about total results. With these thoughts in mind, you can begin!

MAKING YOUR OWN DECISION TO DIET

Before you can be a successful dieter, two important criteria must be met. First, you must make your *own* decision to diet. Second, you must be willing to commit fully to this decision.

The best way to ensure the failure of a diet before even beginning it is to diet for the wrong reasons. Are you dieting because your husband teasingly called you "chubby" or because your friend across the street just bought a brand-new diet book? Before beginning any weight-loss program, make sure it is really your decision to lose weight. You must accept personal responsibility for your decision to diet. No one can motivate you to diet; no one can make you diet. Once you have made the decision to, it will be *your* commitment, *your* motivation and, consequently, *your* success!

MATCHING COMMITMENT WITH DECISION

Commitment keeps you motivated. Commitment is the belief that you can, and will, succeed. Nothing can be more important. One Diet Center dieter, who lost over a hundred pounds, used this sign on her refrigerator to reinforce her commitment to lose weight: "STOP! Is it really worth it? What is several weeks of dieting compared to another 20 years of misery?" Having a strong commitment will keep you on the right track and help you to focus on that final goal — a slim, healthy self. Dieting becomes a commitment when you begin with the right reason. Because YOU want to lose weight!

Motivation makes all the difference! As one dieter recalls:

Diet Center was my last ray of hope in a multitude of weight-loss schemes and dreams. I had been overweight since the age of five. All through my school years, I carried enough extra weight that I was teased by other kids, shunned by the "popular group," and almost dateless in high school and college.

After marriage, I gradually gained more weight and with the birth of our son, I hit over the 200-pound mark. When the doctor confirmed my second pregnancy, it was like a dinner bell ringing in my head. I literally ate myself through the next seven months. After my daughter was born, I told myself that I had all the reasons in the world to get down to my proper weight, but the motivation was not there. I was on the deadly treadmill of depression, eating, and guilt. By the time my daughter was six months old, I was so miserable and overweight that I could not get up from a sitting position with her in my arms. I decided I needed help!

I had seen an old friend who had lost 60 pounds on the Diet Center Program. I knew that I must work extremely hard on the psychological part of losing and maintaining my weight because I had been heavy all my life. I signed up that very day. Today, I have lost 119 pounds, reached my goal and gained poise, self-confidence, a positive self-image and a much greater self-worth. LOOK OUT WORLD, HERE I COME!

Karen Lint
Newton, Iowa

WORK TO MAKE SMALL CHANGES EACH DAY

Once you are ready to diet, you need to focus on HOW. This "plan of action" is given to dieters each day through the Diet Center Four-Phase Diet (see pages 107–166).

Each day, you will encounter new problems to solve and new challenges to overcome. With each new positive decision, you will advance one more step upward to success.

The first positive action is to set a goal. Have you ever gotten in your car without having a final destination in mind? If it was an extended trip, did you plan approximate stopping places to refuel or rest? Setting goals is similar to making the necessary preparations for taking a trip. A long-term goal may be reaching a new ideal weight or achieving improved physical health. Short-term goals usually involve smaller personal successes, such as being able finally to see your toes, fit into a smaller dress size, or exercise daily.

Every dieter has his or her own incentive for losing weight. Your reason is just as valid and important as anyone else's. What is important is that your incentives and goals be your own. For example, one Diet Center dieter needed to lose forty pounds that she had gained over a five-year period. First, she worked to establish an ideal weight goal. Next, she bought a pair of slacks that she would be able to fit into upon reaching her weight goal. Short-term goals were set so that slowly she could fit into those pants: first, over the knees, thighs, hips, waist, and, finally, to be able to zip them up. This dieter tried on her pants after every ten-pound weight loss to judge her progress. Those pants were also her special incentive whenever she felt discouraged. By trying on the pants, she could see how far she had come and how little was left to accomplish.

2

Chart Your Progress

CHARTING your weight loss can be one of the most exciting and reinforcing parts of dieting.

Use the Diet Center Reducing Weight Chart to keep track of your weight loss (see page 51). Follow these steps:

1. Enter date, height (without shoes), and weight goal.
2. Enter your beginning weight above "actual weight" in the left column. For example, your starting weight on Sunday is 143 pounds. Enter 143 in this space.
3. Next, record your daily progress. Each sqaure is equal to one-half pound. (Each square you lose is like losing two sticks of butter!) If you lose one pound, you can color in two squares; if you lose one-quarter pound, color in one-half of a square. For example: On Sunday morning, you began your diet weighing 143 pounds (see the accompanying chart). Fill in 143 above "Actual Weight" on the left-hand column. By Monday morning, you had lost one-half pound. Write your new weight, *142½*, in the "Actual Weight" column and color in one square under M (Monday) on the graph. Then, extend a line from the bottom of the square you filled in to the T (Tuesday) column. By Tuesday, you lost another one-half pound, so fill in *142* and color in one square. Wednesday, you're down to *141* (fill in two squares); Thursday, *140¾* (one-half of a square); Friday, *140½* (one square); Saturday, *140.*
4. The right-hand column provides an easy way to measure total weight loss. Just fill in the boxes as you go!
5. You can also set goals using this weight graph. On the graph you will note two heavy diagonal lines starting at the upper

left-hand corner. One line extends to a seventeen-pound loss at six weeks. Another extends to a twenty-five-pound loss at six weeks. To achieve a weight goal of a seventeen- to twenty-five-pound weight loss in six weeks, you must stay in between these two lines. Above them, you should work harder to achieve a better daily weight loss. In between or below, you're doing great.

6. Buy a box of gold stars and give yourself a "star" for each smaller achievement. (Resisted a piece of birthday cake? Give yourself a star! Make it through a tough weekend? Give yourself TWO!)

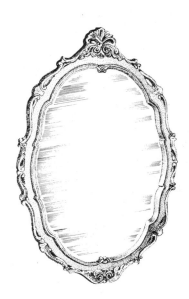

7. As another incentive, take a set of measurements before beginning. Record these measurements in the appropriate area of the weight graph. To obtain the most accurate measurements, have another person take them. Follow this technique:

   (a) Remove bulky clothing (blazers, additional sweaters, coats).
   (b) Stand erect with feet together.
   (c) Measure from the back (optional). Be sure to pull tape taut.
   (d) Make sure you measure from the same place and side each time. Double your extremity measurements to obtain total inch loss from the arms and legs.

THIRTY DIET CENTER IDEAS THAT CAN CHANGE YOUR LIFE!

1. Remember that you alone are responsible for yourself.
2. Concentrate on your goals, not your limitations.
3. Eat on the same schedule each day and eat on time to keep the blood sugar stable.
4. Keep in mind that habits are learned.
5. Reward yourself for each success, no matter how small.
6. Don't let anyone "love" you with food.
7. Remember: YOU create the success in your life.
8. Eat to live; don't live to eat.
9. Shop the outside aisles of the store — avoid tempting food packaging.
10. Avoid going by bakeries and other places where temptation may be too strong to resist.
11. Remember: You can't eat what you don't buy.
12. Remember: You are learning a "way to live," not just a way to diet.
13. Be so strong that nothing can disturb your peace of mind.
14. Diet one day at a time.
15. Don't let a temporary setback discourage you; keep climbing.
16. Say to yourself each day, "To change my life, I must first change my thinking."
17. Set a goal. Print it on a dozen index cards and place them in visible locations throughout your house.
18. Have food prepared "your way" when eating out.
19. Eat slowly in a relaxed manner.
20. Smile — you are a special person!
21. You must begin today what you would like to accomplish tomorrow.
22. Success is both the knowledge of what to do and the commitment to do it.
23. Be in control of your life.
24. Make charts and graphs of your weight loss and eating behaviors. Fill them out EVERY DAY.
25. Tape your weight-loss graph to your refrigerator door.
26. Remember, it takes time — BE PATIENT.
27. Eat fresh fruit and vegetables for "staying power."
28. Visualize what you want to look like tomorrow.
29. It is normal to plateau during weight loss — be patient.
30. WEIGH YOURSELF EVERY MORNING FOR THE REST OF YOUR LIFE.

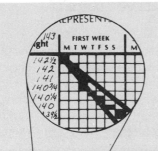

DIET CENTER
REDUCING PROGRAM

Date _____
Height _____
Weight Goal _____

EACH SQUARE REPRESENTS 1/2 POUND   **YOUR PERSONAL WEIGHT GRAPH**

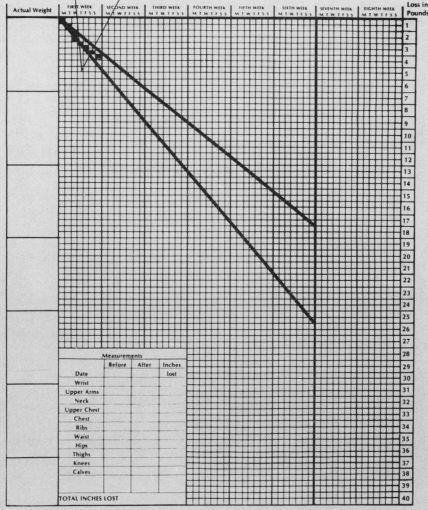

| | Actual Weight | FIRST WEEK M T W T F S S | SECOND WEEK M T W T F S S | THIRD WEEK M T W T F S S | FOURTH WEEK M T W T F S S | FIFTH WEEK M T W T F S S | SIXTH WEEK M T W T F S S | SEVENTH WEEK M T W T F S S | EIGHTH WEEK M T W T F S S | Loss in Pounds |

Loss in Pounds: 1–40

Measurements

	Before	After	Inches lost
Date			
Wrist			
Upper Arms			
Neck			
Upper Chest			
Chest			
Ribs			
Waist			
Hips			
Thighs			
Knees			
Calves			
TOTAL INCHES LOST			

Finishing Date _____

Weighing daily will help you to see the relationship between food and the body. Any potential problems can be solved quickly. Along with graphing your daily progress, you will also need to keep a diary of foods eaten. Exercise and make sure you receive adequate rest. You will see that a recorded history of your progress with all basic ingredients will appear on the graph (page 51) showing your success.

REWARDS

Finally, remember: IT IS IMPORTANT TO REWARD EVEN YOUR SMALLEST SUCCESSES. Be careful, however, not to equate reward with food. (The five pounds you have lost will quickly reappear if your reward is a hot-fudge sundae.) Losing ten pounds means a smaller clothing size! Reward yourself with a pretty new dress. Save that movie you've been wanting to see for a special reward, such as losing five more pounds. Buy yourself a bouquet of fresh flowers when you are halfway to goal. As you lose weight, you will both look and feel better. Others will compliment you on your new appearance, and nothing feels better than a compliment from someone whose opinion is important to you.

3

Relaxation and Visualization

ONE reason many dieters eat out of control is because they are under stress. Learning to set goals, becoming totally relaxed, and visualizing yourself as successful will lead you to permanent weight control, and to becoming the person you want to be. Read this section carefully so you will be able to apply these ideas to your daily dieting routine.

Learn to believe in yourself and your dream. It is easy to believe in yourself and your ability to lose weight when the sun is shining and no one is "pushing your buttons." But most of us do not have days like that very often. Belief in yourself and your ability to succeed is based on your experience. That experience can be real or imagined. Until you actually experience being slim and healthy, you must do the experiencing in your mind.

Diet Center recognizes the importance of building this "slim" experience into our minds by visualization. There are specific steps, however, that you must take to learn how to visualize success.

First, you must learn to relax your body and quiet your mind. Second, you must create graphic mental pictures of a successful, slim you while you are relaxed.

RELAX   Why is the process of relaxing the body and quieting the mind so effective? Relaxation "folds back" the conscious mind and permits your mental images to be fed more effectively into the subconscious. When the conscious mind is "out of the way," it does not interfere with its critical evaluation, subjective attitudes, doubts, or negativity.

Relax, and your mental images are received loudly and clearly by the subconscious. You are reprogramming the mind. The results are instantaneous!

The better and deeper you can relax, the more successful you will be. Your visualized pictures are etched deeper into your mind when you are quiet, in both mind and body. Follow these steps to learn total relaxation:

Diet Center's 10 Steps to Total Relaxation

1. Set aside fifteen minutes for yourself. You will need a private, quiet, dark place away from the hustle and bustle of everyday life. Sit in a comfortable chair (do not lie down); remove your shoes and wiggle your toes (or if conditions do not permit, just close your eyes and proceed). Plant your feet flat on the floor; get comfortable and BEGIN!

2. Take three deep breaths to release all the tension.

3. Tense your left hand by making a fist. Then let go and feel what "limp" really means. Progressively tense all your muscles, starting with the feet and working up. Tighten the muscles in your feet so you can recognize how your body feels when it is under stress. Then, let the tension slowly drain out; work up through the legs, stomach, chest, hands, arms, neck, and face (force a grin, then let go).

4. Enjoy a feeling of limp, relaxed heaviness as it creeps over your entire body, until you are so quieted that you are aware of your breathing.

5. Totally relax. Breathe deeply through your nose. Concentrate on a breathing pattern. Inhale, count to three, then exhale. Repeat. Know that with every breath you take, you go deeper and deeper into this beautiful state of total looseness, agelessness, limpness.

6. Quiet the mind. Let thoughts drift through it until they are gone and your mind is like a clean slate. Empty your mind of any problems or thoughts and continue breathing deeply, letting the blood and oxygen flow to all parts of your body.

7. See yourself as you go into an even deeper state of relaxation. (This happens progressively faster each time you follow this program.)

8. Tell yourself that on the count of three, you will emerge from this quiet state feeling wonderful.

9. Count aloud. One, two, THREE!

10. Write the word RELAX on a card and keep it in a visible place. Every time you see the card, it will remind you to relax.

You may not notice a considerable difference at first; but with continued practice, you will reach a state of relaxation more quickly. Remember, you need to be good to your mind and body if you want them to be good to you. Take time to *relax!*

VISUALIZE

Until recently, visualizing or daydreaming was always considered a waste of time. Traditionally, people were warned that habitual lapses into daydreaming could alienate a person from reality. Today, psychologists agree that to visualize situations (or see them in your mind) helps people gain relief from the stress of the real world, gives a balance to emotions, and helps deal with the pressures of day-to-day existence. Recent research on daydreaming shows that it significantly helps with intellectual growth, the power of concentration, and the ability to communicate with others.

Visualizing is a vital activity. Many successful people actually visualized their successes in full detail before the success was an actual reality. Thomas Alva Edison visualized himself as an inventor; Florence Nightingale visualized herself as a nurse; Harry Truman daydreamed to relieve the stress and tension in his life. Great people throughout the ages have done this.

Why do these visualizations dramatically help you? Scientists have proven that the body's nervous system cannot tell the difference between imagined and real experience. It reacts in exactly the same way to all information you put into the brain. These positive images will improve your self-image. But you should practice for approximately fifteen minutes every day. To get the best results, picture or visualize every detail as if it has already become a fact. Go over every detail several times. This procedure will indelibly impress the image upon your memory. The memory will soon influence your everyday living, and the images of daydreams will have definite effect on your behavior.

To visualize effectively, follow these steps:

1. Find a place where you can be alone and undisturbed. The harassed housewife can escape to a bath filled with tepid water; a busy executive with a private office can isolate himself there. Remember, you need total privacy. Any sudden noise will disturb your success.

2. Allow yourself to become totally relaxed following "Diet Center's 10 Steps to Total Relaxation" (page 54).
3. Now, concentrate on how you will look, feel, and act at your weight goal. Visualize yourself slender, happy, and successful. People compliment you. Your marriage is exciting and you feel like a bride or groom. People of the opposite sex give you a second look. You feel excited and proud of your success, etc. (the more detail, the better!).
4. Visualize wearing a size 10 dress or a new three-piece suit, what color it is, going to the store, selecting the dress, talking to the clerk, trying it on, looking in the mirror, seeing the color, feeling the delightful sense of success. Men, visualize your college days when you were healthy — vibrant, alive, active — wearing the good-looking sweaters tucked in with a belt size 32.
5. Visualize yourself seated at the table selecting a plate of beautifully prepared foods. See the crispness of the salads and the happy expressions of the people you are with. See yourself eating with relish the baked chicken. Savor the crunchiness of each vegetable and the "natural sweetness" of each fruit. You feel full, satisfied, and thin.

IMPORTANT DO'S AND DON'TS IN DIET CENTER

DO:
- Know that you can achieve whatever you "think" you can achieve.
- Make your mind the master of your body.
- Practice becoming a mature person.
- Admit that to maintain your new weight is your choice.
- Be aware that you cannot enjoy life, family, or beauty without good health.
- Know that life is not merely being alive, but being well and happy. (It is up to you.)
- Commit yourself to learning and to improving yourself.
- To not just exist, but live life to the fullest.
- Know that you can do anything you make up your mind to do.

DON'T:
- Become angry (instead, roll with the punches).
- Let unhappiness become your nature.
- Allow adversities to upset you.
- React negatively to situations.
- Put yourself down.
- Hold back love for people — reach out.
- Let indecision become a habit.
- Make angry, quick decisions; they are unsafe.

HOW TO MODIFY YOUR EATING HABITS

1. You are beginning a program to a new, healthier life.
2. Attitudes to try:
   A. I no longer need to be overweight or unhealthy.
   B. I am ready to be active and enjoy a thin, healthy, happy life.
   C. I visualize myself as a more productive person.
3. Let us examine the step-by-step process we will be taking:
   A. The first step — Realize your problem.
   B. The second step — Make a full commitment.
   C. The third step — Set long-term and short-term goals.
   D. The fourth step — Learn the entire five-phase Diet Center Program.
   E. The fifth step — Act.
4. How to condition your subconscious:
   A. Relaxation — Doorway to subconscious.
   B. Visualize — See yourself successful, slender, vibrant, eating and enjoying the proper food and good health.

At 122 pounds overweight, Irene Curtin was crying out for help. Now, at a trim 114 pounds, she is living a dream come true.

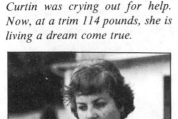

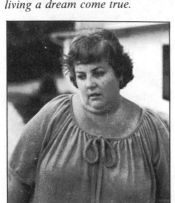

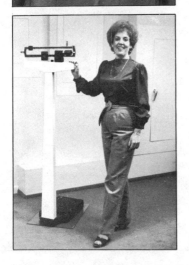

6. You can even visualize negative descriptions of foods or situations you want to avoid. See yourself eating fried chicken. Actually take the meat into your hand and squeeze out the grease. Visualize your greasy hand; see the expression on your face. Feel the grease running down your arm. You feel repulsed!
7. Make up your own!

The process of visualization is safe, harmless, and effective. You do not lose consciousness or go into a trance. You merely approach a sort of sleepy wakefulness. You may stop at any time — if the doorbell rings or the telephone rings or someone enters the room. You can complete this process anywhere you can relax. These thoughts will actually direct you to your goal. If you really want to reach your goal and you believe in it, your subconscious mind will automatically direct you to that goal.

Visualization produces results! As one former dieter recalls:

When I first walked into Diet Center, it wasn't with the commitment to lose my excess 122 pounds, but a cry for help. However, it wasn't until I had been going to Diet Center for five months and lost 67¼ pounds that I realized that I was going to make it; I was going to be thin. The visualization techniques have been important. I had been doing it in every other direction, except in the area of weight loss. Now, in combination with the relaxation exercises, I am spending at least one-half hour a day concentrating on myself and my slim new body. There was nothing that could stop me from reaching my desired weight goal. I have won the biggest battle of my life and I love the new me.

Irene Curtin
Monroe, New York

4

Dieting and Stress

DURING times of increased pressures, we usually hear statements like: "I am under so much stress," or "My boss puts a lot of stress on me." What, however, is stress?

WHAT IS STRESS?

Stress is the general response of the body to any demand made upon it. This is difficult to understand when we know the body responds very specifically to each demand made upon it. When you are cold, you shiver to produce more heat. When you are hot, you sweat to cool the skin. When you exert yourself running up a flight of stairs at full speed, your heart will beat faster to supply more blood to the muscles.

A similar reaction occurs with drugs and hormones. Diuretics increase urine production; adrenaline increases pulse rates and blood pressure; insulin decreases blood sugar.

All these demands have one thing in common: They increase the demand upon the body to readjust itself and return to normal.

It is not important whether the source of stress is pleasant or unpleasant. All that counts is the intensity of the demand. Have you ever experienced thinking you have failed in a special assignment and your job was in jeopardy? The boss calls you in and instead of firing you, he promotes you for doing an outstanding job. Or, have you gone on a ketosis diet where you've robbed your body of essential nutrients to the point of starvation? Two entirely different situations — imagined and physical stress to the body — yet the body physically reacts to both types of stress in the exact same way.

PHYSICAL AND MENTAL SYMPTOMS OF STRESS

The Three Stages of Stress

The body goes through three stages when confronted with a situation or event that causes stress. Let us pretend you are driving a car, and suddenly a child darts out from behind a parked car, directly in front of you. You grab the wheel, slam on your brakes, and, luckily, miss the child. You sit back, totally unable to move. Perspiration breaks out on your forehead. Your heart is beating rapidly, and you feel weak and shaky all over. This is stress. Your body has just instantaneously passed through all three stages of stress.

That's right, there are three stages of stress. In the first stage, adrenaline is released to the body, along with an additional amount of blood sugar, to give the body immediate energy so it can react instantly. In this case, you hit the horn and slammed on your brakes. The body is now in a condition called hyperglycemia, indicating a high level of blood sugar in the system.

The body is now in what is called the "fight-or-flight syndrome" of stress. (This syndrome refers to the immediate reaction most of us have to danger — e.g., an angry bear — to run away or stay and fight.) This is the stage where people often perform seemingly impossible tasks, such as lifting a car off a trapped child.

In the second stage of stress, insulin is released to take care of the increase in blood sugar level. An excess of insulin floods the body, putting it into a state of hyperinsulemia.

The third stage of stress occurs after the stress is over. The insulin leaves the body, pulling out the blood sugar as it goes. This leaves the person weak, trembling, perspiring, with heart beating rapidly and with emotions out of control. The body enters a state of very low blood sugar level called hypoglycemia.

I believe that, when the blood sugar drops, it drains the vitamin B-complex from the body as well. The vitamin B-complex is the body's natural defense against stress. It helps alleviate conditions of stress. When its presence is removed, the body becomes more susceptible to stress. For dieters, this is very important, because B-complex also helps the body to absorb and digest foods. It helps to metabolize food and helps the entire digestive system to function properly. When starvation diets cause physical stress to the body, the person goes through the three stages of stress. Dieters often forgo grain products, thus depriving themselves of a natural source of B-complex and possibly creating serious problems.

The body literally cannot tell the difference between a real or an imagined danger. If you think you are in danger, the reaction is exactly as if you are in fact in danger. For instance, if you are walking down a dark alley at night and you think someone is lurking ready to attack you, you do not need to stop and look behind the garbage cans to see if someone is actually there. Your adrenaline and blood sugar rise to give you immediate energy to get out of the danger.

MENTAL AND EMOTIONAL SYMPTOMS OF STRESS

The body's physiological changes, due to stress, are usually accompanied by some type of emotional or mental change. Stubbing your toe lights up a sign in your head that flashes "PAIN!" Mental and emotional reactions to stress are much harder to judge than physiological reactions for two reasons.

First, the amount of stress varies from one situation to another. Second, no two people react to stress in the same way. While some people are withdrawn and depressed, others become outgoing and hyperactive. Some people lose their appetites; others eat everything in sight!

It is important to remember that a situation cannot make you anxious or depressed; it is your interpretation of the situation that causes the anxiety.

Changes in job performance are often the most reliable indicators of mental and emotional symptoms of stress. Is someone working long hours or sleeping at the office? Does someone who is usually quite friendly seem distant, or very short-tempered? These are psychological warnings that stress is beginning to affect one's behavior.

COPING . . . BUT NOT COPING

People attempt to cope with stress-causing situations in a variety of ways. Unfortunately, some of these solutions are more harmful than the stress itself. One of these "false solutions" is simply to deny: (1) that stress even exists, and (2) that stress is directly affecting you. Denying the fact that stress exists is the first step to a mental and physical "burn-out."

Most people understand that there can be extra pressures on the job and on the executive, but very few people realize how obtrusive a role stress plays in the success of the dieter. It is such a factor, in fact, that it can mean either success or failure for the dieter.

So often, the dieter is totally successful in dealing with everything in life except the diet. Frequently, the overweight person is the otherwise successful executive who can organize entire civic projects or who may be very successful in the political field, but fails totally when it comes to his personal desire to be rid of excess fat. Even though these individuals realize the importance of losing weight for better health, they cannot because of their heavy routine. Often, these people become short of breath, their blood pressure is higher than it should be, and they tire more easily.

The community leader who is overweight may have respect from his or her peer group, and you might think that person can achieve anything, but often that person would love to wear the designer clothes made especially for the slender person. Even though that person appears successful in the eyes of others, his or her own eyes register failure.

Far too often, overweight people feel like personal failures who are undisciplined. How often do we hear people say, "Well, with all her talents and achievements, you would think she would do something about the way she looks." Little do these people know that virtually every overweight person is constantly thinking about dieting, or actually *is* dieting every day of his or her life. I do not remember a single day of my entire adult life that I was not hungry, experiencing that "starved feeling." How could this be when I weighed 186 pounds? Simple! I was always dieting — counting calories; skipping meals; substituting for good nutrition the high-calorie snack food that I could not resist, such as potato chips, a piece of cake, a few cookies; counting calories; skipping food . . . trying to diet.

Dieters everywhere are doing exactly as I just described — counting calories, skipping meals, placing their bodies in starvation conditions, and, therefore, placing their bodies under extreme stress. The B-complex is often depleted; the diet of high-calorie sweets provides little or no foods to replace the Bs, which are so essential in alleviating stress and helping us to remain calm and serene. The blood sugar is erratic because of the constant stress of the starvation diet. The body craves sweets — the dieter eats cookies or cakes, not because they are weak-willed, but rather, because they did not feed their bodies correctly, and the body is literally in a state of shock. The brain knows that energy is found quickly in refined sugars and flour. People eat off their diets not because they are weak-willed but simply because they do not understand how the body functions. This is why it is essential to eat the right foods on time and on a schedule so food stresses can be alleviated.

When dieters begin to relax and visualize, they are learning to cope with stress — then they are able to begin the Diet Center regimen.

III

BEFORE EVEN BEGINNING TO DIET

1

"Be Prepared"

NOTE: **This section deals only with those foods and methods of preparation used in the Conditioning and Reducing phases of the Program.**

How well you *prepare* for dieting is a good indicator of whether your diet will survive the first 48 hours. FOLLOW THESE PREPARATION STEPS FOR SUCCESS.

Plan the time to plan. Starting the diet on Monday? Give yourself two days of advance planning and preparation.

Check your equipment. Food preparation and cooking may be somewhat different for dieting than what you are currently doing. Check for these essential pieces of equipment that make dieting easier:

skillet — preferably with a no-stick surface (e.g., Teflon or Silverstone)
steamer — aluminum or stainless steel
food scale — capable of measuring per ounce
egg slicer — great for salads
blender — helpful when making diet mayonnaise or special fruit drinks and desserts
food processor — especially great for preparing vegetables and fruits for salads or snacks

Constructing a menu. Some dieters never need a menu to follow. Others with more rigid time schedules or those who like more organization would prefer one. Menus do provide an opportunity to explore endless possibilities in creating new dishes or combining foods. Simply eating a chicken salad, apple, fish, and green beans day after day will hinder your efforts just because of boredom, and you will not receive the essential nutrients necessary for overall good health. You may want to examine the menu that follows the explanation of the Diet Center Reducing Diet (pages 130–135) for ideas on how to make your menu both appetizing and appealing, then prepare your own menus.

Make a grocery list. The basics of the Diet Center Reducing Diet are simple natural foods that can be found in any grocery store. You may need, however, to compare the stores in your area to see which one has the greatest selection, freshest fruits and vegetables, and lowest prices. For instance, if large crisp apples and other food items are not available, talk to the store manager. If there is a consistent demand for a certain item, many stores are willing to offer it.

In making a grocery list, take your menu and determine types and amounts of foods you will need. The leftover chicken from Monday's baked chicken can easily be used in Tuesday's noontime salad.

FOOD BUYING — NUTRITIOUS AND ECONOMICAL

Did you know that you fight most of your battle to lose weight long before you sit down to eat? Although you may not realize it, your biggest challenge comes not at the dinner table but at the grocery store.

More than ten thousand food products confront you at the supermarket. Stretching food dollars in today's well-stocked market can be a challenge, particularly for those on tight budgets. Grocery products and packaging are designed to get your attention and trigger impulsive buying.

If you watch television or read magazines and newspapers, you have noticed that not all foods are promoted equally. The term "differentiated" is used to describe those foods that are unique and can be sold by brand names. They also bring a much higher profit to the producer. This in turn allows for a much larger advertising budget. The more an item is promoted, the more likely you are to buy it. In the long run you pay for the whole thing out of your pocket and, more importantly, with your health.

Retailers also influence your food selections. Notice where candy, cookies and other foods that appeal to children are located in markets. The ends of the aisles are also a favorite place for soft drinks and snack chips. It is amazing how food marketers have studied the consumer. They know exactly how to motivate us to buy their products.

But you do have a choice. Diet Center makes the following suggestions to ease the strain on your food dollar:

- Shop the outside aisles of the store. There you will find fresh fruits and vegetables, milk, cheese, eggs, chicken, fish, red meats, bread, etc. There are not many items that are essential for health that cannot be found there. For sundry items, shop quickly so you will not be tempted.
- Prepare a menu ahead of time and use it to make a list specifying exact amounts of each food. You should make a menu plan for a whole week.
- Check your newspaper for "specials." At these prices you may be able to buy meat cuts that are normally beyond your budget.
- Plan your shopping for at least two or three days. (Fresh fruits and vegetables are a must.) The more times you go to the store, the more of those unnecessary "extras" will tempt you.
- Also plan to limit your time in the store. The longer you stay, the more impulsive buying you'll do.
- As a precaution, do your shopping when your stomach is full. Everything looks good when you're hungry.
- Fresh foods in season will be the highest in flavor, quality, and nutrition.
- Select lean cuts of meat, poultry, and fish that provide the most for your money.
- Pass up those aisles full of pasta and pastry. (Remember, they are only good for a few seconds, but they may last a long time as fat.) Stick to the periphery — these outside aisles provide all the fresh produce, dairy products, and meats you need for your diet.
- Portion control begins at the store; buy only the amounts you need, to prevent excesses later when serving or eating.
- Don't buy food that will tempt you once you are at home.
- Look for unit pricing on the products you normally buy. You will find that product quality is similar, but there can be a big price difference.
- Home gardens can provide the very freshest vegetables and can be an enjoyable project for the entire family.

WHEN CHOOSING PROTEIN

Eggs

The color of an egg is unimportant. It doesn't matter if eggs are white or brown, or if their yolks are light or dark. Just avoid eggs with shiny shells. If you're not certain of the freshness of an egg, float it in a bowl of cold water. If it floats, throw it out. A fresh egg has a yolk that stands up when cracked into a pan, and a thick egg white. Stale eggs will run all over the pan. They are still edible, but have lost considerable food value. A spoiled egg can be determined immediately when cracked by the watery appearance and sour smell.

Fish

When shopping, you should look for fish that have the following:

- Clear, bulging eyes, not clouded or sunken
- Reddish gills, with overall good color
- Scales that adhere firmly to the skin
- Firm flesh that springs back when touched; stale fish leave indentations
- Firm scales with a high sheen
- No fishy or offensive odor

The Leanest and Fattest Fish

The fish allowed on Diet Center's Program are the leanest: flat fish, flounder, haddock, halibut, perch, pike, pollock, red snapper, sea bass, sole, and river trout.

The most fatty fish are albacore, bloaters, butterfish, bluefish, chub, eel, herring, mackerel, pompano, salmon, sardine, shad, smelt, sprat, tuna, white fish, and lake trout (lake trout have 74 percent fat while river trout have only 19 percent fat; lake trout and those from a brook or river look basically alike on the outside, but their insides are vastly different, one is almost all muscle and the other is almost all fat).

Chicken

Look for soft legs and feet, bright skin, and a flexible breastbone. If the tip of the breastbone bends easily, it is a young bird; if it is stiff, so is the bird. Avoid birds with skin that is dry, hard, purplish, broken, bruised, scaly, or has hairs protruding from it.

Vegetables

How to Get the Most out of Produce

1. Buy fruits and vegetables in season whenever possible.
2. Buy in small quantities and refrigerate.
3. Choose the darkest and healthiest-looking vegetables. Avoid pale and withered food. Always buy the crisp, dark green leaves and bright yellow and orange varieties. Remember: The darker the vegetable, the more vitamins and minerals.

Note: You may need to shop "specialty" stores to obtain

some items. At your local supermarket, you will find a large variety of herbal teas. Check your local butcher for rabbit, beef heart, and chicken livers. If there is a fish market in your area, see if the types of fish you need can be stocked.

SHOPPING TIP: INTERPRETING THE WEIGHT OF YOUR MEATS

RAW WEIGHT	COOKED WEIGHT	NUMBER OF PORTIONS	RAW WEIGHT DECIMALS
4 oz.	3.5 oz.	One	.25 lb.
8 oz.	7.0 oz.	Two	.50 lb.
12 oz.	10.5 oz.	Three	.75 lb.
16 oz.	14.0 oz.	Four	1.00 lb.

STORING YOUR FOODS . . .

Storing Raw Meat

REFRIGERATOR: Packaged meat in your refrigerator will last longer if commercial wrap is removed and the meat then wrapped loosely so air can circulate through the meat. Store in the coldest part of the refrigerator. Chicken, fish, steaks, chops, and roasts will keep up to three days at a temperature of about 40°F. Ground, chopped, or cubed meat should be used within twenty-four hours.

FREEZER: Freeze meat at 0°F or lower. Inexpensive butcher's paper is the best for meat to protect against drying and freezer burn. Date your meat.

Storing Cooked Meat

REFRIGERATOR: Cool cooked meat an hour before refrigerating, then wrap tightly to prevent drying. Sliced meat spoils more rapidly than roasts, etc. Store in the coldest part of the refrigerator. It will keep from three to five days.

FREEZER: Wrap well in butcher or moisture-proof paper. It will keep three of four months with no loss of flavor.

Shrimp: Parboil shrimp in their shells for two minutes. Drain off water, and put shrimp out into 3½-ounce portion packets.

Chicken breasts: Bone and skin chicken breasts if not already done. Wash, portion out onto foil, and bake eight to twenty portions of chicken breast meat. You may also bake all together in a casserole dish with lemon juice and herbs, and when done, weigh out in 3½-ounce portions to wrap in foil and freeze. Save all juices, cool and skim off fat — a good broth for cooking and soups. Note: Breast meat only takes 35 to 45 minutes to cook at 350 °F.

HOW TO BONE A CHICKEN BREAST

Boning a chicken is a simple process if you follow these basic steps:
1. Place the breast skin side down.
2. Cut through the gristle and bone at the top center of the breast. (You can now flatten the breast and remove the bone.)
3. Cut the meat from the long rib cage bone on both sides up through the joint.
4. Scrape the rest of the meat from the bones.
5. Remove the tendons.
6. Remove the skin. This gives you a whole butterflied breast.

Produce Hints

Wash raw vegetables. Heads of lettuce should then be drained and wrapped in paper towels and cellophane bags. Wash fresh raw mushrooms, dry well, leave whole and store in an air-tight container. Wash two or three bunches of green onions and trim, radishes, the whole celery stalk, etc. Store in plastic bags in the refrigerator.

If you're lucky enough to have a garden, pull only the vegetables you're going to use immediately. If you're buying from the store, buy small quantities and refrigerate immediately.

Vegetables exposed to room temperature and light for several hours lose up to 50 percent of their vitamin C, varying amounts of vitamin B_2, and folic acid.

Leafy greens have more vitamins and minerals per calorie than any other food, but their food value deteriorates rapidly.

Storing Eggs in the Refrigerator

Covered (cartoned) eggs stay fresh longer than uncovered eggs or eggs placed in the refrigerator trays.

To store new egg yolks, cover the yolks with cold water, cover the dish, then refrigerate. These yolks will keep up to four or five days. For longer storage, poach first, then cover and refrigerate. (Chopped or grated poached yolks are delicious as a sandwich spread, or as a garnish for vegetables.)

Store egg whites with a tightly covered lid and use within four days.

Storing Cooked Eggs

The recommended method for hard-boiling eggs is to put a dash of salt in the water to make shelling easier. Put the eggs in cold water in a covered pan and bring to a rapid boil. Continue rolling boil for three to five minutes. Turn the heat off and let eggs sit covered in hot water for 30 to 40 minutes . . . and you will not have a green halo around the yolk and the eggs will peel easier. Boiled eggs can be cut up and added to 2½ ounces of shrimp or crab salad. They also can be deviled for variety. Remember, three to five eggs per week is recommended, but no more than five.

ONE LAST CHECK

Are you "prepared" to diet? Run through this quick checklist to make sure. (Items you are not familiar with will be explained later in this book.)

1. ____Have you designed a menu for the coming week?
2. ____Do you know exactly what you will be eating:
   ____Monday?
   ____Tuesday?
   ____Wednesday?
   ____Thursday?
   ____Friday?
   ____Saturday?
   ____Sunday?
3. ____Are your cupboards, refrigerator, and freezer full of the foods you will need on the diet?
4. ____Are these foods placed in the front where you can easily find them?
5. ____Are there any leftovers? If there are, freeze them.
6. ____Is your cooking equipment ready to go and in easy access?
7. ____Have you divided chicken breasts, ground beef heart, shrimp, crab, fish, etc., into required portion sizes?
8. ____Have you boiled several eggs?
9. ____Is there a batch of Diet Center Bran Muffins (page 314) or Diet Center Apple Cookies (page 314) in the freezer ready to be popped in the oven or microwave?

The following principles cannot be incorporated into your life overnight. Even with your daily efforts and the guidance of this book, permanent changes take time. Work for it, you are worth it!

10. ____Have you made any Pop Squares (page 316)?

11. ____Is your shrimp cooked and ready to be tossed into a salad?

12. ____Have you prepared a large fresh salad and stored it in the refrigerator for lunches or dinners?

13. ____Do you have veggie snacks in plastic bags — ready to be eaten in case of emergency attacks?

14. ____Do you have a bowl of fruit on your kitchen table?

15. ____Do you have a two-quart pitcher of ice water cooling in your refrigerator?

2

Mental Preparation for Dieting

No diet can succeed without *you.* A diet only works when you do. Reaffirm your personal decision and commitment to diet before beginning. Make sure that it is *your* decision, not anyone else's.

Take a quiet thirty minutes to prepare mentally to diet. Your outlook before even beginning can determine your success. This will be the LAST diet you will ever have to go on. You can succeed! Nothing is more important!

Have some morale boosters throughout your house for extra incentive and encouragement. Try these ideas:

1. Pick out a favorite pair of pants or jeans that you have been avoiding because you just can't seem to fit into them anymore. Hang them at the front of your closet where you can see them every day. Then, try them on. Don't be discouraged at any bulged, straining seams or even if you can't quite get that zipper zipped up. Just visualize yourself as thin and slim. Soon, these pants will be too loose!

2. Take a picture. No one likes a "fat" picture, but nothing is a better incentive to start your diet and stick to it! Pictures seem to reveal everything, especially that extra ten pounds we all seem to rationalize away. If you're brave, post the picture on your refrigerator or next to the cupboard you used to keep the cookies in. Or, put it in a place you will see it each day. Try your underwear drawer, bathroom cabinet, a kitchen drawer. Just make sure you see it!

3. Make a bet with a friend or fellow employee. Allow yourself an average weight loss of three pounds per week. Set a goal for a special day or event approaching in the near future.

4. Post this sign on your bathroom scale: "I won't stop until I reach my goal."
5. Ignore any past successes or failures. Be determined, but excited. Eliminate words like "quit" and "failure" and phrases like "I give up" from your vocabulary. YOU CAN DO WHATEVER YOU SET YOUR MIND TO DO.

3

Designing a Schedule That Works for You

FEW people realize how important a schedule can be for weight loss success. Take a minute to review your own eating habits.

Your body needs a daily supply of nutrients to function at peak efficiency. The mid-morning let-down for the executive or the mid-afternoon snacking by the housewife results from the body's demanding energy to keep on going. Unfortunately, the foods most of us resort to in these situations are composed of refined sugars, flours, and saturated fats — foods, as you have learned previously, that lack the "staying power" to provide the lasting energy you need.

Learn the importance of scheduling what and how much food is eaten. The Reducing Diet schedule is designed to provide adequate amounts of food throughout the day to ensure that the blood sugar level remains stable. With a stable blood sugar level, you feel energetic and satisfied. You are not constantly craving sweets or fighting the temptation to head into the kitchen for a snack. When you give food the importance it deserves in your life, your body will function more efficiently and effectively.

Remember to eat on time and on a schedule. If your day doesn't coincide with the schedule outlined on pages 130–135, then readjust the times so that they parallel the basic schedule presented. Do not wait to eat until you are hungry. If you do, you may be out of control. By eating to feed your body before you are hungry, you can select what you know you should eat without feeling persecuted and deprived. It is essential that you maintain this schedule SEVEN DAYS A WEEK. You may want to take a "vacation" on the weekends, but your body doesn't.

Vital Nutrients and the Diet Center Program

OUR approach to vital nutrients is essential for your good health. This section has been prepared so you can study why each type of food, in exact amounts, with the correct method of preparation is so important to both your dieting success and your permanent good health.

PROTEIN

Protein is the life substance of the body and is considered the "building blocks of life." It is the only nutrient capable of building and repairing the cells and tissues of the body. Protein is the major building material for muscles, blood, skin, hair, nails, and internal organs, including the heart and brain. It also helps to keep the elasticity in the skin as dieters lose fat from their cells. By eating the correct amount of protein, the body will stay healthy and satisfied. Next to water, protein is the most abundant substance in the body. When your body is not provided with an adequate amount of protein, you may experience problems with hunger, loss of stomach muscle tone (which can result in poor posture), and possible problems with irregularity and water imbalances. On the other hand, too much protein will be stored on the body in the form of adipose tissue, better known as "fat." The RDA states that women aged twenty-three to fifty need 44 grams of protein per day. The protein is important in this amount to keep the skin and body from deteriorating.

PROTEIN FOODS

Two cooked servings, 3½ ounces each, are required per day. (Weigh food 4 ounces raw.) This group contains approximately 20 to 30 grams of protein and 5 to 10 grams of fat per serving.

Cooking   Broiling, pan-broiling, pan-frying, oven-roasting, baking, stewing, using slow cookers, simmering, braising and pot-roasting are all recommended methods, but remember, use no added oils or fats.

Portion Size   Dieters should eat their two servings of protein — 3½ ounces, each, cooked — for lunch and dinner. When you prefer protein at breakfast, use one egg (equaling one ounce protein) and then reduce protein allotment to 2½ ounces for lunch *or* dinner.

How you prepare foods high in protein can be just as important as whether they are eaten. Dieters *must* weigh exact protein portions. Even though you think you can accurately judge four ounces of raw chicken livers or ground beef heart only by dividing one pound into four equal parts, it is best to use a scale. It is easy to misjudge without measuring. By adding or subtracting just one ounce of protein per day, you will create an adverse affect on weight loss. For true and accurate measurement, purchase a small food scale.

Preparation Hints *Chicken breasts:* These must be skinned and boned. Fat deposits in all animals lay along bones, as well as underneath the skin. Examine a chicken breast and you will actually be able to see the deposits of yellow fat. Cut away all visible fat.

Fish: Halibut, or any other fatty fish, should be trimmed of fat and skin and be boned. You may skin river trout if desired.

Beef heart: Remove all fat and veins before grinding or baking.

Shellfish: Use fresh whenever possible, with frozen as a second choice. Canned shellfish contain large amounts of sodium. If used, rinse thoroughly with water several times and drain.

Rabbit, deer, and elk: Remove bone and any obvious fat. If broiling, blot off any excess fat on surface before eating.

Tofu: See special instructions and suggestions on page 80.

Diet Center Crunchies or *Textured Vegetable Protein* (*TVP*): If you use these, rehydrate in warm water. Crunchies may be used in soup or with eggs, in salads, or eaten alone. Remember, because Crunchies are a soybean product, people over twenty-five years of age do not experience optimum weight loss by eating them. Diet Center Crunchies are available at any Diet Center location.

THINGS YOU SHOULD KNOW ABOUT TOFU

Although sometimes referred to as the "meat without a bone," tofu is not meant to be a meat-tasting substitute. Actually, tofu has no taste at all. In fact, tofu's lack of flavor is one of its most fascinating properties. Tofu is very versatile, as it takes the taste of any food it is combined with.

Tofu is packed full of nutrients. It actually provides more calcium than dairy milk, along with a lengthy list of other vitamins and minerals. Tofu contains the eight essential amino acids, thus making it a "complete protein." Because of its high-protein quality and easy digestibility, tofu makes an inexpensive protein choice for most elderly dieters and those who have difficulty chewing and digesting meat. Often, the elderly and very young adults find meat far too expensive for their budgets. Tofu is surprisingly inexpensive. It is also a good alternative for dieters who are vegetarians. (Eight ounces of tofu is equivalent to approximately 164 calories; 18 grams protein; 5 grams carbohydrates; 10 grams fat.)

The grams of protein may differ with brands of tofu. Read the label to confirm you are eating 18 grams of protein per serving. Although 8 ounces are usually equivalent to one protein serving, the tofu may not contain this amount of protein and more should be eaten to compensate for the difference. Be sure to check the "purchase by date." The fresher the tofu is, the better the texture. Also, check the label to avoid preservatives.

Tofu should be kept refrigerated under water. The water should be changed daily. This will ensure that the tofu will last for seven to ten days.

Many recipes call for the tofu to be pressed; and in most recipes, pressed tofu gives a superior product. The exception is if tofu is added to liquid, such as in soup or as a drink. Some people prefer that tofu, if added to salads and eaten cold, not be pressed. Experiment to find your preference.

TO PRESS: Place tofu in towel and twist ends of towel in opposite directions (hold over sink — a lot of moisture will come out).

REMEMBER, tofu is a soybean product, and if your weight loss is slow, use another recommended source of protein.

EGGS

Even though we do not count calories, we must be aware of them. Three eggs have 121 more calories than one chicken breast, but supply only 19.5 grams of protein compared to 26 grams provided by the chicken breast. Therefore, use only a maximum of five eggs per week. Combine one egg with 2½ ounces of another protein selection. DO NOT USE EGGS AS A SOLE SOURCE OF PROTEIN AT ONE MEAL!

For the best weight loss, use hard-boiled eggs. Boil several eggs and keep them on hand for convenience.

FISH

The key to preparing fish is to make sure that it is done. Use the easy "fork and eye" test. When the flesh flakes easily with the fork and the fish no longer looks translucent, it is ready to eat.

Fish is a wonderful protein source. It contains little cholesterol and fat while providing abundant amounts of vitamins and minerals. Fish offers a vast selection for varied tastes and is delicious when baked with lemon juice and herbs, broiled, or pan-fried in a no-stick pan or poached with lemon and herbs.

MEAT

Typically, red meat is not allowed on the Women's or Children's Reducing Diet (with the exception of elk and deer). We live in a society that has abundant quantities and varieties of meats. Americans now eat record amounts of red meats in their diets. Unfortunately, along with meat comes large amounts of hidden animal fats that contain more calories per gram than any other food. Did you know that 80 percent of the calories in a hot dog can be attributed to fats, or that 64 percent of the calories in a hamburger are due to fat? A combination of saturated animal fats comprises nearly half of the calories in an average American's diet.

For example, a 16-ounce broiled sirloin steak yields 1,281 calories, 104.3 grams of protein, and 136.8 grams of saturated and unsaturated fats. Diet Center suggests frequent use of fish and chicken as alternative meat entrées. The same 16 ounces of halibut have approximately 500 less calories than red meat, yet contain 114.3 grams of protein! To lower your consumption of animal fats, Diet Center recommends that you switch to lean sources of protein such as fish, chicken breasts, or tofu.

REMEMBER:

- Measure exactly. One pound of raw meat equals four cooked servings.
- Remove all visible fat.
- Cook well-done to ensure low-fat content.
- Do not substitute!

CARBOHYDRATES — VEGETABLES, FRUITS, AND BREADS

Carbohydrates are the body's main energy supplier. The brain relies almost exclusively on one carbohydrate, glucose, to provide it with fuel to operate. The brain *must* receive this glucose on a daily basis. Without carbohydrates, the body is forced into an emergency situation. Over a prolonged period of time, it can develop into a potentially dangerous condition called ketosis (see page 26). Carbohydrates also assist in bodily functions, digestion, and muscle exertion while helping a person to think more clearly and to maintain a good energy level. It is important to consume the right kind of carbohydrates (unrefined, natural foods) to help maintain a stable blood sugar concentration and keep you from destructive snacking. Usually, a good test to determine if a carbohydrate is the right kind is whether it appears in "Mother Nature's wrapper" or one from a manufacturer (after the food has been refined). The RDA states that the average woman needs 300 grams of carbohydrates. When restricting your diet for weight loss, it is essential to eat more than 60 grams in order to avoid ketosis. The Reducing Diets for Women and Children provide an average daily allowance of 90 to 156 grams of carbohydrates. (The Men's Reducing Diet provides a substantially higher daily intake of carbohydrates.)

Carbohydrates on the Reducing Program come from fruits, vegetables, and whole grains (breads). These foods also provide the body with another important element, fiber. Fiber helps keep the body satiated longer and aids in proper digestion and elimination.

Vegetables

Vegetables make up a large part of the total volume of foods you eat each day while dieting. Who doesn't believe in the importance of salads for losing weight? The list of vegetables on the Reducing Diet is designed to provide maximum "staying power" and nutrients, yet with the lowest levels of calories. Dieters are instructed to eat one large salad daily, consisting of five to seven different vegetables, to ensure a wide variety of vitamins and minerals daily. Don't limit yourself just to lettuce. Watch the produce section at your local grocery for the "unusual" vegetables on the Reducing List that you may not normally use. Dieters are also encouraged to eat a one-cup serving of cooked vegetables every day. Again, try a variety of vegetables for a unique blend of flavor and texture.

The cooking process alters nutrient states of some types of vegetables. In achieving a balanced diet, it is important to eat both raw and cooked vegetables! Women dieters are cautioned not to eat both raw and cooked vegetables at the same meal. (I know that I promised at the beginning of this book to tell you not only "what" to do, but "why" you should do it.

This is one exception to that promise. Personal experience and years of monitoring the progress of other women dieters has proven to me that eating raw and cooked vegetables at the same meal inhibits weight loss. I can find no biological or logical explanation for this, but I know it to be true. Men, however, are not affected by this phenomenon. In any case, it is an important principle in the Diet Center Reducing Diet for Women.)

Fresh vegetables are suggested as an excellent mid-morning and mid-afternoon snack. Prepare "veggie-treats" ahead of time, including: celery sticks, mushroom caps, cucumber and zucchini rounds, green onions, radish roses, and cauliflowerettes. Even raw green beans are a crunchy treat. Along with fresh spinach, store these treats in individual sealed sandwich bags in your refrigerator, ready to be eaten anytime as a snack or to use for a large, crisp salad.

While the majority of vegetables on the Reducing Diet for Women list (see page 125) may be familiar, some may be ones you have never even considered trying! The additional following list also provides not only a description of these "unusual" varieties of vegetables, but gives suggestions on how to use them and the important nutrients you can find in them.

Beet greens: The leafy tops of beets taken from young plants are very good when prepared as steamed greens with lemon and Diet Center "Buttery Flavor Salt." They also provide a unique addition to salads. Beet greens are an excellent source of iron and contain vitamins A, B_1, B_2, B_6, and C, potassium, and calcium.

Chard: Swiss chard has long been a favorite because of its versatility. Its leaves complement any salad and are just as delicious cooked, tasting similar to spinach. Swiss chard is easy to grow and can be found when lettuce and spinach are unavailable. It contains vitamins A, B_1, B_2, B_6, C, and E. Iron and calcium are also found in chard.

Chicory: Chicory may be referred to in several ways — French or Belgian endive or chicory Witloof. The leaves grow into an elongated stalk and are bleached white. The French prefer the looser-leaved variety for winter salads, while elsewhere the more compact crowns are favored. Chicory provides vitamin A, calcium, iron, phosphorus, and potassium.

Chinese cabbage: Like most types of cabbage, Chinese cabbage (also called *Bok Choy*) is an excellent salad plant. It can be used alone or combined with other vegetables. Chinese cabbage has a milder flavor than other varieties, and if kept cool will store well. It is good either cooked or eaten raw. This cabbage contains vitamins B, B_2, B_6, and C, phosphorus, and calcium.

Endive (escarole): Endive and escarole are very similar and often are grouped together and referred to as endive. Both plants are leafy greens, but escarole has a broader leaf and does not curl as much at the tips. As a general rule, endive is used in salads, and escarole for cooking. Endive and escarole provide vitamins A, B_1, B_2, and E, phosphorus, potassium, and iron.

Fennel: Fennel grows from two to four feet in height. All parts of the plant are usable and supply an "aromatic taste" to foods. Fennel is often used as an herb. It is a source of vitamins A and C, calcium, iron, potassium, and phosphorus.

Kale and Collards: Kale and collards are pleasing both to the eye and palate. Their colorful leaves are often used to complement flower arrangements. At the same time, they resemble cabbage that has not formed into heads. Kale and collards supply vitamins A, B_1, B_2, B_6, C, and E, phosphorus, potassium, iron, and calcium.

Mung bean sprouts: Sprouts are becoming increasingly popular as a salad ingredient. Mung bean sprouts were developed by the Chinese and are a good source of vitamins A, B_1, B_2, and C, phosphorus, potassium, and calcium.

Okra: Okra is best tasting when its seedpods are picked unripe. It can be used in soups, stews, or as a cooked vegetable. Okra furnishes vitamins A, B_1, B_2, B_6, and E, phosphorus, potassium, and iron.

Peppers: Peppers come in a variety of shapes, sizes, and colors. They are a great salad ingredient, adding flavor and color. Green peppers are a rich source of vitamin C while also providing vitamins B_1 and B_2, potassium, phosphorus, and calcium.

Zucchini: A member of the squash family, zucchini livens up a salad or is a tasty dish served on the side. Its versatility has made it one of my favorites. Zucchini is a source of vitamins A, C, and B_1, niacin, iron, calcium, and potassium. While you may have thought of zucchini only as a cooked vegetable, it's delicious raw.

How you prepare vegetables can be an important factor in weight control. For example, it is interesting to note that a potato and a carrot have approximately the same number of calories, but most people think of potatoes as being fattening and carrots as a diet food. Why? An ordinary potato, baked or boiled, may contain only 100 calories. Mashed, with some milk, takes it up to 250 calories. If you french fry it, you make it 200 to 250 calories, and if you make it hashbrowned in bacon fat, you can build calorie count to 400 to 450 calories. Still potatoes! It really depends much more on how the food is prepared than what it is. On the Reducing Diet for Women, neither potatoes nor carrots are allowed because dieters do not lose as rapidly as they do when eating other vegetables. However, after weight goal is reached we recommend that they be included in your diet.

Dieters are advised to use FRESH vegetables whenever possible. Although sometimes available on only a seasonal basis, fresh vegetables are the BEST! Frozen vegetables have already been somewhat processed and consequently drained of vital nutrients and fiber. Your last resort should be canned vegetables. Canned vegetables can contain large amounts of

Use the following suggestions to avoid the "produce enemies."
1. Keep fresh produce out of light and air. Oxygen is an enemy of vitamins A and C. Light is an enemy of vitamins A, C, and B_2 (riboflavin); B_2 resists heat, but deteriorates when exposed to light.
2. Water is an enemy of B vitamins. Never soak fruits and vegetables, because water-soluble vitamins leach away rapidly. Wash produce quickly, and never throw away cooking water. Drink it or use in soups, vegetable juices, etc.
3. Don't peel unless absolutely necessary. The peel is loaded with nutrients. If you must peel, never overpeel. Use a vegetable peeler rather than a knife.
4. Inexpensive steamers, waterless cookware, or double-boilers are excellent for cooking produce. Never start vegetables in cold water, and always use tiny amounts of water.
5. Select cooking utensils wisely. Glass, unchipped enamel, or stainless steel are best for cooking food. Copper destroys vitamin C on contact, and aluminum leaves metal residue in food.
6. Always use lids when cooking produce. Open pans let in air and light, and allow steam to escape. Steam is excellent as it cooks produce quickly. Pressure cookers destroy many of the nutrients in foods. Avoid them, except for canning certain vegetables.
7. "When you see the boil, you see the spoil," is a good motto in cooking any food. Never let foods continually boil — always steam or cook briefly on low heat.
8. Never overcook food. Cook on low heat for the shortest length of time possible. Cook vegetables so they still have a crunch.
9. Don't salt vegetables before or during cooking. Spinach salted during cooking loses up to 50 percent of its iron. Salt used during cooking destroys nutrients!
10. Use your microwave to cook vegetables. Wash and cut the selection. Place in a seal-locking baggie and cook 2 minutes or until done. Your vegetables will be crisp, tender, and delicious.

sugar, sodium (salt), and chemicals used to create long shelf-life. You will also note that cauliflower is allowed only in the raw form. Some vegetables during cooking undergo changes that can impair weight loss. Cauliflower is one example. As cauliflower is cooked, it becomes sweet. You will lose less weight with cooked cauliflower than if it is eaten raw. For some individuals, this also may happen with cabbage. Remember that dieting is different with every individual. Keep careful track of what you eat and what you weigh EACH DAY, and you will be able to determine the best foods for you!

Fruits

After three exhausting hours in the hot afternoon sun, you are ready for a quick-energy "pick-me-up." Few foods can provide the natural burst of energy found in a crisp, cold apple or the tangy brillance of a luscious orange. Fruits are probably the most enjoyable item on any dieter's list.

On the Reducing Diet, two fruits are eaten per day. One of these must be a large apple. It is recommended that fruits be used as in-between-meal snacks. The natural fruit sugar (fructose) provides an instant burst of energy to remedy mid-morning and mid-afternoon blahs. Some dieters prefer to save one fruit as a snack for after dinner while watching television or relaxing.

Dieters are not allowed to substitute juices for whole fruits. Raw fruits (also vegetables) have more "staying power" than either fruit puree or fruit juice. Whole fruits are bulky and fibrous; therefore, they take longer to eat, are digested more slowly, satisfy hunger longer, and are excellent sources of energy. Fruit puree and juice contain fiber, but have the opposite effect because the fiber is pulverized and requires no chewing, so it digests more quickly and is less satisfying. One small glass of puree or one-half glass of juice contains the equivalent of three whole fruits, so whole fruits have greater "staying power," and fewer calories than puree or juices.

Dried fruits are also not allowed as substitutes for whole fruits. They contain a high concentration of sugar and lack the fiber found in fresh fruits.

Like vegetables, fresh fruits are best! Whenever fruits are canned or frozen, they lose some of the fiber and bulk needed by dieters. Fruits canned in "heavy sauce" contain large amounts of sweeteners for taste and chemicals for preservation. Even fruits "canned in their own juices" require addi-

THINGS YOU SHOULD KNOW ABOUT APPLES

A LARGE APPLE MUST BE EATEN EVERY DAY AS ONE OF YOUR FRUIT CHOICES!

1. Whether reducing or not, you should eat an apple every day. True/False

True. Apples help to satisfy the dieter's hunger while dieting. They have what we call "staying power." In addition to this quality, apples are surprisingly loaded with essential vitamins, minerals, and nutrients.

2. An average apple is approximately 50 percent water. True/False

False. An apple consists of almost 85 percent water — the explanation of why this delectable fruit is so juicy!

3. Research has revealed that the pectin in an apple helps to lower the amount of sugar absorbed by the body. True/False

False. However, there has been some evidence to indicate that pectin assists in lowering the body's absorption of cholesterol. If so, "an apple a day keeps the doctor away" may be more than just an old adage, especially in some types of heart disease.

4. Apples are a natural way to supply your body with quick energy. True/False

True. The natural sugars in fruits are absorbed at a more even rate than refined sugars. Therefore, they yield quick energy with a gradual and moderate increase in the blood sugar concentration, instead of the rapid "skyrocket" effect that results from the refined sugar in a candy bar.

5. Apples should not be eaten if a person has diarrhea because of the high-quality fiber they contain. True/False

False. Although apples do provide a good source of fiber, which aids in proper elimination, they can be helpful in correcting diarrhea. Mild acids and pectin assist the body in ridding itself of toxins (which can be responsible for the diarrhea).

6. Apples are often referred to as "Nature's toothbrush," and are helpful as one form of preventive dentistry. True/False

True. The fiber in an apple requires extra chewing. Consequently, prolonged chewing increases production of salivary juices and also massages the gums. When combined with the fact that apples do not stick to tooth enamel, they produce a brushing effect. However, apples were not meant to replace the toothbrush — just the sweet, sticky treats that contribute to dental caries!

7. Apples may be beneficial in relieving tension-related headaches and illnesses. True/False

True. Current research has indicated that people who regularly consume apples suffer less from headaches and illnesses due to tension. Although no specific factor has been isolated, assumptions regarding the better digestion and toxin removal, which result from eating apples, have been cited as possible reasons. (The stabilizing effect on the blood sugar concentration may be another explanation.)

8. Wax naturally exists on an apple as its own form of protection. True/False

True. Granted, many apples are waxed in stores to appeal to the customer's eyes. However, the apple does produce its own wax that protects it from moisture loss, disease, insects, and injury. Neither wax is harmful.

9. Skins should be removed from apples when used in cooking or eaten fresh. True/False

False. Apple peels and the flesh directly under them contain nutrients, and should be eaten. The skin takes longer to digest and gives prolonged "staying power," which prevents hunger and satiates the appetite. The skin also provides additional bulk and fiber in the diet. It requires thorough chewing, which starts the enzymes working in the mouth and throughout the system.

10. Dieters on the program should eat at least one large apple a day for a fruit choice. True/False

True. The high nutritional benefits, combined with its fiber and bulk ("staying power"), make an apple an ideal choice for people who are dieting. It also promotes a healthy digestive system and proper elimination.

tional sodium and additives for preservation. Use only fruits found in "Nature's own wrapper."

Eat the entire fruit — peel and pulp included! Many important nutrients lie directly below the peel. The pulp has a role in maintaining normal digestion and elimination.

When eating your fruit "snack," cut it into small sections and eat slowly, one piece at a time. Savor the "natural sweetness" found in fruits. Amazingly, once refined sugar has been removed from the diet, dieters report actually being able to "taste" the sugars in fruits and find them deliciously sweet!

To achieve a proper nutritional balance, vary the type of fruit in your daily diet. Don't just eat an apple and orange every day! Be brave and try some of those fruits on the Reducing Diet for Women (page 128) that may not be familiar to you. You may find a new favorite!

The end result will be a change in attitude toward fruit, and your children will learn to enjoy it in place of sweet, processed foods. This will be an extremely beneficial change in your children's eating habits, which are now being formed for the rest of their lives.

Breads

When examining those foods which helped them gain weight initially, many dieters blame breads rather than "sweets." One dieter explained how she would have three or four slices of toast for breakfast, two or three sandwiches for lunch (two slices of bread each), another sandwich in the late afternoon, and then biscuits for dinner. "I never even ate sweets!" she said. What this dieter didn't realize is that many of the same ingredients found in "sweets" are also found in breads: refined sugars and white flour. Refined sugar, as well as many other types of sugar, is used to make foods "taste good." Refined white flour holds many other products together. Preservatives create a longer shelf-life. The "preprocessed" ingredients fail to contain the "staying power" found in whole grains. In contrast, the breads on the Reducing list (page 127) help provide necessary fiber for proper digestion and elimination. These breads are made of whole grains, which take much longer to digest than breads made from refined, white flour. Either six Diet Center Thins or two Lite Rye Wasa Brod must be eaten each day. (Note: Only the "Lite Rye" variety of Wasa Brod is allowed.)

OIL

The main objective of any diet is to rid your body of its excess fat; yet, the nutrient fat is essential to the body. Fat is the last nutrient to be digested and, therefore, helps provide the body with the "staying power" that is so important to a dieter. It also lubricates the skin and keeps the organs and glands functioning smoothly. Most dieters want to eliminate oil totally from their diets. This is not advisable because dieters will experience hunger and feel less satiated. It is important that the oil be measured very carefully — only 2 teaspoonfuls a day. OIL IS AN ESSENTIAL COMPONENT IN THE DIET.

The importance of the daily oil requirement cannot be overstated. When dieters switch from the diet of highly refined and preprocessed foods to one of natural foods high in roughage, both the digestive and excretory systems must adjust. The daily oil requirement helps with smooth digestion and elimination. Constipation will occur if the daily oil requirement is not met.

The oils on the Reducing list are all polyunsaturates from natural plant sources. It is recommended that dieters use the oil in a dressing with apple cider vinegar for salads or as a marinade. (Some dieters just use oil with Diet Center "buttery flavor salt" and herbs and pour it over heated vegetables, or dip crab, lobster, shrimp, or fish in it. Your method is up to you. Just get it in!) DO NOT use commercial diet dressings — the calorie content may be low; but the levels of sodium, sugar, additives, and preservatives are high. Remember, the best way to achieve maximum weight loss on this diet is directly related to controlling all foods that you eat each day!

A final recommendation — DO NOT HEAT OIL. Heating the oil may cause compositional changes that directly affect weight loss.

SEASONINGS

DO NOT OVERUSE SALT! Any seasonings or spices that do not contain oil or sugar are permitted in moderation. Read the label! (See pages 278–280.) Diet Center makes a variety of seasonings that can be used to enhance the flavor of your foods. Herbal seasonings are recommended to be used in place of salt. If salt is included in seasonings, Diet Center recommends using it sparingly (¼ teaspoonful of salt retains ½ pound of water).

Seasonings can spice up an ordinary chicken breast or fish

fillet. Use spice moderately to create interest. DO NOT OVER-SEASON.

Any leaf or herbal seasoning is allowed. *Watch out* for all packaged, mixed seasonings. Read the labels for sugar (dextrose, lactose), salt, or starch or fats. Any ingredient ending in *"ose"* is a form of sugar and should be avoided. Also, use sodium sparingly. In addition to the above, lemon or lime juice can also be used to bring out the "natural goodness" in foods.

SWEETENERS

Recommended: Diet Center sweetener has less than 2 percent saccharin.

Dieters are advised to check labels carefully before using any product other than Diet Center sweetener. Other products may contain sugars (including fructose, maltose, or dextrose) not so labeled, which will adversely affect weight loss.

VITAMIN C

During times of physical or emotional stress, the body requires vitamin C to replace that which is lost. Because vitamin C is a water-soluble vitamin, the increased water you are drinking may flush out this vitamin. Vitamin C is not stored in the body and therefore must be replenished each day. It helps in the healing of wounds and maintenance of bones. Vitamin C also assists in the absorption of calcium.

This daily supply of vitamin C is supplied to dieters both through natural food sources (fruits and vegetables) and an additional supplement. Dieters need additional vitamin C in their diets because of increased stress and increased fluid intake. Dieting, like smoking, and even environmental conditions (heavy smog areas), is a stressor that causes the body to lose vitamin C more rapidly. At the same time, your body will retain vitamin C for only a short period before flushing it out through the urine. This action can even be increased as greater amounts of fluids are drunk.

Consequently, dieters are advised to take 1,000 mg. of supplemental vitamin C per day while on the Reducing Diet. This supplement should be formulated from only natural sources, e.g., rose hips. (Many chewable vitamin C tablets contain various forms of sugar for "better taste.") This amount should be taken in equal intervals during the day. It is recommended that if taken twice per day (500 mg. each time), the tablet be in a time-release form.

CALCIUM

Calcium is the most plentiful mineral in the body and is found mostly in the bones and teeth. It is also found in small quantities in the soft tissues surrounding the nerve endings. Calcium has been called "Nature's natural tranquilizer." It is also involved in the body's metabolism (the rate at which the resting body uses energy). If inadequate calcium is supplied in the diet, the person may become irritable and nervous. When this happens, dieters may think they are hungry and eat. Calcium can also be obtained through many of the foods on the diet (e.g., vegetables and tofu).

A well-known source of calcium is milk. However, milk is not allowed on the Diet Center Reducing Diet because of its high content of milk sugar (lactose), which interferes with optimum weight loss. Instead, dieters can meet normal calcium requirements from natural foods and supplements. Did you realize large amounts of calcium are also found in dark green, leafy vegetables? As further fortification, Diet Center dieters also take 750 mg. of calcium per day. This amount can be taken in the morning or at three separate intervals (250 mg. each time) during the day. Individuals who suffer from periodic insomnia or severe muscle strain and cramps can take the entire amount shortly before going to sleep. (Did your mother ever give you a warm glass of milk right before going to bed to "help you sleep"?)

WATER

The body itself is comprised of 50 to 75 percent water. This remarkable fluid is not only the major constituent of the blood, but is also involved in almost every bodily function. It serves as a supplier and carrier of nutrients, a medium and participant in chemical reactions, a disposer of waste products, and a regulator of body temperature by its continual bathing of the body's cells.

Although most people never suffer from severe dehydration, they may still not be supplying their bodies with adequate amounts of water. When there is insufficient water in-

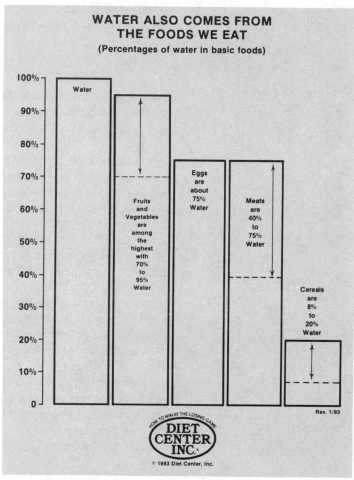

WATER ALSO COMES FROM THE FOODS WE EAT
(Percentages of water in basic foods)

take, organs and glands cannot function properly and the body's impurities are not washed out of the system. The body may manifest this water shortage by the development of a poor complexion, and eventually the individual may experience a feeling of sluggishness.

Every day, the body loses 2½ to 3 quarts (approximately ten to twelve glasses) of water through breathing, perspiration, urination, and other bodily processes. Under normal circumstances, no matter what the amount of intake, the body will still excrete at least that minimum amount of fluid. Therefore, it is only reasonable to replace the same amount of water daily to maintain a balance.

Water is one of the main ingredients for success in dieting. Remember the last time you drank a big glass of water and your stomach felt as if you had eaten a seven-course meal? Water can keep the stomach feeling full and satiated between meals, thus helping to prevent it from signaling the brain that it is hungry. When water is drunk in conjunction with foods high in fiber (whole grain, fruit, and vegetables), this satiated feeling is increased because the fiber found in these foods actually absorbs the water and swells in size.

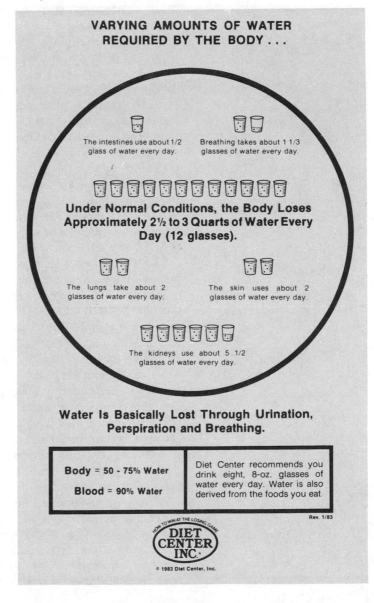

VARYING AMOUNTS OF WATER REQUIRED BY THE BODY...

The intestines use about 1/2 glass of water every day.

Breathing takes about 1 1/3 glasses of water every day.

Under Normal Conditions, the Body Loses Approximately 2½ to 3 Quarts of Water Every Day (12 glasses).

The lungs take about 2 glasses of water every day.

The skin uses about 2 glasses of water every day.

The kidneys use about 5 1/2 glasses of water every day.

Water Is Basically Lost Through Urination, Perspiration and Breathing.

Body = 50 - 75% Water

Blood = 90% Water

Diet Center recommends you drink eight, 8-oz. glasses of water every day. Water is also derived from the foods you eat.

Rev. 1/83

HOW TO WIN AT THE LOSING GAME

DIET CENTER INC.

© 1983 Diet Center, Inc.

When you experience hunger pangs or cravings for food, think before you eat the first thing in sight. That signal may actually be the body expressing a need for additional fluid. So, don't misinterpret it — try a glass of water before eating.

While dieting, water is extremely important. It is the skin's natural moisturizer, and is partially responsible for the skin's elasticity. To help the skin stay healthy and have the ability to "shrink" normally when weight is lost, you must have sufficient water in the diet.

Oxidation also plays an important part in weight loss. When the body is losing its stores of fat, extra water from the breaking-down process is left over. This is a crucial time for dieters because they experience what is referred to as a plateau. They may go for several days or even weeks without losing any weight until the body naturally rids itself of this excess fluid. This process of oxidation is explained here to give you encouragement and understanding should you encounter a plateau.

If you experience a plateau, take your measurements. Even though you may not be losing weight during this time, you will lose inches because water is more compact than fat. So, just because the weight stops coming off, don't throw in the glass! Water retention can't be countered by reducing water intake. Getting enough water during a plateau will actually help the body dispose of the extra water.

Whether dieting or not, keep in mind that drinking water is one of the easiest and least expensive things that can be done to improve overall health. Start the water-drinking habit and feel the difference it can make in your life!

Dieters are instructed to drink eight 8-ounce glasses of water throughout each day. (This amount may be decreased to six 8-ounce glasses for women under 5′2″ and children.) Drinking 64 ounces of water sounds like a lot to most people, but only because they have not made it a habit to drink eight glasses a day. At first, it will take a conscious effort to incorporate that amount of water into your daily routine, but in no time at all water will seem like the natural choice and will replace other beverages.

Dieters are encouraged not to exceed an intake of ten 8-ounce glasses per day under normal circumstances. (Extra water may be needed under conditions of heavy physical exertion or an extremely hot climate.) Too much water, drunk in too short a time period, can flush out vital vitamins and minerals essential for good health. When this happens, the body may experience an "electrolyte imbalance." This imbalance, when continued for an extended period of time, can result in dangerous physical consequences.

It is important to understand that waiting to drink water only when you feel thirsty is not sufficient to meet the body's need for water. It's the only way of telling the brain that it has not been receiving adequate amounts of fluids for a period of time. But, by drinking eight glasses of water every day, you can be certain that your body is receiving sufficient liquids. Dieters are instructed to sip at a glass of water throughout the entire day. If this isn't possible, follow an exact schedule such as the typical schedule for one day of the Diet Center Reducing Diet. All water should be drunk before 8:00 P.M. each night.

TIP THE GLASS

Experiment with the following helpful tips while acquiring the healthful habit of drinking water.

- Fill a two-quart pitcher with water and ice. Always keep your glass filled. By the end of the day, if the pitcher is empty, you'll have drunk 64 ounces.
- Start by drinking your water on a schedule (e.g., one glass every two hours). It will soon become a habit to drink eight glasses without even thinking about it. It is important to drink the water throughout the day, rather than trying to do it all at once.
- When socializing, choose seltzer with a twist of lemon or lime. Not only is it a wise choice for your health, but also for your waistline.
- Make sure to get in adequate water while traveling. If traveling by car, carry a thermos for easy access. You'll find you won't feel as sluggish at the journey's end.
- Don't cut down on drinking water when the seasons change. Drink a minimum of 8 glasses daily, winter or summer.
- If you find the water in your area unpalatable, add lemon juice to it to improve the flavor. You may also prefer to use bottled water. However, be sure that you are getting natural spring or mineral water and not just reprocessed tap water. Distilled water is not recommended because it does not contain those essential trace minerals.

LEMONS   Lemons are an important part of dieting. Lemon juice is high in vitamin C and acts as a "cleansing agent" for the skin, hair, digestive tract, and excretory system. Dieters must drink 2 tablespoonfuls of pure lemon juice in 8 ounces of hot water each morning (add some artificial sweetener if too tart!). Lemon juice helps break that "first-cup-of-coffee" habit many of us seem to depend on in the morning. The hot lemon drink is a good "waker-upper" and gets you started for the day. It is best to use pure lemon juice only! Fresh lemons are the best. If not available, however, use a pure frozen concentrate. Shelf products contain preservatives, chemicals, and additives.

OTHER FLUIDS — COFFEE, TEA, AND DIET DRINKS

Americans are substituting coffee, tea, and soft drinks for water. Without realizing it, they are compromising their good health. THERE IS NO SUBSTITUTE FOR WATER! Diet Center does not recommend overconsumption of these drinks. Although other diets may allow unlimited amounts, they are talking about calories instead of good health and sound nutrition.

These fluids are now considered "extras" in your diet. NO LIQUID CAN TOTALLY REPLACE WATER IN A NUTRITIOUS DIET. You will be amazed that as you drink eight glasses of water per day, your intake of these other fluids will drop substantially.

Any drink with caffeine causes an immediate reaction in your body. (Many adults and children are unknowingly addicted to caffeine.) Caffeine acts as a stimulant, which makes your heart beat faster and harder, causes nerves to become more jittery, and increases basic metabolic rate. And when dieters are nervous, they tend to think they are hungry. This increased activity wreaks havoc on a stable blood sugar level, drastically increasing and then lowering it, which causes the dieter to crave sweets. These changes can hinder a dieter trying to control hunger and sustain energy through maintaining a constant blood sugar level.

Coffee

Coffee is probably the most abused liquid in the American diet today. It is not unusual for dieters to drink from twelve to twenty-four cups of coffee per *day*. Dieters learn to reduce this amount gradually to approximately two cups per day. Heavy coffee drinkers tend to be slower weight losers as they frequently skip meals, only to become famished as the effects of caffeine subside.

Decaffeinated Coffee

Decaffeinated coffee is often offered as an alternative to coffee. In reality, it is not much better. A combination of over twenty different acids are used in decaffeination. Again, dieters are urged to reduce consumption of even decaffeinated coffee to no more than two cups per day.

Tea

Tea is made from a variety of methods, and these methods can adversely affect your weight loss. Black teas are the basis from which all flavored and decaffeinated teas are made. Black teas contain large amounts of caffeine and tannins (also referred to as tannic acids). Some types of black teas even contain as much caffeine as coffee! Flavored teas may sound better because they come in an array of flavors: orange, brandy, rum, blackberry, etc. These teas, however, are simply black teas with flavorings added.

Decaffeinated Teas

Decaffeinated teas are made through a process similar to that for decaffeinated coffees. In many cases, the solvent used only partially removes this caffeine. Dieters are not allowed to drink black, flavored, or decaffeinated teas on the Diet Center Program.

Herbal Teas

Herbal teas are allowed. These teas are produced from natural plant sources and contain no caffeine. Dieters who consume large amounts of coffee are often urged to switch to herbal teas. An 8-ounce cup of herbal tea can be used to replace an 8-ounce glass of water. Dieters are allowed to substitute herbal tea for water, but are cautioned not to exceed a limit of two cups per day.

Soft Drinks

Americans drank more than *8.9 billion gallons* of soft drinks last year, an amazing average of 212 cans per person! If soft drinks just contained their first ingredient, water, there would be no problem. However, if you examine the ingredients on a can label, you can find sodium, artificial colorings and flavorings, preservatives, caffeine, sugar or saccharin: the ingredients for a "nutritional disaster."

Regular sodas are definitely off any dieter's list. In fact, children can actually become "addicted" to the large amounts of sugar (up to six teaspoonfuls) found in each can. The high levels of phosphorus impair the body's ability to use calcium effectively. Ironically, sugar-laden sodas actually increase the body's need for additional water instead of eliminating thirst.

Diet Sodas

Diet sodas are allowed on the Diet Center Reducing Diet. Some dieters even use them as a "crutch" at parties or other

THINGS YOU SHOULD KNOW ABOUT LIQUIDS

For a quick review on liquids, try this quiz to test your knowledge

1. The body regulates its temperature by:
   A. Craving cold drinks when overheated, and craving something to eat when too cold.
   B. Burning up less fat during cold weather when fat is needed as insulation and using more fat when the weather is hot.
   C. Sweating.
      (C) Sweating. The body can stay within a reasonably normal temperature range by perspiring when it is working hard or the outside temperature is high. Replacing water lost while exercising is vitally important. Failure to do so can result in stroke caused by water depletion, which can even result in coma and death. Heat stroke symptoms are pronounced thirst, fatigue, muscle cramps, rapid heart rate, giddiness, and frequent urination.

2. Under normal conditions, the body requires _____ quarts of water per day. While some of this water comes from internal metabolic processes and the foods you eat, it is still recommended you drink _____ eight-ounce glasses of water per day.
   A. 1 to 2; 1 to 2
   B. 2 to 2½; 3 to 4
   C. 2½ to 3; 6 to 8
   D. 3½ to 4; 5 to 6
      (C) 2½ to 3, 6 to 8. The body requires this amount of water to function efficiently. This amount must be increased (as high as four quarts) with heavy physical activity or a hotter climate.

3. Which of the following foods are not more than 50 percent water?
   A. Cereals
   B. Meats
   C. Eggs
   D. Fruits and vegetables
   E. Milk
      (A) Cereals. While cereals are the logical answer, even they are high in water (8 to 20 percent). Meats are between 40 and 75 percent; fruits and vegetables, 70 to 95 percent; eggs, 75 percent; milk, 87 percent.

4. Which of the following types of vinegar is the most nutritional?
   A. Distilled
   B. Malt
   C. Synthetic
   D. Apple cider
      (D) Apple cider vinegar, of course! Apple cider vinegar is made from crushed apples in which the juice is allowed to mature. Regular use of apple cider vinegar, high in potassium and other trace minerals, is reported to help attain and maintain better health. In processing distilled vinegar, steam is used to remove the dark color and residue, resulting in the clear vinegar seen on the grocery store shelf. Unfortunately, this process also leaches out vital minerals. Malt vinegar is just another refined processed form. Synthetic vinegar, the cheapest shelf product, is simply an imitation produced from coal tar!

5. At a cocktail party, you have the choice of the following beverages. Which would be the best for both your health and waistline?
   A. Diet soda
   B. Club soda
   C. Seltzer
      (C) Seltzer. Seltzer is simply thrice-filtered water with added carbonation containing no added salts, flavorings, preservatives, and sugars. (Bottled water with natural carbonation, such as Perrier, falls into this category.) Of course, if you don't care for seltzer, you can always depend on water. Club soda, on the other hand, is tap water containing a mixture of such additives as sodium bicarbonate (baking soda), sodium chloride, sodium phosphate, and

sodium citrate. This high-sodium content produces edema (water retention) in some individuals. Diet sodas are "nutritional disasters" in the form of water, saccharin, and a heavy dose of chemicals in the form of flavorings, colorings, and preservatives.

6. Pure lemon juice:
   A. Acts as a natural diuretic.
   B. Is high in ascorbic acid (vitamin C).
   C. Can be used to coat pared fruit and prevent discoloration because of its high acidity.
   D. Should be purchased in "100% Pure Lemon" or "Natural" form to avoid adulteration with synthetic citric acid.
   E. All of the above.
   (E) All of the above. All of these facts about lemon juice are TRUE. At only 20 calories each, and high in ascorbic acid (vitamin C) and pulp, lemons are a recommended fruit choice.

7. John is a heavy coffee drinker (10 to 12 cups per day). Will this influence his attempts to diet successfully?
   A. Yes
   B. No
   (A) Yes. The high level of caffeine found in coffee can be both physically and psychologically addicting. As a stimulant, caffeine works to make the heart beat faster and harder, and your nerves are more "jittery." It increases your basic metabolic rate, which burns up available glucose more quickly and results in a subsequent lowering of blood sugar. This can produce a feeling of hunger. John should slowly decrease his consumption of coffee by substituting water or other caffeine-free alternatives.

8. After several hours of gardening and lawn work in the hot sun, you are ready to quench your thirst. You should reach for:
   A. A glass of water
   B. A can of soda pop
   C. A glass of fruit juice
   D. A glass of Gatorade (or other "athletic" thirst quencher)
   (A) A glass of water. A glass of water is by far your best choice. All these other beverages contain sugar, which slows the rate of gastric emptying and can actually make you more thirsty! For example, one can of soda may contain up to *six teaspoonfuls* of sugar. Orange and grapefruit juices have over *four* teaspoonfuls of sugar per quart, and even drinks specially formulated for athletes contain at least *two* teaspoonfuls of sugar per quart.

9. Which type of tea is best for you?
   A. Black tea
   B. Flavored tea
   C. Herbal tea
   D. Decaffeinated tea
   (C) Herbal tea. Black teas are the basic tea from which flavored teas are made. Black teas can be high in both caffeine and tannins (tannic acid, which is suspected to cause lip cancer). Flavored teas are simply black teas with a variety of flavorings added, including spice, orange, brandy, rum, and blackberry. Herbal teas contain no caffeine and are produced from natural plant sources, however; many herbal teas are medicinal. Moderation is the key. Consumption of herbal teas is recommended, but herbal teas *should not* be substituted for more than two glasses of water daily. Select green teas over black teas and either tea over coffee. Herbal teas, such as rose hips, are preferable to green teas. Water is the best of all. THERE IS NO SUBSTITUTE FOR WATER.

How do you rate? Give yourself one point for each correct answer.
9 Correct: You know your liquids.
8 Correct: Read through the answers one more time.
7 Correct: Check to make sure you are drinking enough water each day.
Below 7: You may be affecting both your diet and your health.

social occasions when they might be tempted to eat off the diet. However, dieters are cautioned that diet sodas cannot be substituted for the required 64 ounces of water. Also, the chemical and sodium levels in some sodas are hard on the kidneys and may cause water retention. Dieters are limited to two diet sodas or less per day. A limit of five cans or less per week is better yet.

Alcohol

No alcoholic beverages are allowed on the Diet Center Reducing Diet. Because alcohol has a diuretic effect, there may be a weight loss (fluid) the next day, but actually, the body will not lose weight for three days if beer, wine, or any type of alcohol is drunk. Alcohol is absorbed immediately into the bloodstream and it will definitely retard your progress.

REMEMBER:
- Although coffee and tea are made with water, they contain caffeine, tars, and chemicals that may be harmful to the body in excessive amounts. Coffee acts as a diuretic, causing the kidneys to excrete more water than normal.
- Drinking alcohol will stop a steady weight loss for up to *three days!* The day after drinking, a weight loss may occur due to the diuretic effect, but it will be three days before the body returns to normal. The high calorie content of alcoholic beverages cannot be overlooked either.
- Soda has just the opposite effect on the body. If several cans are drunk a day, the sodium content may create water retention. Although diet sodas are free from the high-sugar content found in normal soda, they too may cause the body to retain fluids.
- A large number of sodas also contain caffeine. Caffeine may even be in some fruit juices, so it's prudent to read the label.
- Overconsumption of these beverages usually decreases the amount of water a person drinks. Set a goal to limit your consumption of "all other fluids" to TWO servings per day.
- There is no other beverage that is a comparable substitute for water. It contains no chemical additives that will disrupt the body's delicate balance, but does contain essential trace minerals. Water is inexpensive and is calorie-free, making it the perfect drink for dieting.

IV

HOW TO SELECT A WEIGHT-LOSS PROGRAM
by
Dr. Lester J. Petersen

BEFORE selecting any reducing diet, examine the specific needs you expect the diet to satisfy. Of course, the diet should allow you to lose weight. However, at the same time, it should sustain the principles of sound nutrition to ensure good health. No reducing diet plan should deprive the body of its required nutrient intake to achieve weight loss.

Carefully consider the following list of criteria. Unless you can answer a definite "yes" to each question, in my opinion, this form of dieting should not be considered a sensible or recommended approach to weight loss.

1. Is this a program that your doctor would appove?

Review your proposed dieting plans with your doctor. He will be able to advise you as to the positive and negative aspects of any diet and foresee the possible effects it could have on your health.

NOTE: Dr. Petersen has been affiliated with the Diet Center Program since its inception. He was medical adviser during the formulation of the Diet Center Program and continues to serve as a consultant.

Dr. Petersen is a member of: Madison Memorial Hospital Medical Staff; Upper Snake River Medical Society; Idaho State Medical Association; American Medical Association; American Academy of Family Practice. He is Clinical Instructor, University of Utah Medical School, Department of Family and Community Medicine.

He has served as President of Madison Memorial Hospital Staff; President of Upper Snake River Medical Association; Member of Idaho State Board of Health, appointed by the governor, from 1971 to 1977; Member of House of Delegates, Idaho Medical Association.

2. *If any health problems exist, will these factors be taken into consideration?*

The majority of reducing diet plans do not take into consideration that many potential dieters have health problems. Serious complications may result if these diets are undertaken without consulting your doctor. Be sure that your reducing plan can be adjusted to conform to any specific health needs, if they exist.

3. *Are you satisfied that no dangerous physical condition could result from this diet?*

Many fad diets rely upon ketosis or dangerously low caloric levels for rapid weight reduction. Others employ the use of artificial stimulants that can result in hypertension, insomnia, or a variety of other unhealthful physical conditions. Again, consult your doctor.

4. *Has this diet really worked for other people?*

Ask to be referred to others who have been on this plan. No sales presentation or published advertisement can be as credible or reassuring as the comments from one "who has been there," and maintained his or her weight for a reasonable period of time.

5. *Is this a diet you can live with?*

Look beyond your immediate desire to lose weight. Can you realistically stay on this diet long enough to reach your goal? Does this diet provide the permanent eating patterns necessary to weight maintenance?

6. *Does this diet actually result in the loss of nonessential fat?*

There are several ways to reduce body weight. To be effective, a weight-loss program must reduce nonessential body fat. Many diets employ diuretics or laxatives to promote rapid weight loss. As soon as metabolic balance is restored, the weight returns.

7. *Does this diet provide an adequate volume and variety of familiar foods?*

A safe and effective reducing diet plan must provide adequate intake of the required nutrients as outlined by the RDAs. Foods should be inexpensive and easy to obtain and prepare.

8. *Is this reducing plan flexible enough to meet your particular needs?*

Consider your life-style, your eating schedule, your frequency of dining out. Unless this diet is adaptable to your situation, it is NOT a realistic solution to your weight problem.

9. *Does this diet provide for long-term changes that will make it possible for you to keep the weight off, once you have lost it?*

Unless you are making permanent changes in your eating habits, the likelihood of long-term weight maintenance is bleak. If, for example, you are relying upon prepackaged foods for weight reduction, what will you do when the responsibility for food selection and preparation reverts to you? Are you learning to make your own food choices?

10. *Does this weight-loss program teach you how to change your eating habits and provide nutrition education?*

Until you know how your body functions and how it is affected by the foods you eat, you will not be able to make informed decisions necessary for weight maintenance. Unless you change your eating habits, *permanently,* you will regain excess weight.

> Be extremely selective and cautious in your decision. Choose a weight-loss program that is nutritionally sound, realistic in its demands, and medically safe.

V

THE *TOTAL* DIET CENTER PROGRAM

THE Diet Center Program is unique. Based on a "common-sense" approach to dieting and nutrition, the Diet Center Program is one that has been the solution for millions of men, women, and children.

Success to Diet Center means PERMANENT WEIGHT CONTROL. The Diet Center Program is not a diet plan that achieves instant weight loss by depleting the body of fluids or essential nutrients. Instead, it is a sound, nutritionally balanced program that can be adjusted to the health needs of all dieters. The Diet Center Program takes into consideration all of the physical, emotional, and psychological needs of each dieter. Most diets ignore important emotional and mental changes that must take place. Other dieting programs do not address the important physical and emotional needs of a dieter. Perhaps this is the reason most dieters fail miserably at keeping off any weight they do lose.

Diet Center has created a *total* approach that will help you lose weight quickly, yet safely, and keep it off forever. You will be guided to a totally new life-style. The Diet Center Total Program consists of a four-phase diet regimen:

The CONDITIONING DIET (Phase One) prepares you to diet.

The REDUCING DIET (Phase Two) promotes rapid, yet safe, weight loss.

The STABILIZATION DIET (Phase Three) provides a "resting point" in the transition back to everyday eating.

And the MAINTENANCE DIET (Phase Four) is the "blueprint" for a lifetime of nutritious eating and permanent weight control.

THE DIET CENTER
FIVE-PHASE PROGRAM

OVERWEIGHT
AND
OBESITY

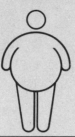

Poor eating habits + an unbalanced diet + rich and refined foods + lack of exercise = **obesity.**

PHASE I
CONDITIONING

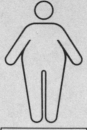

Dieter begins transition from diet typically high in rich, refined foods to natural foods; lean meats, fresh fruits and vegetables. Daily caloric intake is reduced from up to 3500 to approximately 1500. This phase cleanses the body and prepares it for dieting.

PHASE II
REDUCING

Reducing phase includes a natural-food diet consisting of a nutritional balance of proteins, fats, complex carbohydrates and naturally occurring sugars. Daily caloric intake; women 950 to 1200; men 1350 to 1500. Reducing Diet phase provides all micronutrients as outlined by RDA. Progress is monitored and charted daily during private counseling sessions.

PHASE III
STABILIZATION

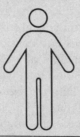

A stabilizing period with new varieties and larger quantities of food. Body continues to tone and firm. This phase continues one week for each two weeks spent in the Reducing phase, up to a maximum of three weeks. Supportive counseling continues on a twice-weekly basis.

PHASE IV
MAINTENANCE

Nutritional eating habits are established for lifelong weight maintenance. This phase parallels the (U.S.) Dietary Guidelines and continues under Diet Center Counselor's supervision for one full year.

PHASE V
NUTRITION/
BEHAVIOR
MODIFICATION

Through all phases of the Diet Center Program, weekly classes are taught in nutrition, behavior modification, self-direction, stress management and sensible exercise. These principles are reinforced daily during private, counseling sessions. This education enables dieters to make informed decisions for permanent weight control.

Rev. 1/83

HOW TO WIN AT THE LOSING GAME
DIET CENTER INC.

The Total Diet Center Program also addresses an additional dimension in a fifth phase — NUTRITION/BEHAVIOR MODIFICATION AND NUTRITION EDUCATION. This phase teaches the principles of sound nutrition. You will learn to identify those factors that caused your initial weight gain and your previous dieting failures. This phase also incorporates the importance of goals, visualization, coping with stress, and other issues that are vital to dieting success.

This section of the book explains each facet of the Total Diet Center Program in detail and provides examples, charts, and graphs and directions for incorporating these principles and concepts into your own life.

In providing a specific reducing phase, we know that the nutritional needs of men, women, and children are different.

Before beginning the Diet Center Reducing Program, you will want to study these charts. Diet Center has based its program on nutrients by using the Recommended Dietary Allowances (RDA). Please compare the Diet Center Program and note that because we are on a reducing program using approximately 1,000 calories, some nutrients are supplied by supplementation. In order to obtain all essential nutrients required by the body (according to the RDAs) on a 1,000-calorie diet, additional vitamins and minerals are required.

The Diet Center Reducing Diet is not a high-protein diet nor is it a high-carbohydrate diet. It is a well-balanced program providing correct percentage of proteins, carbohydrates, and fats within the needed maximum number of calories.

It is also important to note that the Diet Center Program meets or surpasses every RDA micronutrient recommendation.

DIET CENTER RECOMMENDS WORKING CLOSELY WITH YOUR PERSONAL PHYSICIAN

Before beginning any restricted dieting regimen, dieters should consult their personal physicans.

At Diet Center, dieters are encouraged to obtain a complete physical examination by their own physician before beginning the Diet Center Program. At Diet Centers, dieters with medical conditions, such as diabetes, heart problems, or cancer, and those who are pregnant must have written approval from their physicians before beginning the program. If dieters have multiple illnesses, use heavy doses of medications, or are fifty or more pounds overweight, prior physician approval is required before beginning the program.

Our dieters are also required to have a checkup following a forty-pound weight loss, because of chemical changes that occur in the body following significant weight loss. Blood workups of triglycerides, cholesterol, hemoglobin, and uric acid levels are conducted. Written permission from the physician is necessary before the dieter may continue. Further checkups are recommended after each additional forty-pound loss. We strongly recommend that you consult your physician concerning these matters.

1

The Diet Center Conditioning
Diet — Phase One

NOTE: Before beginning this or any weight reduction program, consult your doctor. It will also be helpful to read this entire book before beginning the diet itself. The Diet Center Program, as represented here, provides a nutritionally balanced diet that will result in natural weight reduction.

For more information on the additional features that Diet Center offers to help you be even more successful, please read section XI, "If You Need Further Help, Don't Give Up," beginning on page 297.

You are now ready to begin Phase One of the Diet Center Program, the Conditioning Diet. This diet is unlike any other. It has a specific purpose, so read and follow every step of this program exactly!

Are you a dedicated Monday-morning dieter? Do you gather together all your enthusiasm and motivation to start that new diet each Monday? Do you find, however, that you begin to falter on Thursday, and that by Friday you feel too exhausted, drained, and hungry to continue?

Recall your last "Monday-I'll-start" diet. What foods did you eat on Saturday and Sunday in "preparation" for your diet? Did you cram in pizza, ice cream, cookies, or candy because after Monday they weren't on your diet? Or, perhaps you're the type of dieter who has literally starved your body of its essential nutrients by going on one fad diet after another. Fad diets are ANY diets that deprive the body of one of more essential nutrients.

As explained previously, the foods mentioned above lack the staying power necessary to sustain your body during times of stress, including dieting. They are also very high in calories from refined sugars and fats. When you drastically reduce the amount, your body, which has become accustomed to the larger intake, begins to starve. It is no wonder that just four or five days after starting on a diet you feel too exhausted to continue.

The Diet Center Conditioning Diet conditions and prepares the body for the Reducing Phase of the Program. This is not a diet where we are concerned with calories, but rather the focus is on how the food and nutrients interact in the body. Processed foods high in refined sugars and starches are replaced by natural foods high in nutrients, fiber and bulk, and complex carbohydrates. Fruits help to keep the blood sugar level stable and produce a full, satisfied feeling. The natural sugars found in fruits provide the dieter with a high energy level. You do not have to fear becoming hungry, weak, or tired; you will feel full and energetic. Also, dieters do not experience the terrible headache or irritable jumpiness associated with fad dieting.

As the diet "conditions" the body for dieting, the body is flooded with low-cholesterol proteins. Proteins are the only nutrient that rebuilds cells and tissue. Proteins are also slow in digesting and, therefore, add to the feeling of satiation. Building up the body with a supply of protein prevents the fatigue and hunger that usually plague a fad dieter.

Finally, the abundance of fresh vegetables available on the Conditioning Diet helps each dieter adjust to the carefully controlled reduction in calories. Before beginning this diet, some overweight people may consume up to 3,500 calories per day! The Conditioning Diet is especially designed to ease the individual down to a lower level of calories before beginning the Reducing Diet.

THIS DIET IS TO BE USED FOR TWO DAYS ONLY.

TWO-DAY CONDITIONING DIET

To prepare properly for the Reducing Phase, a two-day Conditioning Diet is used. Remember it is for two days only. This diet is designed to help your body adjust from eating highly refined, rich foods to eating an abundance of lean meats, fresh fruits and vegetables. You may think you are eating too much, but *conditioning* is essential to your success on the Reducing Diet. The order of foods is important while on the Conditioning Phase. At each meal, eat fruits first, then proteins, then vegetables and breads.

Do not leave the table hungry. At breakfast, lunch, and dinner, eat until satisfied, but not stuffed. You should finish eating and drinking before 8 P.M., each day. Eat on time, on a schedule. Do not substitute any other foods.

Vitamin C

Take 1,000 mg. of vitamin C daily.

| Calcium | Take 750 mg. of calcium daily. |

| Water | Drink eight 8-ounce glasses of water throughout the day. (Do not drink more than two glasses at a time.) There is no substitute for water; it is essential for good health. |

| Lemon Juice | Every day you must have the juice of one lemon. Diet Center recommends 2 tablespoons of pure lemon juice daily. Mixed with hot water and a no-calorie sweetener, this drink counts as part of your water. The lemon can be used on a salad or protein entrée if desired. |

Coffee, Tea, and Diet Drinks

Any food or drink containing caffeine tends to make a person nervous. Decaffeinated coffee has over twenty-nine different acids; black and green teas have caffeine and tannic acid, many herbal teas are medicinal, and diet drinks contain high levels of additives and preservatives.

DIET DRINKS, COFFEE, AND GREEN AND BLACK TEAS DO NOT COUNT AS PART OF YOUR DAILY EIGHT GLASSES OF WATER.

Herbal teas may be counted as part of your water. (Use in moderation.)

Diet Center recommends you limit your intake of these beverages to no more than two per day.

ALCOHOLIC BEVERAGES ARE ABSOLUTELY NOT ALLOWED!

Fruits

It is important that you eat five to seven fresh fruits each day of the Conditioning Diet.

All fruits must be eaten fresh. No juices or canned fruits are allowed at this time. Choices on the Conditioning Diet include a combination only of apples, oranges, and grapefruit (one-half grapefruit equals one fruit). DO NOT substitute any other fruit choices for the next two days.

Protein Foods

On the Conditioning Diet, you should have protein throughout the entire day, eating as much as you would like of any of the protein foods on this list. Remember, eat until comfortable. The lean meats should be broiled, baked, boiled, steamed, grilled, or cooked in a no-stick pan. All visible fats must be removed. Blot extra fat off broiled meats. Use no fats or gravies in cooking. Eggs may be poached, boiled, or cooked in a no-stick pan with no added fats.

You may eat all you want of the following foods:

Beef (lean, well-done)	Liver
Chicken	Rabbit
Cottage cheese (low-fat)	Shellfish, any type
Deer or elk	Tofu
Eggs	Tuna (water packed)
Fish, any type	Turkey
Heart (beef)	Veal
Lamb	

Vegetables

On the Conditioning Diet, you can have all you want of the following vegetables, as long as they do not reduce your appetite for fruit and protein foods.

Asparagus	Mushrooms
Beans (green and yellow wax)	Mustard greens
	Okra
Beet greens	Onions (maximum allowed, 2 Tbsp.)
Cabbage	
Cauliflower (raw)	Parsley
Celery	Peppers (all types)
Chard	Potato (baked)
Chicory	Radishes
Chinese cabbage	Spinach
Collard	Sprouts, alfalfa, radish, and mung beans
Cucumbers	
Endive	Squash (crookneck, scallop varieties, yellow, zucchini)
Escarole	
Fennel	Tomatoes
Green onions	Turnip greens
Kale	Watercress
Lettuce	

Breads

Two bread servings are allowed each day. One of these servings must be either 6 Diet Center Thins or 2 Lite Rye Wasa Brod. You may choose your other serving from the list on page 116:

(6) Diet Center Thins
(2) Wasa Brod (Lite Rye)
(1) Ak-Mak cracker
(1) Finn Crisp cracker
(1) Italian (Grissini) breadstick
(2) Melba rounds
(1) Melba toast
(1) Norwegian flatbread

Oil

Each day you must have two teaspoons of corn, cottonseed, safflower, soybean, or sunflower oil. You may eat the oil as a salad dressing by adding the oil to as much apple cider vinegar or lemon juice as desired, or you may use the Diet Center Salad Dressing* packets. Each packet equals 1 teaspoon of oil. (Two packets allowed daily.) DO NOT HEAT OIL!

* Diet Center products have been especially developed for convenience of use. They are available at your local Diet Center if you wish to purchase them.

Sweeteners

Any no-calorie sweetener may be used. Recommended: Diet Center "Diet Lite" sweetener has less than 2 percent saccharin.

Seasonings

DO NOT OVERUSE SALT! Any seasonings or spices that do not contain oil or sugar are permitted in moderation. Read the label! Diet Center makes a variety of seasonings, including a variety of herbal seasonings, that can be used to enhance the flavor of your foods.

SUGGESTED SCHEDULE FOR THE CONDITIONING DIET: USE THIS DIET FOR TWO DAYS ONLY!

7:30 A.M. 1 (500 mg. time-release) vitamin C
750 mg. calcium tablet(s)
Hot lemonade (2 Tbsp. pure lemon juice in 8 oz. hot water)

8:00 A.M. 1 grapefruit
2 eggs
1 glass (8 oz.) water

10:00 A.M.	1 orange 3 Diet Center Thins or 1 Wasa Brod 1 glass (8 oz.) water
11:30 A.M.	1 glass water
12:00 noon	1 apple (eat entire apple before you eat meal) Chicken breast Salad of mixed vegetables (1 packet Diet Center Dressing or oil and vinegar dressing) Steamed green beans 3 Diet Center Thins or 1 Wasa Brod 1 glass (8 oz.) water
2:30 P.M.	1 orange ½ cup low-fat cottage cheese 1 glass (8 oz.) water
3:30 P.M.	1 apple 1 glass (8 oz.) water
6:30 P.M.	Steak, well-done, all fat removed Baked potato Salad (1 packet Diet Center Dressing or oil and vinegar dressing) Asparagus (steamed) 1 bread choice 1 orange
7:30 P.M.	1 (500 mg. time-release) vitamin C ½ grapefruit 1 glass (8 oz.) water

NOTE: This suggested Conditioning Diet contains eight glasses of water and seven fruits.

Remember on the Conditioning Diet:

1. Fruits are of the first importance;
2. Proteins are second; and
3. Vegetables and breads rank third.

Eat only until satisfied.

2

The Diet Center Reducing
Diet — Phase Two

ONCE the body has been properly conditioned for dieting, you can move on to the Diet Center Reducing Diet. The Reducing Diet forms the basic foundation for all other diets in the Diet Center Program.

This diet is based on controlled portions of low-fat proteins; complex carbohydrates containing naturally occurring sugars, bulk, and fiber; polyunsaturated fats; vitamins; minerals; and water. Every nutrient that the body needs for good health is included on this plan. We are counting and working with nutrients; and while we are well aware of the calories involved, we are not concerned about them. A wide variety of food choices are to be eaten throughout the entire week to ensure good health and proper intake of nutrients.

The Reducing Diet also combines exact amounts and types of specific nutrients needed for rapid weight loss, yet you'll find it supplies the body with the energy it needs. This chemical balance is a fragile one. "Cheating" even by eating just one candy bar can impair weight loss for up to three days. Adding a new food or subtracting a particular amount will drastically affect weight loss. An extra serving of protein is still "extra," and can inhibit your weight loss or make you gain.

You are now ready to begin the Reducing Phase of our program. Diet Center's Program offers a well-balanced diet that has no white sugars, and is low in fats, cholesterol, and calories, yet provides the body with all the necessary nutrients for optimum health. Below is a chart that compares a typical week of the Diet Center Program to the Recommended Dietary Allowances.

DIET CENTER'S REDUCING AND MAINTENANCE DIETS COMPARED TO THE RDA

Diet Center's Program offers a well-balanced diet, low in refined sugars, fats, and calories; yet it provides all the necessary nutrients for optimum health. Below is a safe nutritional range of macronutrients (protein, fats and carbohydrates) and calories plus a five-day average of micronutrients comparing Diet Center's Program to the Recommended Dietary Allowances (RDA) established by the Food and Nutrition Board of the National Academy of Science, National Research Council. (All statistics pertinent to women between the ages of 23-50.)

In order to obtain all essential nutrients (according to the RDA's) on a reducing diet, supplemental vitamins and minerals may be required.

Rev. 5/83

	RDA	Diet Center's Reducing Diet	Diet Center's Maintenance Diet
Calories	1600-2400	950-1200	1600-2400
Protein g.	44	55-106	44+
Fat g.	66	22-34[1]	66 or less
Carbohydrates g.	300	90-156[2]	300+
Calcium mg.	800	1400	800+
Iron mg.	18	25	18+
Magnesium mg.	300	693	300+
Phosphorus mg.	800	1099	800+
Potassium mg.	1875-5625	3007	1875+
Sodium mg.	1100-3300	1100+[3]	1100+
Zinc mg.	15	17	15+
Manganese mg.	2.5-5.0	2.8	2.5+
Copper mg.	2.0-3.0	2.9	2.0+
Vitamin K mg.	.70-1.40	.70-1.40[4]	.70+
Vitamin A IU	4000 (0.8 mcg.)	4000+ (0.8 mcg.)	4000+
Thiamine B_1 mg.	1.0	1.0+	1.0+
Riboflavin B_2 mg.	1.2	1.2+	1.2+
Vitamin B_6 mg.	2.0	2.0+	2.0+
Vitamin B_{12} mcg.	3	3+	3+
Biotin mcg.	100-200	100-200[4]	100+
Folic Acid mg.	0.4	0.4	0.4+
Niacin and Niacinamide mg.	13	13+	13+
Pantothenic Acid mg.	4-7	5+	4+
Vitamin D IU	200 (5 ug)	412	400+
Vitamin C mg.	60	1352	60+
Vitamin E mg.	8	15	8+
Selenium mg.	.05-0.2	.2+	.05+

The Diet Center Supplement adds additional thiamine, riboflavin, niacin, vitamin B_6, vitamin B_{12}, biotin, folic acid and panthothenic acid.

[1] In order to lose weight, the Reducing Diet has less carbohydrates and fats than the RDA.

[2] Eating less than 60 grams of "digestible" carbohydrates per day can result in ketosis, which is potentially dangerous to health.

[3] Sodium intake can vary drastically according to how heavily you salt your foods. One teaspoon of salt adds 2,132 mg. of sodium.

[4] Because of the lack of food-composition information available for vitamin K and biotin, accurate values cannot be established. However, our diet provides an abundance of foods rich in each of these nutrients. We are, therefore, confident we meet the Recommended Dietary Allowances (RDA).

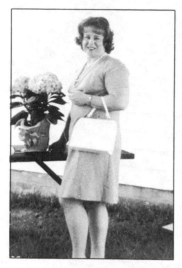

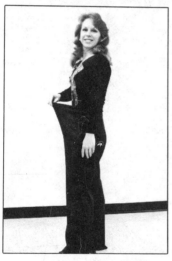

Lynda Huebel's interests changed from soap operas and sweets to maintaining a healthful life-style at an ideal weight.

The Diet Center Reducing Diet also uses those foods you eat on an everyday basis. Not only can you "diet" from the Reducing list of foods, but you can also prepare meals for your family from these same foods. A diet based on prepackaged and prepared foods, or foods so exotic that the only time you would ever eat them is on that diet, does not teach lifelong weight maintenance.

Dieters are often amazed by the difference a well-balanced, nutritionally sound diet can have on their lives. For one woman, the experience of "dieting" was both physically and mentally rewarding.

When I started the Reducing Program, I was really surprised when I suddenly realized that I was no longer hungry. I certainly had more energy — I left the soap operas and started swimming and playing tennis. In time, I was able to get off tranquilizers. And the biggest thrill was — I no longer craved sweets and if I saw anyone eating candy or ice cream, I didn't feel like a martyr if somebody ate something I couldn't eat.

When I started losing weight, my mental attitude changed, and I started liking myself. And then I started liking others. All of a sudden, I had friends! As the pounds came off, the compliments came on. As I started looking better physically and feeling better mentally, I felt much more secure as a woman, and this helped in all areas of my life — as a wife, mother and employee.

On the Diet Center Program, I learned that refined carbohydrates quickly digest and a person can become very hungry. No wonder I had always been so hungry. I was eating sugared cereals, cookies, candies, noodles, spaghetti, pizza and loads of white bread.

Lynda Huebel
Marshall, Texas

Diet Center dieters remain on this Reducing Phase until they reach an ideal weight goal as determined by the "Desirable Weight Chart" (page 20). Achieving this personal weight goal is one of the most important psychological barriers any dieter can overcome.

EXPLANATION OF THE DIET CENTER REDUCING DIET

Each of the foods, vitamins, and minerals on the Diet Center Reducing Diet performs a vital function in maintaining a healthy body while producing optimum weight loss. There is much more, however, to a diet than just following a list of foods. Recall any other diet you have recently tried. Did you know the exact reasons for eating each of these foods in the proper amounts? Did you understand the process by which each of these foods helped you lose weight, yet kept you healthy? Knowledge is the key. Remember, permanent weight control comes from understanding how foods interact with your body.

Also included within this book are instructions on how to prepare and cook the appropriate foods for dieting. The way you prepare and cook foods is just as important as what foods are used. Did you know that you should remove the skin and bones from chicken breasts before cooking? Or, that certain vegetables are fine when raw, but when cooked, undergo a sugar conversion and become sweet, triggering water retention? Carefully study this book. It provides invaluable information and ideas that can make weight loss not only easy, but enjoyable!

Do you know how important it is to get necessary amounts of vital nutrients from your diet? The following tables illustrate the importance of a balanced, nutritional diet provided by Diet Center. Compare these tables with your own life-style. What foods, in what quantities, are you eating now? Then, read the explanations for each of the nutrients listed. A well-balanced, nutritionally sound diet does make sense!

The Diet Center Program provides the nutrients your body needs to maintain good health. You will feel great and have good energy. It is important to feed your body properly in order to achieve optimum weight loss. Remember, on this diet, you will lose only the excess fat, not the muscle tissue. Every nutrient has been carefully calculated to ensure the best results.

The Diet Center Reducing Phase is approximately 1,000 calories for women, with the correct percentage of protein, carbohydrates, and fat for a healthy program.

THE DIET CENTER REDUCING DIET FOR WOMEN

The Diet Center Program counts nutrients, not calories. It is the chemistry of the food that helps you to lose weight quickly while maintaining good energy.

- Remember to eat on a schedule and on time. Do not eat or drink later than 8:00 P.M.
- FOODS NOT ON THE LIST ARE STRICTLY FORBIDDEN!!!! DO NOT SUBSTITUTE ANY FOODS!

DIET CENTER'S REDUCING PROGRAM NUTRIENT BREAKDOWN

The Diet Center Reducing Program provides all the micronutrients as outlined by the Recommended Dietary Allowances (RDA), and parallels the (U.S.) Dietary Guidelines. It provides a nutritionally sound diet with a balance of proteins, fats, carbohydrates, vitamins, minerals, fiber, bulk and water.

PROTEIN

Men ....75-140 gm.
Women ....55-106 gm.

Protein, sometimes referred to as the "body's building blocks," is responsible for cell maintenance and growth. Protein is obtained from meats, vegetables, whole-grain products and fruits.

FATS

Men ....25-52 gm.
Women ....22-34 gm.

Fats are essential to health because they create energy, aid in digestion, soften the skin and are transporters of the fat-soluble vitamins A, D, E and K.

CARBOHYDRATES

Men .... 110-170 gm.
Women ....90-156 gm.

Complex carbohydrates and naturally occurring sugars (found in fresh fruits, vegetables and whole grains) are the best sources of energy. (Eating less than 60 grams of "digestible" carbohydrates per day can result in ketosis, which is potentially dangerous to health.)

WATER

8 (8-oz.) glasses

Water, a source of minerals, is the most valuable nutrient. Water carries nourishment to the cells, aids in digestion and elimination, and flushes waste from the body.

CALORIES (Daily Caloric Levels)

Men .... 1350-1500 calories
Women .... 950-1200 calories

VITAMINS AND MINERALS

Vitamins and minerals are essential for sustaining optimum health. A diet composed of a wide variety of wholesome, natural foods in the proper amounts provides the body with an adequate supply of these vital nutrients.

FIBER & BULK

Diet Center's Diets provide an abundance of fiber and bulk, which are necessary for "staying power" and proper elimination. The fiber contained in natural whole-grain products, fresh fruits and vegetables supplies the body with the necessary bulk. Although meats contain no fiber, they do provide additional bulk.

Rev. 1/83

HOW TO WIN AT THE LOSING GAME

DIET CENTER INC.

© 1983 Diet Center, Inc.

Water

Every day drink eight (8 oz.) glasses of water. DRINK YOUR WATER! Drink your water throughout the day. Drink no later than 8:00 P.M.

Vitamin C

Take 1,000 mg. of vitamin C daily. Take 250 mg. at 7:30 A.M., 11:30 A.M., 3:30 P.M., 7:30 P.M., or take time-release vitamin C capsules (500 mg.) two times a day.

Calcium

Take 750 mg. of calcium daily.

Lemon Juice

Every day you must have the juice of one lemon. Diet Center recommends 2 tablespoons of pure lemon juice daily. Mixed with hot water and a no-calorie sweetener, this drink counts as part of your water. The lemon can be used on a salad or protein entrée if desired.

Coffee, Tea, and Diet Drinks

Any food or drink containing caffeine tends to make a person nervous. Decaffeinated coffee has over twenty-nine different acids; black and green teas have caffeine and tannic acid,

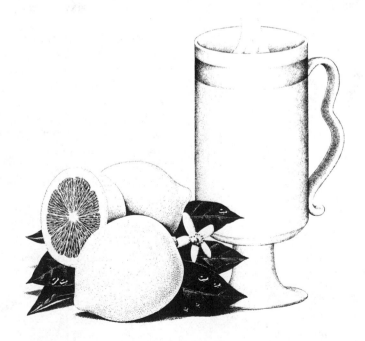

many herbal teas are medicinal, and diet drinks contain high levels of additives and preservatives.

DIET DRINKS, COFFEE, AND GREEN AND BLACK TEAS DO NOT COUNT AS PART OF YOUR DAILY EIGHT GLASSES OF WATER.

Herbal teas may be counted as part of your water. (Use in moderation.)

Diet Center recommends you limit your intake of these beverages to no more than two per day.

ALCOHOLIC BEVERAGES ARE NOT ALLOWED!

Protein Foods

Each serving of protein has approximately 21 grams of protein, 4 grams of fat, and 1 gram of carbohydrates.

Seven ounces of protein foods are required per day, two 3½-ounce cooked servings. (Weigh food 4 ounces raw to ensure 3½ ounces after cooked.) These foods are to be broiled, baked, poached, boiled or pan-fried (no grease). See schedule of Diet, pages 130–135.

Select protein from the following:

Chicken breast — remove bone and skin before cooking.
Chicken livers — bake or broil.
Deer or elk — bake or cook in a no-stick pan.
Eggs — 3 eggs equals 1 meat serving. (Do not use eggs as your total protein for the day.) 1 egg equals a 1-ounce protein serving. Do not exceed 5 eggs per week.
Fish — flatfish, flounder, haddock, halibut, perch, pike, pollock, red snapper, sea bass, sole, river trout.
Heart (*beef*)
Rabbit
Shellfish — crab, crawdad (crayfish), lobster, shrimp.
Tofu — 1 (8 oz.) cake.
*Diet Center Crunchies** or *TVP* (*textured vegetable protein*) — ⅓ cup (1½ oz.) equals 1 cooked protein serving.

* Two tablespoonfuls of Crunchies are allowed as a free food. Crunchies can be purchased at your local Diet Center, or use 1½ oz. textured vegetable protein.

Do NOT eat cod, salmon, tuna, turbot, or any other protein not on this list. This type of fish and any red meat is high in fat content.

THESE MEATS ARE CALCULATED FOR OPTIMUM WEIGHT LOSS!! DO NOT SUBSTITUTE!

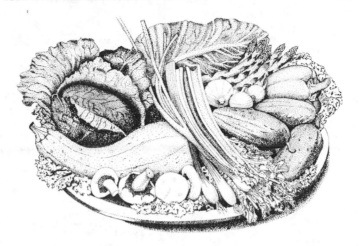

Vegetables

Each cup of vegetables has approximately 2 grams of protein, ⅓ gram of fat, and 5 grams of carbohydrates.

Unlimited amounts of fresh raw vegetables, plus one cup cooked vegetables are allowed each day. Do not have raw vegetables and cooked vegetables at the same meal.

A crisp, fresh vegetable salad provides the bulk and fiber your body requires for optimum weight loss. Each day, you may have up to half a head lettuce with five to seven additional kinds of raw vegetables (including one cup dark, leafy greens).

Select vegetables from the following:

Asparagus	Kale
Beans (green and yellow wax)	Lettuce
	Mushrooms
Beet greens	Mustard greens
Cabbage	Okra
Cauliflower (raw)	Onions
Celery	(maximum allowed, 2 Tbsp.)
Chard	Parsley
Chicory	Peppers (all types)
Chinese cabbage	Radishes
Collard	Spinach
Cucumbers	Sprouts, alfalfa, radish, and
Endive	mung beans
Escarole	Squash (yellow, crooknecked,
Fennel	scallop varieties, zucchini)
Green onions	Watercress

It is recommended that you alternate your choice of vegetables at each meal. Always use fresh vegetables whenever pos-

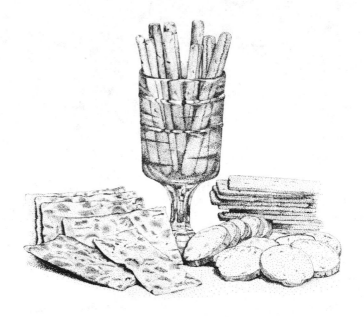

sible, using frozen vegetables as your second choice, and canned only as a last resort, due to a higher sodium content and loss of natural nutrients.

Oil

Daily oil allowance has approximately 9 grams of fat.

Have 2 teaspoonfuls of oil (corn, cottonseed, soybean, sunflower, safflower) per day. Be sure to measure the exact amount of oil. To minimize oil intake, DO NOT HEAT THE OIL. (You can make the oil into a salad dressing by adding the oil to as much apple cider vinegar or lemon juice as desired.) For salad dressing recipes, see pages 329–330.

You may want to use Diet Center dressings for a great taste. Each packet equals 1 teaspoon of oil. In place of the oil requirement, two packets of Diet Center dressings may be used (available from your local Diet Center). Lobster, chicken, fish, and shrimp may be dipped in Diet Center dressings or lemon for a tasty variety.

Breads

Two bread servings are allowed each day. ONE OF THESE SERVINGS MUST BE EITHER 6 DIET CENTER THINS OR 2 LITE RYE WASA BROD. You may choose your other serving from the list below.

(6) Diet Center Thins
(2) Wasa Brod (Lite Rye)
(1) Ak-Mak cracker
(1) Finn Crisp cracker
(1) Italian (Grissini) breadstick
(2) Melba rounds
(1) Melba toast
(1) Norwegian Flatbread

Fruits

One extra-large apple has approximately ½ gram of protein, 1½ grams of fat, and 37 grams of carbohydrates. The remain-

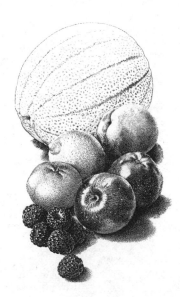

ing fruit serving is approximately 2 grams of protein, ½ gram of fat, and 22 grams of carbohydrates.

HAVE ONE APPLE PLUS ONE OTHER FRUIT CHOICE DAILY.

Two fruits (preferably fresh) are allowed, and one of the fruits must be an apple. *Only one* apple is allowed, so eat the biggest one you can find. (Two small apples cannot be eaten in place of an extra-large one.) No juices.

Eat a variety throughout the week, but avoid overripe fruits, as their sugar content is too high. One cup mixed fruit equals 1 fruit serving. Select fruits from the following:

Apple (1 large, approximately 5″ diameter, *daily*)
Apricots (3 fresh, or ½ cup raw or water-packed)
Blackberries (1 cup)
Blueberries (1 cup)
Cantaloupe (⅓ to ½ melon, depending on size)
Grapefruit
Honeydew (⅓ to ½ melon, depending on size)
Nectarine (1 large, fresh)
Orange (1 whole)
Papaya (½ whole)
Peach (1 fresh, or 1 cup water-packed)
Persimmon (½ whole)
Raspberries, red or black (1 cup)
Rhubarb (½ cup, cooked without sugar)
Strawberries (1 cup)
Tangerines (2)

Sweeteners

Any no-calorie sweetener may be used. Recommended: Diet Center "Diet Lite" sweetener has less than 2 percent saccharin.

Seasonings

The following seasonings may be used to enhance natural food flavors in place of table salt. Use sparingly.

Herbs	*Spices*
Basil	Chili powder
Bay leaves	Cinnamon
Dillweed	Curry
Marjoram	Ginger
Parsley	Mustard
Rosemary	Nutmeg
Sage	Paprika
Savory	Pepper (all types)
Tarragon	
Thyme	

Sauces
Kikkoman soy sauce*
Tabasco
Wicker's Barbeque sauce*
Worcestershire*

Miscellaneous
Garlic
Horseradish
Mustard (prepared)
Liquid Smoke*
Onion
Pimento
Vanilla

* Use in moderation (just a drop). DO NOT USE KETCHUP because of high sugar and salt content. Bouillon cubes, sauerkraut, and dill pickles are not allowed because of salt content.

For your convenience, a variety of seasonings that can be used enhance the flavor of your foods are available for sale from a local Diet Center. A complete line of herbal seasonings are available and recommended to be used in place of salt.

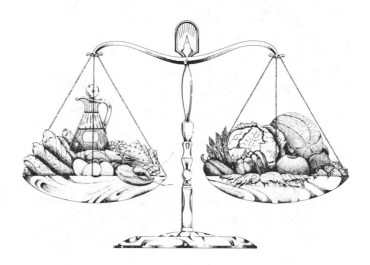

Additional Foods   You can have these additional foods each day if desired:

Diet Center Protein Powder (2 Tbsp.)
Unflavored gelatin
Lemons and limes
Unprocessed bran (2 Tbsp.)
Apple cider vinegar
Skim milk (2 Tbsp.) *or* Powdered skim milk (1½ tsp.)
Diet Center Crunchies (2 Tbsp.) *or* Textured vegetable protein

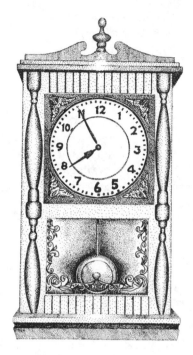

WHILE ON THE DIET CENTER REDUCING DIET, REMEMBER THESE IMPORTANT TIPS:

- Focus on counting nutrients, not calories.
- Do not make any substitutions! Check your list.
- Eat on time.
- Follow the same schedule each day.
- You must drink the required amount of water each day.
- Be prepared ahead of time.
- Make a large salad with a variety of five to seven types of vegetables. Keep this in your refrigerator at all times.
- Keep sealed bags of cleaned vegetables available in your refrigerator for "snack attacks."
- Place a large bowl filled with fruits on your kitchen table.
- You will lose better weight by eating fish than chicken.
- Be sure to get enough exercise and plenty of sleep.
- Use little or no salt.
- Set goals.
- Visualize your success.
- Relax.
- Learn to cope with stress.
- Eat half of all vegetables raw.
- Trim all fats from meat.
- Cook all meats well-done.
- Steam vegetables.

SUGGESTED TIMES AND FOODS FOR THE REDUCING PHASE OF THE PROGRAM

Remember:

- Eat on time, on a schedule.
- Be prepared with foods.
- Eat an apple every day.
- Drink eight 8-ounce glasses of water each day.
- Do not substitute with any foods NOT LISTED on Reducing Diet.

NOTE: This menu planner incorporates many recipes that can be found in section XII, "Diet Center's Reducing Recipes for Women and Men." These recipes are indicated by page numbers. For variation, you may want to try some of the other delicious reducing recipes not featured in this menu planner.

MONDAY

7:30 A.M. 1 (500 mg. time-release) vitamin C
750 mg. calcium tablet(s)
Hot lemonade (2 Tbsp. pure lemon juice in 8 oz. hot water)

8:00 A.M.	1 scrambled egg (no oil, use no-stick pan) 3 Diet Center Thins or 1 Wasa Brod (Lite Rye), toasted 1 Tbsp. Blackberry Jam (page 313) 1 glass (8 oz.) water
10:00 A.M.	½ large orange 1 glass (8 oz.) water
12:00 noon	Herb-baked Haddock (2½ oz. cooked) (page 322) 1 cup Stir-Fry Vegetables (page 331) 1 Bran Muffin (page 314) 1 Diet Center Custard (page 317) 1 glass (8 oz.) water
2:30 P.M.	3 Diet Center Thins or 1 Wasa Brod (Lite Rye) ½ orange 1 glass (8 oz.) water
6:00 P.M.	3 cups Chicken-Salad Supreme (2 tsp. oil in dressing) (page 326) 2 Melba rounds 1 cup herb tea 1 glass (8 oz.) water
7:30 P.M.	1 (500 mg. time-release) vitamin C 1 glass (8 oz.) water 1 Baked Apple (page 315)

TUESDAY

7:30 A.M.	1 (500 mg. time-release) vitamin C 750 mg. calcium tablet(s) Hot lemonade (2 Tbsp. pure lemon juice in 8 oz. hot water)
8:00 A.M.	Apple-Bran Pancakes (1 oz. serving protein) (page 313) 1 Tbsp. Blackberry Jam (page 313) 1 cup herb tea
10:00 A.M.	¼ cantaloupe serving 1 glass (8 oz.) water
12:00 noon	Crockpot Chicken (2½ oz. cooked chicken) (page 320) Tasty Spinach Salad (eat until full; save remainder until 3:30 P.M.) (page 328) 3 Diet Center Thins or 1 Wasa Brod (Lite Rye) 1 glass (8 oz.) water
3:30 P.M.	Salad (remainder from lunch) ¼ cantaloupe serving 1 glass (8 oz.) water

4:00 P.M.   1 glass (8 oz.) water

6:00 P.M.   Shrimp and Vegetable Kabobs (page 323) with Diet Center
               French Dressing (2 pkgs. equals 2 tsp. oil) or own dressing
               (page 331)
               1 Melba Toast
               1 glass (8 oz.) water

7:30 P.M.   1 (500 mg. time-release) vitamin C
               Pop Squares (page 316)
               1 large apple
               1 glass (8 oz.) water

WEDNESDAY

7:30 A.M.   1 (500 mg. time-release) vitamin C
               750 mg. calcium tablet(s)
               Hot lemonade (2 Tbsp. pure lemon juice in 8 oz. hot water)

8:00 A.M.   1-egg Mushroom Omelet (page 318) (use Pam or similar prod-
               uct and a no-stick pan)
               3 Diet Center Thins or 1 Wasa Brod (Lite Rye)
               1 glass (8 oz.) water

10:00 A.M.   ½ cup strawberries (no sugar)
               1 glass (8 oz.) water

12:00 noon   Stuffed Chicken Breasts (2½ oz. cooked chicken) (page 320)
               with
               Sage Stuffing (page 313)
               "French-Style" Green Bean Medley (1 cup) (page 331)
               Garlic-Vinaigrette Dressing (1 tsp. oil) (page 329)
               1 Norwegian flatbread
               1 glass (8 oz.) water

2:30 P.M.   ½ cup Strawberry Parfait (page 317)

3:30 P.M.   1 glass (8 oz.) water

4:30 P.M.   1 glass (8 oz.) water

6:00 P.M.   Baked halibut steak (3½ oz.)
               Vegetable salad, large (5 to 7 types of vegetables)
               1 glass (8 oz.) water

7:30 P.M.   1 (500 mg. time-release) vitamin C
               1 glass (8 oz.) water
               1 large Baked Apple (page 315)

THURSDAY

7:30 A.M.   1 (500 mg. time-release) vitamin C

	750 mg. calcium tablet(s) Hot lemonade (2 Tbsp. pure lemon juice in 8 oz. hot water)
8:00 A.M.	Eggnog (page 317) 1 Bran Muffin (page 314) 1 Tbsp. Blackberry Jam (page 313)
10:00 A.M.	½ grapefruit 1 cup herb tea
11:30 A.M.	1 glass (8 oz.) water
12:00 noon	Taco Salad (2½ oz. cooked beef heart in 3 cup lettuce salad) (page 325) Mayonnaise (page 312) 3 Diet Center Thins or 1 Wasa Brod (Lite Rye, break up in salad as chips) 1 glass (8 oz.) water
2:30 P.M.	Fruit Ambrosia (½ cup) (page 316) 1 cinnamon Wasa Brod (Lite Rye), toasted 1 glass (8 oz.) water
3:30 P.M.	1 glass (8 oz.) water
6:00 P.M.	Sweet-and-Sour Chicken (page 321) 1 breadstick 1 glass (8 oz.) water
7:30 P.M.	1 (500 mg. time-release) vitamin C 1 glass (8 oz.) water 1 large apple

FRIDAY

7:30 A.M.	1 (500 mg. time-release) vitamin C 750 mg. calcium tablet(s) Hot lemonade (2 Tbsp. pure lemon juice in 8 oz. hot water)
8:00 A.M.	1 boiled egg 1 Bran Muffin (page 314) 1 Tbsp. Blackberry Jam (page 313) 1 glass (8 oz.) water
10:00 A.M.	1 orange (sectioned) 1 glass (8 oz.) water
11:30 A.M.	1 glass (8 oz.) water
12:00 noon	1 trout, barbecued (2½ oz. cooked; leave skin on to cook, remove skin to eat; drench in lemon and add Diet Center "buttery flavor salt" sparingly) 3 cups Red-Cabbage Salad (page 327) 1 package Diet Center Dressing (1 tsp. oil allowance) *or*

12:00 (con't) Vinegar and Oil Dressing (page 330)
     6 Diet Center Thins or 2 Wasa Brod (Lite Rye)
     1 glass (8 oz.) water

3:30 P.M. Remainder of Red-Cabbage Salad, *and*
     Vegetable sticks
     1 cup herb tea

6:00 P.M. Tofu Quiche (page 318)
     1 breadstick
     1 glass (8 oz.) water

7:30 P.M. 1 (500 mg. time-release) vitamin C
     1 glass (8 oz.) water
     1 Baked Apple, large (page 315)

SATURDAY

7:30 A.M. 1 (500 mg. time-release) vitamin C
     750 mg. calcium tablet(s)
     Hot lemonade (2 Tbsp. pure lemon juice in 8 oz. hot water)

8:00 A.M. 1 poached egg on 1 toasted Wasa Brod (Lite Rye)
     1 glass (8 oz.) water

10:00 A.M. ½ broiled grapefruit

11:30 A.M. 1 glass (8 oz.) water

12:00 noon Chicken-Salad Supreme (2½ oz. cooked chicken in 3 cups
     salad) (page 326)
     2 Tbsp. Vinegar and Oil Dressing (page 330)
     3 Diet Center Thins or 1 Wasa Brod (Lite Rye)
     1 glass (8 oz.) water

2:30 P.M. Baked Apple, large (page 315)
     3 Diet Center Thins or 1 Wasa Brod (Lite Rye)
     1 glass (8 oz.) water

3:30 P.M. 1 glass (8 oz.) water

6:00 P.M. Broiled halibut
     1 cup asparagus, frozen (use salt sparingly)
     1 Bran Muffin (page 314)
     1 Tbsp. Blackberry Jam (page 313)
     1 glass (8 oz.) water

7:30 P.M. 1 (500 mg. time-release) vitamin C
     1 glass (8 oz.) water
     ½ serving Peach "Ice Cream" (page 317)
     1 serving Diet Center Custard (page 317)

SUNDAY

7:30 A.M.   1 (500 mg. time-release) vitamin C
750 mg. calcium tablet(s)
Hot lemonade (2 Tbsp. pure lemon juice in 8 oz. hot water)

8:00 A.M.   1 Bran Muffin (page 314)
1 ounce protein
3 Diet Center Thins or 1 Wasa Brod (Lite Rye)
1 glass (8 oz.) water

10:00 A.M.   ½ cup strawberries
1 cup herb tea

11:30 A.M.   1 glass (8 oz.) water

12:00 noon   Chicken Chow Mein (2½ oz. cooked chicken in 1 cup cooked
vegetables) (page 319)
3 Diet Center Thins or 1 Wasa Brod (Lite Rye)
1 glass (8 oz.) water

3:30 P.M.   1 glass (8 oz.) water
1 serving Pop Squares (page 316)

6:00 P.M.   Broiled halibut with herbs
3 cup salad (5 to 7 varieties of vegetables), *with*
2 packages Diet Center Italian Salad Dressing *or* Garlic-Vinaigrette Dressing (page 329)
1 Bran Muffin (page 314)
1 glass (8 oz.) water

7:30 P.M.   1 (500 mg. time-release) vitamin C
1 glass (8 oz.) water
1 large apple

This is only a sample menu planner. You may wish to develop your own, using the same quantities, but different recipes.

3

Plateaus

"PLATEAUS" are experienced by almost everyone who diets. Plateaus are those times when no matter how faithfully you follow your diet, the scale doesn't show a loss. During these times, the body may be adjusting to new physiological changes that are taking place. At other times, the body "pulls in" water as a defense mechanism. This happens when you become extremely tired, ill, or experience severe muscle strain or sunburn. Consequently, you may be losing excess adipose tissue, but extra water weight seems to obliterate your efforts.

Remember the discussion about the "panic points" of gaining weight. When a dieter over 200 pounds begins to lose weight, there is a tendency to plateau at those panic points or following every twenty-five-pound loss (approximately). Believe in yourself during these rough times. Plateaus are normal. One "morale booster" to use during a plateau is to take measurements and see that although the scale is showing no drop, the tape measure can be tightened.

It is interesting to note that while dieting on the Diet Center Reducing Diet, you can expect to lose one measured inch for every pound lost. Plateaus are one of the main reasons that you should be sure to take your measurements before beginning the diet. (See page 19 to review how to take your measurements.)

If your weight loss does slow down, DON'T GIVE UP! The most important part of permanent weight loss is to reach your weight goal. Stopping just ten pounds shy may be a physical victory, but it is a psychological defeat. No matter how close you are, achieving goal will increase your success at permanent weight control.

I have found that when you achieve your ideal weight goal, you are at a healthy lean weight. You will be able to make the correct food choices and yet maintain your weight. However, if you quit dieting at 150 pounds after losing fifty pounds, instead of reaching your weight goal of 130, you have only achieved a "relative success." You may feel successful, and you are; but you will not be at a lean healthy weight. You would be twenty pounds from it. Your heart is still pumping through miles of extra blood vessels to feed this additional tissue.

Imagine carrying around a twenty-pound bag of potatoes every day. You cannot put it down when you get tired. It would not take very long before you would realize the type of stress that you place on your body, and especially your heart, by those extra twenty pounds.

Even though a dieter is relatively successful, it is important to continue until reaching weight goal. Then, the body can function at a healthy and productive level, and every gland and organ will operate at peak efficiency. Activity is increased; the mind is more alert; you will have learned to select lean foods with staying power; and your weight can be maintained more easily.

If you are about to give up, try these techniques used by Diet Center Counselors to help dieters successfully achieve weight goal:

1. *Measure!* Every inch you lose is equivalent to another pound lost. This is especially helpful when you are retaining excess water.
2. *Remember the yo-yo!* Breaking the "yo-yo syndrome" comes only by eating correct nutrients and by reaching goal. Stopping ten pounds early invariably results in gaining back all the weight you lost. It means you haven't really seen yourself as a thin person yet.
3. *Don't lose your self-discipline!* Successful dieters have conditioned their thinking. Once an exception has been made, it is impossible to regain the momentum of a disciplined state of thinking. Remember to eat on time on your schedule, and to maintain discipline.
4. *Get excited!* Has your diet become boring or do you feel that you will never reach goal? Stop for a minute to realize just how far you have actually come. Pull out one of your "formerly fat" outfits or photos. Congratulate yourself for the accomplishments you have achieved so far.

Dieting takes time, commitment, and effort. Yet, as important as it is to reach ideal weight goal, we have found that when dieters lose below their weight goals, they can slip into anorexia nervosa, which can be fatal. We firmly state no one should go below the recommended weight goal.

With the Diet Center Program, we know that THE SUCCESS OF ATTAINING GOAL IS AN ACCOMPLISHMENT ANY DIETER CAN REACH!

4

The Diet Center Stabilization Diet — Phase Three

THE Stabilization Diet provides dieters with a "resting point" in the transition from the discipline and restriction of reducing to everyday eating. Stabilization also provides an increased intake of proteins essential for continued retoning and refirming soft body tissue. Throughout the Reducing Phase, dieters will have lost approximately one inch per pound where needed and desired from their bodies. Increased protein intake rebuilds body tissue, and by the end of Stabilization, the body is firm and toned.

The Stabilization Diet allows larger variety and greater quantities of foods, yet maintains the disciplined schedule of the Reducing Phase. Added quantities of new, nutritious foods, however, prevent giving in to the temptation to "let loose and eat everything in sight." At the same time, these foods will maintain your new weight.

Stabilization also requires that you reprogram your thinking. An increase in foods may at first be threatening after being used to such a strict Reducing Diet. But you will learn to adjust slowly by adding new foods, one or two at a time.

A schedule is also very important on the Stabilization Phase of the program. (See the suggested Stabilization schedule on pages 146–149.) You should eat three main meals each day: breakfast, lunch, and dinner. Don't skip!

Introduce the new foods one at a time. Weigh yourself the next morning to see if a weight change has occurred. Continue to add a new variety of foods — one day at a time. If a gain does occur, cut back on the new food.

The Stabilization Diet should be followed one week for each two weeks of Reducing. To calculate length of time on the Stabilization Phase, use the following timetable.

REDUCING	STABILIZATION
1–3 weeks	1 week
4–5 weeks	2 weeks
over 6 weeks	3 weeks

Stabilization SHOULD NEVER EXCEED THREE WEEKS. An initial weight gain may occur on Stabilization (up to three pounds) as you begin to eat more foods in greater quantities. This weight gain is ENTIRELY NORMAL and will disappear by the end of the third week. Remember, however, that the function of the Stabilization Phase is not to lose weight, but to adjust to new foods and continue rebuilding of body tissue. This diet must be followed *exactly*. Protein is high in calories and ANY INTAKE OF EXTRA REFINED SUGARS WILL RESULT IN A DRASTIC WEIGHT GAIN. This Stabilization Diet is chemically balanced and must be followed exactly to ensure the best results.

Remember these important thoughts when stabilizing:

- "The Stabilization Phase of the program is just as important as the Reducing Diet."
- "Even though new types of proteins and vegetables have been allowed, I must continue to be very careful to follow this diet exactly!"
- "I must stabilize, or I will gain my weight back."
- "I am satisfying my body with three meals and protein snacks."
- "I am weighing daily and will continue to do so each day."
- "I am introducing new foods, giving my body a chance to refirm and retone."
- "I still need to eat on time and on a schedule."
- "I must drink eight glasses of water each day."
- "I must continue to exercise for a healthy body and mind."
- "If I eat any sugars, I might gain weight."
- "I must prepare my salads and foods ahead of time."

Stabilization is an integral step to attaining permanent weight control. One Diet Center dieter discovered the remarkable difference of stabilizing at an ideal weight goal. Losing weight on the Diet Center Program was easy. However, she had also lost on other programs, but *never* permanently. With Diet Center, she not only learned how to lose, but how to maintain that weight loss. After stabilizing, she experienced a small weight gain, but instead of letting it mushroom into a problem, she dieted right back down to goal. As she states:

I had tried other programs, but just couldn't stick with them long enough to do any good. Diet Center made losing weight easy, and I've never felt better! Best of all, I feel good about me. Diet Center taught me how to get slim and stay that way for the rest of my life!

Amanda Garcia
San Benito, Texas

DIET CENTER'S STABILIZATION DIET FOR WOMEN

This diet is just as important to the total program as the Reducing Diet. Follow it carefully. Stabilize one week for every two weeks on the Reducing Diet. Stabilization should never exceed three weeks.

Remember: no sugar and no flour; trim all fat off meat.

Vitamin C

Take one 250 mg. tablet each day.

Calcium

Take 750 mg. of supplemental calcium daily.

Water

Drink eight 8-ounce glasses of water throughout the day. (Do not drink more than two glasses at a time.) Do not drink after 8 P.M. There is no substitute for water; it is essential for good health.

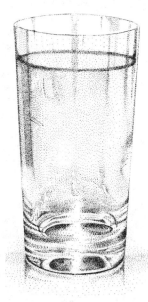

Coffee, Tea, and Diet Drinks

Any food or drink containing caffeine tends to make a person nervous. Decaffeinated coffee has over twenty-nine different acids; black and green teas have caffeine and tannic acid, many herbal teas are medicinal, and diet drinks contain high levels of additives and preservatives.

DIET DRINKS, COFFEE, AND GREEN AND BLACK TEAS DO NOT COUNT AS PART OF YOUR DAILY EIGHT GLASSES OF WATER.

Herbal tea may be counted as part of your water. (Use in moderation.)

Diet Center recommends you limit your intake of these beverages to no more than two per day.

ALCOHOLIC BEVERAGES ARE ABSOLUTELY NOT ALLOWED!

Protein Foods

Do not go hungry. Eat until satisfied. Eat small quantities of lean meat, low-fat cottage cheese (listed as a protein food), and eggs throughout the day. Have snacks, if desired, of additional protein foods. Diet Center Crunchies are a good source of protein. They may be eaten dry, or added to low-fat cottage cheese, in scrambled eggs, or in salads.

Select protein from the following:

Beef (well-done)
Chicken breast (remove bone and skin before cooking)
Chicken livers (baked or broiled)
Cottage cheese (low-fat)
Deer or elk
Eggs (1 egg equals 1-oz. protein serving. Do not use eggs as your total protein for the day. Do not exceed 5 eggs a week.)
Fish (all types)
Heart (beef)
Lamb
Liver (beef or veal)
Rabbit
Shellfish (all types)
Tofu (one 8-oz. cake equals one 3½-oz. protein serving)
Turkey
Veal
Diet Center Crunchies (⅓ cup equals 3½-oz. protein serving)
PLUS, you may have 2 Tbsp. Crunchies free a day (unless weight loss is slow).

These meats (and all others) should be broiled, baked, boiled, steamed, grilled, or poached. They may also be cooked in a no-stick pan, microwave, or crockpot. All visible fats must be removed. Eggs may be poached, boiled, or cooked in a no-stick pan with no added fat.

Vegetables

Have two to four servings of vegetables daily. Have at least one raw and one cooked. To ensure a wide variety of vegetables daily, Diet Center recommends a variety of five to seven fresh vegetables in your salad each day.

Asparagus	Mushrooms
Beans (green and yellow)	Mustard greens
	Parsley
Beet greens	Okra
Cabbage	Onions (maximum allowed,
Cauliflower (raw)	2 Tbsp.)
Celery	Peppers (all types)
Chard	Potato (baked)
Chicory	Radishes
Chinese cabbage	Spinach
Collard	Sprouts, alfalfa, radish, and
Cucumbers	mung beans
Endive	Squash (crookneck, scallop
Escarole	varieties, yellow, zucchini)
Fennel	Tomatoes
Green onions	Turnip greens
Kale	Watercress
Lettuce	

You may have a cooked vegetable and a salad both at lunch and dinner. You may add broccoli, brussels sprouts, carrots, eggplant, pickles, and tomatoes. Potatoes may be eaten twice a week.

Alternate your selection of vegetables at each meal so a larger variety is eaten. Always use *fresh* vegetables whenever possible, using frozen vegetables as your second choice and canned only as a last resort, becaue of a higher salt content and loss of natural nutrients. Steam your vegetables lightly when cooking. Each day add one new vegetable at a time, and weigh yourself, every morning. If you begin to gain weight, cut back on new additions and eat smaller quantities of foods that create weight gain.

Fruits

One fruit choice is allowed daily. DO NOT eat more than one fruit a day.

Eat a variety, but avoid overripe fruits. One cup mixed fruit equals 1 fruit serving.

Select from among the following:

Apples (large, approximately 5″ diameter, do not peel!)
Apricots (3 raw or ½ cup water-packed)
Blackberries (1 cup)
Blueberries (1 cup)
Cantaloupe (⅓ to ½ melon)
Gooseberries (1 cup)
Grapefruit (½ per serving)
Honeydew (⅓ to ½, depending on size)
Nectarine (1 large)
Orange (1)
Papaya (½)
Peach (1 whole or 1 cup water-packed)
Persimmon (½)
Raspberries, red or black (1 cup)
Rhubarb (½ cup cooked, sweetened with "Diet Lite")
Strawberries (1 cup)
Tangerines (2)

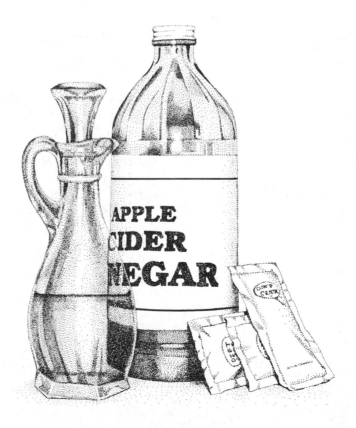

Breads

Two bread servings are allowed each day. One of these servings must be either 6 Diet Center Thins or 2 Lite Rye Wasa Brod. You may choose your other serving from the list below:

(6) Diet Center Thins
(2) (Lite Rye) Wasa Brod
(1) Ak-Mak cracker
(1) Finn Crisp cracker
(1) Italian (Grissini) breadstick
(2) Melba rounds
(1) Melba toast
(1) Norwegian flatbread

Oil

Each day you must have 2 teaspoons of corn, cottonseed, safflower, soybean, or sunflower oil. You may eat the oil in a salad dressing by adding the oil to as much apple cider vinegar or lemon juice as desired, or you may use the Diet Center Salad Dressing packets. Each packet equals 1 teaspoon of oil. (Two packets allowed daily in place of oil.) Oil is treated as a seasoning that makes food taste good. To minimize oil intake in foods, DO NOT HEAT OIL!

Dairy Products

Choose one 1-cup serving from the following list:

Buttermilk
Low-fat milk
Skim milk
Plain, low-fat yogurt

Sweeteners

Any no-calorie sweetener may be used. Recommended: Diet Center "Diet Lite" sweetener has less than 2 percent saccharin.

Seasonings

DO NOT OVERUSE SALT! Any seasonings or spices that do not contain oil or sugar are permitted in moderation. Read the label! Diet Center makes a variety of seasonings that can be used to enhance the flavor of your foods. Herbal seasonings are recommended to be used in place of salt. If salt is included in seasonings, Diet Center recommends using it sparingly (¼ teaspoon of salt retains ½ pound of water).

Additional Foods

You can have these additional foods each day if desired:

Apple cider vinegar
Unflavored gelatin
Lemons and limes
Unprocessed bran (2 Tbsp.)
Diet Center Bran Muffin (page 314)
2 Tbsp. Diet Center
   Crunchies or 1½ oz.
   textured vegetable protein
2 Tbsp. Diet Center Protein Powder

A SUGGESTED DIET FOR STABILIZING

The purpose of the Stabilization Diet is to flood your body with protein. Protein is the only nutrient that will rebuild and retone the body's muscles and cells. We do not count calories at this time. As you begin to stabilize, and to change your eating patterns, it's not unusual to gain one to three pounds the first week. If you begin stabilization on Monday and gain three pounds, do not worry. By Friday, you will have lost those pounds and will have returned to your previous ideal weight. Do not plan to lose weight while stabilizing.

Prepare a turkey or a rolled beef roast ahead of time. You may eat as much of this meat and low-fat cottage cheese as you like. Eat eggs in moderation.

Plan to eat fish and seafoods at noon.

Eat whatever the family eats in the evenings.

Do not go hungry, yet do not stuff yourself.

REMEMBER — ONLY EAT THE EQUIVALENT OF ONE FRUIT! You may eat both raw and cooked vegetables at your meals.

FOUR-DAY SAMPLE MENU PLANNER FOR STABILIZATION

DAY ONE

7:30 A.M.   Hot lemonade (2 Tbsp. pure lemon juice in 8 oz. hot water)
   Calcium (750 mg.)
   Vitamin C (250 mg.)
   Vitamin B-complex

8:00 A.M.   Scramble 1 egg and add:
   1 Tbsp. Crunchies
   2 Tbsp. cottage cheese
   (Cook together in no-stick pan)
   Apple-Bran Pancakes (page 313)
   1 glass (8 oz.) water

10:00 A.M.   ½ cup plain, low-fat yogurt
              1 glass (8 oz.) water

12:00 noon   4 oz. crab salad with 5- to 7-vegetable salad (save uneaten
              salad for 3:00 snack)
              2 tsp. oil and vinegar dressing
              3 Diet Center Thins or 1 Wasa Brod (Lite Rye)
              1 glass (8 oz.) water

3:00 P.M.   Remainder of crab salad
              Pop Squares (page 316)
              1 cup herb tea or diet drink

6:00 P.M.   4 oz. turkey
              1 cup cottage cheese (sprinkle with Crunchies, on
                 sliced tomatoes and lettuce)
              1 cup broccoli (steamed)
              1 Bran Muffin (page 314)
              1 glass (8 oz.) water

8:00 P.M.   1 oz. turkey if hungry
              3 Diet Center Thins or 1 Wasa Brod (Lite Rye)
              1 large Baked Apple (page 315)
              1 glass (8 oz.) water

DAY TWO

7:30 A.M.   Hot lemonade (2 Tbsp. pure lemon juice in 8 oz. hot water)
              Calcium (750 mg.)
              Vitamin C (250 mg.)
              Vitamin B-complex

8:00 A.M.   1-egg Mushroom Omelet (page 318)
              1 Wasa Brod cinnamon toast
              1 glass (8 oz.) water

12:00 noon   4 oz. tuna in large 5- to 7-vegetable salad (3 cups)
              2 tsp. oil and vinegar dressing (eat until full, save
                 remainder of salad for afternoon snack)
              1 breadstick
              1 glass (8 oz.) water

2:00 P.M.   Remainder of tuna salad
              ½ large apple
              1 glass (8 oz.) water

6:00 P.M.   4 oz. broiled lean hamburger patty
              Cottage cheese salad on bed of lettuce
              Baked potato (use cottage cheese dressing)
              1 cup green beans

| 6:00 (con't) | 3 Diet Center Thins or 1 Wasa Brod (Lite Rye)
1 glass (8 oz.) water |
| 8:00 P.M. | ½ cup Fruit Ambrosia (page 316)
1 glass (8 oz.) water |

DAY THREE

7:30 A.M.	Hot lemonade (2 Tbsp. pure lemon juice in 8 oz. hot water) Calcium (750 mg.) Vitamin C (250 mg.) Vitamin B-complex
8:00 A.M.	1 scrambled egg (with 1 Tbsp. Crunchies) 1 Tbsp. cottage cheese 1 Wasa Brod, toasted, *with* 1 tsp. Wildberry Jam (page 313) 1 glass (8 oz.) water
10:00 A.M.	⅓ cup cottage cheese, *with* ½ cup peaches on a bed of lettuce 1 glass (8 oz.) herb tea
12:00 noon	4 oz. shrimp, in Shrimp and Egg Salad (page 329; eat salad until full, save remainder to eat at 2:00 P.M.) Vinegar and Oil dressing (page 330) 1 breadstick 1 glass (8 oz.) water
2:00 P.M.	¼ cantaloupe Remainder of Shrimp and Egg Salad 1 glass (8 oz.) water
6:00 P.M.	4 oz. roast beef Cooked asparagus Vegetable plate (cucumbers, sliced tomatoes, cauliflowerettes) ½ cup cottage cheese 1 Bran Muffin (page 314) 1 cup milk (2%)
8:00 P.M.	2 oz. roast beef if hungry 1 cup Diet Center Custard (page 317) 3 Diet Center Thins or 1 Wasa Brod (Lite Rye) 1 glass (8 oz.) water

DAY FOUR

| 7:30 A.M. | Hot lemonade (2 Tbsp. pure lemon juice in 8 oz. hot water)
Calcium (750 mg.) |

	Vitamin C (250 mg.)
	Vitamin B-complex
8:00 A.M.	1 Bran Muffin (page 314)
	1 tsp. Blackberry Jam (page 313)
	1 glass (8 oz.) water
10:00 A.M.	1 glass buttermilk
12:00 noon	Broiled halibut
	Tasty Spinach Salad (page 328)
	½ cup stewed tomatoes
	½ cup cottage cheese
	6 Diet Center Thins or 2 Wasa Brod (Lite Rye)
	1 glass (8 oz.) water
2:00 P.M.	¼ honeydew melon sprinkled with lime
	1 glass (8 oz.) water
6:00 P.M.	Stuffed Chicken Breast (page 320)
	Sliced tomatoes, cucumbers, lettuce, celery sticks
	Baked potato (cottage cheese dressing)
	Cooked spinach (¼ cup)
	1 Bran Muffin (page 314)
	1 glass (8 oz.) water
8:00 P.M.	Strawberry Parfait (page 317)

5

The Diet Center Maintenance Diet — Phase Four

LEARNING how to leave a restricted reducing diet and return to the challenges of everyday eating, yet maintain that new weight, is not as difficult as it sounds. It does require, however, a basic program. This program should act as a "blueprint" that you can follow for the rest of your life!

This plan requires the important skills of preparing food ahead of time, as you learned to do while reducing. Having a large salad and fresh fruit on hand will make the "intelligent" decision to chose the "right" foods easy. (For example, remember how an apple can maintain a stable blood sugar concentration?) The same principles you learned while reducing should be used every day for the rest of your life! Prevent overeating by making the correct choices of *what* and *when*. This is the key for controlling the blood sugar concentration, and, thereby, conquering obesity.

Remember the basics: Eat on time on the same schedule; be prepared; eat three fresh fruits daily and a wide variety of vegetables; eat no more than 7 ounces of protein servings daily, which has been trimmed of excess fat and skin. Plan to eat 3½ ounces of fish and seafood at the noon meal, and a 3½-ounce serving of protein for the dinner meal. As you begin to incorporate these ideas into everyday eating, you will gain a whole new nutritious life-style. Add each new type of food choice, one at a time, and see how your body tolerates it. If you gain weight, avoid that particular food. These foods may include spaghetti, macaroni, pizza, pie, or hamburgers. You may be able to tolerate these foods once in a while, or you may

NEVER be able to include these foods in your diet. Most important, be in control and learn to know your body.

The foundation of your Maintenance Diet should be based on lean meats, fresh fruits, vegetables, unsaturated fats, low-fat milk products, and whole grains. By limiting consumption to these basic foods, you will always insure that you receive an adequate intake of nutrients and fiber. Whole grains are especially vital for this fiber intake. Few people, however, realize that commercial breads and cereal products contain few whole grains. Consequently, a special section of recipes has been created to show you how to prepare whole grain cereals and breads at home. (See "Diet Center Whole-Grain Bread and Cereal Recipes for Maintenance Diet," pages 337–341.)

I've had dieters ask me, "Do you have to diet forever?" The answer is, "Yes, you have to be on a program for the rest of your life!" I used to diet every day when I weighed 186, so I wouldn't reach 200 pounds. Now, I eat on a program every day so I don't weigh over 140 pounds. Dieting is a word that has negative connotation for many people. However, following a lifelong program of weight maintenance is one of the most positive things that you can do for yourself! When you eat fresh fruits and vegetables, you no longer even *want* the rich, gooey foods you once craved simply because your body was starving for energy. I can honestly say today that I am never hungry — with that starved feeling. I no longer wring my hands and pace the floor trying to understand why I have no control and feel like a failure.

Today, I eat on time and on a schedule. It doesn't matter if I am in a taxi in New York or Washington, D.C., I simply have the driver stop for a minute at a store so I can buy fresh fruit.

You don't need to be afraid that you will never eat a particular favorite food again. But, go slowly. Take a taste. Is it good enough to eat all of it? You may be surprised: a favorite dessert may no longer taste as good as it used to. Remember how hard you worked to lose each pound. Is it really worth it? If you do want it, enjoy it. Don't feel guilty. BUT NEVER OVEREAT TWO DAYS IN A ROW! Be ready to diet the next day.

WEIGH EVERY DAY! Weighing every day is an absolute must in total weight control. Don't skip even one day or you will lose control. Weighing every day also gives you the personal knowledge as to which foods are an absolute NO! Do you have a certain favorite that has always been your downfall in the past? Why overtempt yourself by even buying it? It may take a while to put this philosophy to use. For instance, take the example of a birthday. Your daughter's birthday may be approaching and you plan to make a cake. What is your favorite kind of cake? Chocolate? It may not even be her favorite, but it is yours! Make a white cake that you can easily resist and that will still look festive for the occasion. DON'T OVER-TEMPT YOURSELF! DON'T BUY THOSE FOODS YOU CAN'T RESIST! DON'T EVEN ALLOW THEM IN YOUR HOUSE!

Do you feel "sorry for yourself" for not eating those foods? DON'T! Remember, you have an incurable illness, as detrimental to your health as diabetes. Like the diabetic, you can control this disease. But, it is up to you. IT IS SOLELY YOUR RESPONSIBILITY! No one else can do it for you. When you want a certain food that you know will lead to trouble, remember the whole cycle that leads to obesity. The diabetic also wants favorite foods, but has learned to live with the illness. Diabetics receive an instant reminder, through insulin shock, that what they ate was wrong. The illness of obesity, however, is a slower process, although it can be just as deadly. Recall what was it like to be overweight or obese? Fat cells never disappear; they shrink, but they are still there. This is why obesity is an incurable illness. You may not have felt physical pain, but the emotional feelings should be unforgettable — lack of self-worth, humiliation, retreating to the point of just existing. Then, remember the miracle of permanently gaining control and reaching your goal. The excitement of loving yourself, your life, and everything around you! Is letting yourself get out of control worth it? ABSOLUTELY NOT! Remember self-discipline. With the Diet Center Program, you will not be hungry or crave foods. You must, however, make your own personal decision to follow the program. It is up to you!

Just as important as what foods are eaten is the method by which these foods are prepared. Steam vegetables; broil meats. Retain the "natural goodness" in your food whenever possible. Reverting to deep-fat frying, creamy sauces, and thick gravies will cause your figure to revert back to its fat shape!

Now that you are on the Maintenance Diet, you will need to ease yourself carefully into new food choices. Records of your food intake must be kept during each week and should be closely reviewed.

Sign the Maintenance Contract (see page 154), pledging to remain "true" to nutritious eating forever. Also make a list of those foods or behaviors that are the most difficult for you.

FOLLOW THESE STEPS FOR PERMANENT WEIGHT CONTROL AND A HEALTHY, NUTRITIONALLY SOUND LIFE-STYLE FOREVER!

1. Weigh every day! Do not even let one day go by without weighing. Be sure to weigh even after you have "indulged" so you will know exactly which foods you can enjoy and which foods you should avoid.

   Do not panic if you experience a small weight gain. This is essential for your continued success!

2. Be on a program! Don't follow a "diet" for the rest of your life. Instead, follow a "program" designed to ensure your good health.

3. Eat on time, on a schedule! Eat on the same schedule, both weekdays and weekends. If you eat fish and seafood meals at noon, then eat 3½ ounces of other types of proteins with your evening meal.

4. Eat fresh fruits! Women should eat three to five fresh fruits every day. Men can eat five or more. Remember that fruits are the key for controlling blood sugar level. Eat fruits so you are in control and don't feel deprived or persecuted. Because you won't crave sweets, you will be able to make intelligent food choices.

5. Eat fresh vegetables! Always have cleaned, fresh vegetables on hand. Keep small air-tight bags of a variety of vegetables in your refrigerator for snacks and "instant" salads.

6. Eat salads! Eat a large, fresh salad every day. Be sure to combine at least five to seven different vegetables into your salad for proper nutrients and variation.

7. Steam your vegetables for maximum nutrient retention. It is the easiest method available. Have both a raw and cooked vegetable every day.

8. Drink water! Every day, you should drink eight glasses of water. Remember, there is no better beverage than pure, fresh water.

9. Keep foods basic and simple! Avoid fattening combinations of food. Rely on salads, fresh fruits and vegetables, whole-grain crackers, and simply prepared meats for basic menus. Those casseroles and deluxe desserts probably caused your weight gain! "Keeping it simple" is one of the easiest ways to maintain an ideal weight and stay healthy. Remember, "simple" doesn't have to be bland or boring!

10. Eat protein, but don't eat too much! For good health, women should eat approximately seven ounces of protein per day; men, ten ounces. Choose primarily those meats lowest in fats and highest in protein content. Remember, extra protein turns to fat!

11. Be selective! Taste food before eating. Eat only those "extra" foods that you really want; avoid those you eat just for the sake of "eating." Refuse foods you don't want. Stay in control! NEVER OVEREAT TWO DAYS IN A ROW!

12. Eat whole wheat and whole grains! Gain the "staying power" from these grains that will satisfy you for a long time and keep you from becoming hungry. These foods also supply the vitamin B-complex that aids digestion and helps to calm nerves. The fiber and bulk present in these foods will keep your digestive system regular for good health.

13. Study the subjects of food and nutrition! Become interested in these topics, which can affect your life so drastically. Spread this knowledge to others. Apply these concepts to your own family, feeding them the same basic, natural foods that you eat.

14. Eat an apple and drink water before going out and you will not be hungry. You can now be selective and are now in control.

Then, place this contract and list in a place where you can see them each day. At the end of every week, evaluate your progress.

You will now need to adjust to a new physical appearance and self-image. Finding yourself weighing a healthy, slim and trim twenty pounds less than you can ever remember or weighing less than you did in high school can be very exciting, but it can also be a very traumatic experience when you are left alone at the end of the diet. Attaining a new ideal weight produces feelings of self-discovery and self-evaluation. Dealing with these new feelings as well as a rash of compliments can often be unnerving. You may need a special friendship and support system that will help you through this emotional time.

Now that you have lost your excess weight and will be on a well-balanced program, you will be able to maintain this de-

MAINTENANCE CONTRACT

I WILL:

1. Set daily, monthly, and long-term goals.
2. Weigh myself every morning.
3. Be aware of which foods I can eat and which foods I will need to avoid.
4. Not allow myself to become nervous or anxious when I gain two pounds, but will relax and visualize my success.
5. Eat on time and on a schedule.
6. Be prepared — fix foods ahead of time.
7. Sit down to eat.
8. Eat slowly and chew foods thoroughly.
9. Eat a variety of fresh fruits and vegetables for staying power.
10. Limit caffeinated drinks to two a day.
11. Eat before 8 P.M., if possible.
12. Never overeat two days in a row.
13. Exercise for optimum health every day.
14. Avoid refined sugar and flour; avoid foods made with either.
15. Eat foods as close to "natural" as possible, avoiding prepackaged or precooked foods.
16. Prepare fruit and vegetable snacks ahead of time for myself and/or my family.
17. Eat a 3-cup salad (containing five to seven vegetables and proteins) daily.
18. Steam vegetables.
19. Drink eight glasses of water daily.
20. Eat three to five fresh fruits each day.
21. Eat mostly fish and poultry; eat red meats only occasionally.
22. Use little salt.
23. Eat whole-grain cereals three to five times a week.
24. Not be afraid to eat, but I will eat correct foods.

SIGNED: _____

DATE: _____

sired weight. Diet Center does not recommend vitamin supplements on this diet as you will receive adequate nutrients from your food.

Vitamins are not recommended unless you live in a high-smog area, you smoke, or you are under extreme stress or are ill. Check with your personal physician.

DIET CENTER'S MAINTENANCE DIET FOR WOMEN

This is a suggested diet to help you eat correctly for the rest of your life. Don't skip meals, and eat a balanced diet.

Water

Drink eight 8-ounce glasses of water throughout the day. (Do not drink more than two glasses at a time.) Do not drink after 8 P.M. There is no substitute for water; it is essential for good health.

Coffee, Tea, and Diet Drinks

Any food or drink containing caffeine tends to make a person nervous. Decaffeinated coffee has over twenty-nine different acids; black and green teas have caffeine and tannic acid, many herbal teas are medicinal, and diet drinks contain high levels of additives and preservatives.

DIET DRINKS, COFFEE, AND GREEN AND BLACK TEAS DO NOT COUNT AS PART OF YOUR DAILY EIGHT GLASSES OF WATER.

Herbal teas may be counted as part of your water. (Use in moderation.)

Diet Center recommends you limit your intake of these beverages to no more than two per day.

Alcoholic beverages are allowed *in moderation.*

Protein Foods

Select your protein foods from the following list. Eat seven ounces of protein daily. A variety of lean meats, cooked well-done, is recommended. Always plan your weekly menus from a wide variety of protein choices in order to obtain the highest nutritional value.

Meat and Poultry. Eat 3½-ounce portions (cooked weight) of lean meat: beef, lamb, veal, poultry, pork, deer, elk, rabbit, or beef heart every day. Have liver once a week. Pat any excess fat off with a paper towel.

Fish. Eat a 3½-ounce portion (cooked weight) of seafood for

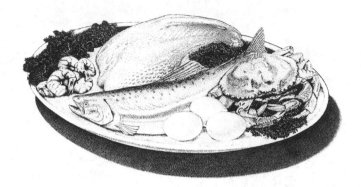

one meal each day or at least five times each week. Seafoods are delicious in salads and make good noon meals, such as a crab or shrimp salad or a tuna sandwich, salmon patties, etc. You may use any type of seafood; however, your best choices are: flatfish, flounder, haddock, halibut, perch, pike, pollock, red snapper, sand dabs (baby halibut), salmon, sea bass, sole, river trout, tuna, and white fish. Also, shellfish: crab, crawdad (crayfish), lobster, and shrimp (rinse canned tuna and shrimp).

Chicken, turkey, and other fowl. Remove bone and skin before cooking.

Chicken livers. Bake, broil, or steam-fry.

Cottage cheese. One-half cup, low-fat, may be eaten in addition to these other protein foods.

Eggs. 1 egg equals a 1-ounce protein serving. Do not use eggs as your total protein for the day. Do not exceed five eggs a week.

Tofu. One 8-ounce cake equals one 3½-ounce protein serving.

Diet Center Crunchies or *TVP.* One-third cup equals one 3½-ounce protein serving.

Plus, you may have 2 tablespoons TVP as a snack.

Remember: All meats should be broiled, baked, boiled, steamed, grilled, poached, or cooked in a microwave, crockpot, or no-stick pan totally eliminating all oils and fats in frying and cooking. Pans may be sprayed with Pam or similar product. All visible fats must be removed. Eggs may be poached, boiled, or cooked in a pan with no added fat.

Vegetables

Unlimited amounts of raw vegetables plus 1 cup cooked vegetables are allowed each day. Unlimited vegetables include those listed below and any with 15 grams or less of carbohydrates a serving.

Artichokes	Kale
Asparagus	Lettuce
Beans (green and yellow wax)	Mushrooms
Beet greens	Mustard greens
Broccoli	Brussel sprouts
Cabbage	Okra
Carrots	Onions
Cauliflower (raw)	Parsley
Celery	Potatoes
Chard	Peppers (all types)
Chicory	Radishes
Chinese cabbage	Spinach
Collard	Sprouts, any kind
Cucumbers	Pickles (in moderation)
Eggplant	Squash (crookneck, scallop
Endive	varieties, yellow, zucchini)
Escarole	Tomatoes
Fennel	Watercress
Green onions	

Limited vegetables include: those higher in carbohydrates, such as corn, lima beans, peas, and hubbard squash. These may be eaten two or three times a week. Alternate your selection of vegetables at each meal so a larger variety is eaten. Always use fresh vegetables whenever possible, using frozen vegetables as your second choice and canned only as a last resort, because of a higher salt content and loss of natural nutrients. Steam your vegetables lightly when cooking. Each day add one new vegetable at a time, and weigh yourself every morning. If you begin to gain weight, cut back on new additions and eat smaller quantities of foods that create weight gain.

Fruits

Have three fruits each day. Eat sparingly of fruits high in sugar: bananas, dates, dried fruit, figs, grapes, pineapple, raisins, watermelon, and cherries. One cup mixed fruit equals 1 fruit serving. Add each new fruit, one at a time. Weigh yourself each day, and if your weight is up, cut back on the fruit.

Apples (large, 5″ diameter, do not peel!)
Apricots (3 raw or ½ cup water-packed)
Blackberries (1 cup)
Blueberries (1 cup)
Cantaloupe (⅓ to ½ melon)
Casaba (½ melon)

Gooseberries (1 cup)
Grapefruit (½ per serving)
Honeydew melon (⅓ to ½, depending on size)
Nectarine (1 large)
Orange (1)
Papaya (½)
Peach (1 whole or 1 cup water-packed)
Persimmon (½)
Raspberries, red or black (1 cup)
Rhubarb (½ cup cooked, with no-calorie sweetener)
Strawberries (1 cup)
Tangerines (3)

Breads

Whole grains are excellent sources of complex carbohydrates, protein, and the B vitamins plus valuable bulk and fiber. You may have two servings of 100-percent whole-wheat, whole-grain, or multi-grain bread each day. (Remember, go easy on the butter or margarine, a total of 2 pats or 2 teaspoonfuls per day can be used on bread or vegetables.)

Whole-grain cooked or dry cereals. In addition to two bread servings, you may have ½ cup of cooked or dry cereals three times per week with 1 teaspoonful of honey. Read labels: do not buy sugared cereals. Try old-fashioned oatmeal, whole or cracked wheat, Cream of Wheat Farina or Roman Meal. Avoid breads, pastries, and cereals made of refined white flour and sugar, as they lack the nutrients and the bulk and fiber necessary for a healthy, well-balanced diet.

Milk

Drink two glasses of skim milk, 2-percent low-fat milk, or buttermilk each day. Plain, low-fat yogurt, low-fat cottage cheese (approximately ½-cup serving), or one ounce of hard cheese can be substituted for one milk serving.

Oil and Fats

Each day you must have 2 teaspoons of corn, cottonseed, safflower, soybean, or sunflower oil, and can have 2 teaspoons of butter or margarine. You may eat the oil in a salad dressing by adding the oil to as much apple cider vinegar or lemon juice as desired, or you may use the Diet Center Salad Dressing packets. Each packet equals 1 teaspoon of oil. (Two packets allowed daily in place of oil.) Oil is treated as a seasoning that makes foods taste good. To minimize oil intake, DO NOT HEAT OIL!

Sweeteners

Any no-calorie sweetener may be used. Recommended: Diet Center "Diet Lite" sweetener has less than 2 percent saccharin.

Seasonings

DO NOT OVERUSE SALT! Any seasonings or spices that do not contain oil or sugar are permitted in moderation. Read the label! Diet Center has a complete line of herbal seasonings that can be used to enhance the flavor of your foods. Herbal seasonings are recommended to be used in place of salt. If salt is included in seasonings, Diet Center recommends using it sparingly (¼ teaspoon of salt retains ½ pound of water).

Remember, the Diet Center Maintenance Diet is actually a "blueprint" on which you can base your eating habits for the rest of your life. Now that you understand how specific foods affect your body, you can add in many new foods. For example, you may even want to use commercial salad dressings instead of just vinegar and oil. The bottom line is WEIGHT MAINTENANCE. Weigh yourself daily. If a gain occurs, review the previous day's intake and reduce or eliminate those new foods which have had an averse affect on your weight loss.

Things to Remember on Maintenance

At noon:

- Eat five to seven fish or seafood meals a week.
- Eat one liver meal a week.
- We suggest seafood salads or fish at noon.

At dinner:

- Eat chicken, lean beef, pork chops, hamburgers (lean); approximately 3½ ounces.

Every day:

- Eat three to five fruits per day; ONE APPLE PER DAY!
- Do not use fruit juice.
- Eat all the fresh vegetables you would like.
- Eat 1 cup or more of cooked vegetables per day.

SEVEN-DAY MAINTENANCE MENU PLANNER

DAY ONE

7:30 A.M.	Hot lemonade (2 Tbsp. pure lemon juice in 8 oz. hot water)
8:00 A.M.	Scrambled egg
	1 slice whole-wheat toast
	½ tsp. butter
	1 Tbsp. Wildberry Jam (page 313)
	1 glass (8 oz.) water
10:00 A.M.	1 cup herb tea
	½ grapefruit
12:00 noon	3 oz. salmon patty
	Tossed 5- to 7-vegetable salad (3 cups)
	½ cup green beans
	1 slice whole-wheat bread
	½ pat butter
	1 apple
	1 glass (8 oz.) water
3:00 P.M.	Strawberry Parfait (page 317)
	1 glass (8 oz.) water
6:00 P.M.	3½ oz. meat (see pages 155–156)
	Asparagus
	Salad–vegetable plate (cucumber, carrot sticks, cauliflower, radishes, green onions)
	Baked potato (½ tsp. butter and 1 tsp. sour cream)
	Diet Center Custard (page 317)
	1 glass (8 oz.) water
8:00 P.M.	1 cup strawberries (with 8 oz. milk)
	1 glass (8 oz.) water

DAY TWO

7:30 A.M.	Hot lemonade (2 Tbsp. pure lemon juice in 8 oz. hot water)
8:00 A.M.	½ cup cracked-wheat cereal
	Taste of honey
	½ cup milk (use on cereal)
	1 slice whole-wheat toast
	½ pat butter
	1 Tbsp. Wildberry Jam (page 313)
	1 glass (8 oz.) water
10:00 A.M.	½ grapefruit
	1 cup of herb tea

12:00 noon	Large Middle-Eastern Tuna Salad (page 335) 3 cups 5- to 7-vegetable tossed green salad (eat until full, save remainder for 3:00 snack) 2 tsp. salad dressing (Diet Center dressing or see page 335) 1 slice whole-wheat toast ½ pat butter 1 glass (8 oz.) water
3:00 P.M.	Remainder of Tuna Salad 1 apple 3 Diet Center Thins or 1 Wasa Brod 1 glass (8 oz.) water
6:00 P.M.	3½ oz. protein (turkey, pork chop, ½ chicken breast, sliced roast beef, large, well-done hamburger patty) Green beans Sliced tomatoes ½ cup cottage cheese (on sliced tomatoes, with bib lettuce) Vegetable plate (celery sticks, radishes, etc.) 3 Diet Center Thins or 1 Wasa Brod 1 glass (8 oz.) water
8:00 P.M.	1 Apricot Fluff (page 315) 1 glass (8 oz.) water

DAY THREE

7:30 A.M.	Hot lemonade (2 Tbsp. pure lemon juice in 8 oz. hot water)
8:00 A.M.	1 slice French Toast (whole-wheat) (page 338) ½ pat butter 1 tsp. Wildberry Jam (page 313) 1 glass (8 oz.) milk 1 glass (8 oz.) water
10:00 A.M.	1 sectioned orange 1 glass (8 oz.) water
12:00 noon	Crab Casserole (page 322) (eat until full, save remainder for 4:00 snack) 5- to 7-vegetable salad 2 tsp. Vinegar and Oil dressing (page 330) 1 slice whole-wheat toast ½ pat butter 1 cup Fruit Ambrosia (page 316) 1 glass (8 oz.) water
4:00 P.M.	1 apple Remainder of Crab Casserole

4:00 (con't)	3 Diet Center Thins or 1 Wasa Brod 1 glass (8 oz.) water
6:00 P.M.	3½ oz. protein (pages 155–156) ½ cup steamed broccoli ½ cup steamed carrots 3 Diet Center Thins or 1 Wasa Brod 1 cup Diet Center Cole Slaw (page 326) 1 Diet Center Custard (page 317) 1 glass (8 oz.) water
8:00 P.M.	Dish (1 cup) of sliced peaches 1 glass (8 oz.) water

DAY FOUR

7:30 A.M.	Hot lemonade (2 Tbsp. pure lemon juice in 8 oz. hot water)
8:00 A.M.	½ cup cracked-wheat cereal (sweeten with 1 tsp. brown sugar)
10:00 A.M.	1 glass peppermint tea 1 Melba toast ½ cantaloupe
12:00 noon	Herb-Baked Haddock (page 322) 1 cup brussels sprouts ½ cup Diet Center Cole Slaw (page 326) 1 slice whole-wheat bread 1 glass (8 oz.) water
3:00 P.M.	1 large apple 1 glass (8 oz.) water
6:00 P.M.	3½ oz. protein serving 1 cup asparagus Fresh tossed green salad, with 2 tsp. Vinegar and Oil dressing (page 330) 1 Bran Muffin (page 314) Pop Squares (page 316) 1 glass (8 oz.) water
8:00 P.M.	1 glass (8 oz.) water Strawberry Parfait (page 317) 3 Diet Center Thins or 1 Wasa Brod

DAY FIVE

7:30 A.M.	Hot lemonade (2 Tbsp. pure lemon juice in 8 oz. hot water)
8:00 A.M.	Boiled egg 1 Wheat Waffle (see Sourdough Starter, page 339)

1 tsp. honey syrup
1 glass (8 oz.) milk

10:00 A.M.
1 glass (8 oz.) water
1 cup orange and banana slices
1 toasted Wasa Brod

12:00 noon
Broiled or baked halibut
1 cup broccoli with 1 slice cheese
5- to 7-vegetable salad, with 2 tsp. dressing (Diet Center dressing or Vinegar and Oil, page 330)
1 slice whole-wheat toast
1 glass (8 oz.) water
Apricot Fluff (page 315)

3:00 P.M.
½ large apple
1 glass (8 oz.) water

6:00 P.M.
Crockpot Chicken (page 320)
1 baked potato with 2 heaping Tbsp. cottage cheese
Stir-Fry Vegetables (page 331)
1 glass (8 oz.) water

8:00 P.M.
Strawberry Parfait (page 317)
1 glass (8 oz.) water

DAY SIX

7:30 A.M.
Hot lemonade (2 Tbsp. pure lemon juice in 8 oz. hot water)

8:00 A.M.
Eggnog (page 317)
1 Bran Muffin (page 314)
1 glass (8 oz.) water

10:00 A.M.
1 orange, sectioned

12:00 noon
Toasted tuna (½ can) on whole-wheat bread
Pickles, celery, radishes, carrot strips, cauliflowerettes
1 large Diet Center Cole Slaw (page 326)
1 Diet Center Custard (page 317)
1 glass (8 oz.) water

3:00 P.M.
Baked Apple (page 315)
1 glass (8 oz.) water

6:00 P.M.
Sweet-and-Sour Chicken (page 321)
½ cup rice
½ cup green beans
1 large serving Tasty Spinach Salad (page 328)
1 glass (8 oz.) water

8:00 P.M.
Fresh Fruit Cup (page 316)
1 Bran Muffin (page 314)
1 glass (8 oz.) water

DAY SEVEN

7:30 A.M.	Hot lemonade (2 Tbsp. pure lemon juice in 8 oz. hot water)
8:00 A.M.	1 scrambled egg 1 Tbsp. Wildberry Jam (page 313) ½ cup shredded wheat or grapenuts 1 cup milk 1 glass (8 oz.) water
10:00 A.M.	¼ cantaloupe 1 glass (8 oz.) water
12:00 noon	3½ oz. fried liver (lightly flour and season, grease sparingly) Large serving of 5- to 7-vegetable salad ½ cup Italian Zucchini Bake (page 333) 1 slice whole-wheat bread 1 glass (8 oz.) water
3:00 P.M.	1 large apple 1 cup peppermint tea
6:00 P.M.	Chicken Salad Supreme (page 326), *with* 2 tsp. oil (as dressing) Fruit salad on lettuce 1 breadstick 1 glass (8 oz.) water
8:00 P.M.	Peach "Ice Cream" (page 317) 1 Apple Cookie (page 314) 1 glass (8 oz.) water

HOPE'S STORY

The story of Hope Salazar could be that of many dieters. How many diets have you tried? How many types of pills? Perhaps, in desperation, you even tried jaw wiring or stomach stapling? Hope's story can inspire any dieter. Meet Hope Salazar, an incredible woman, who now spreads her own knowledge, inspiration, and caring as a Diet Center Counselor.

I have now experienced true happiness. My goal is to use the knowledge I have learned from the last thirteen years of fad dieting to help others lose weight at Diet Center. I have learned the wonderful lessons of overcoming the dreaded disease, obesity, for I have successfully lost 101 pounds and I feel terrific! I'd like to tell you my own true story.

I wasn't the poor, unloved, overweight child, which is typical of many overweight adults. I had a wonderful childhood, and my years as a teenager were filled with love and happiness. As a result, I developed into a happy, slim outgoing adult.

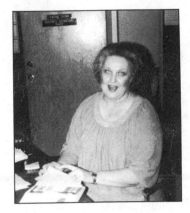

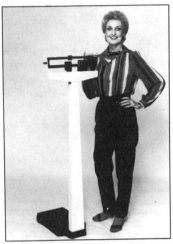

Hope Salazar had tried virtually every diet on the market, but it was the Diet Center Program that finally helped her lose 101 pounds and taught her to keep them off.

In my mid-twenties, I married Rudy Salazar, a U.S. Air Force Military Policeman at that time. Our life was one of travel and adventure. We even lived in Spain for one tour of duty.

I never even thought of the word "diet" until I was almost thirty years old. But after giving birth to three sons, I noticed one day that I was starting to look a little plump. At 5'9", 179 pounds didn't show too badly; but I went on my first diet. Little did I know then that I had embarked on a thirteen-year dieting career that would rob me of the most precious years of my life.

At first I tried the diet-pill routine. I took any over-the-counter pill I could get my hands on. I also started my career of joining health studios and exercise clubs. The lowest weight I achieved during this time was 142 pounds. I reached this weight while my husband was assigned to a tour of duty in Turkey, and I was forced to remain in the United States. The happiness of being together after his release from the Air Force and the return to a normal life caught me off guard. I soon found myself weighing 180 pounds.

I joined a national weight-loss program and started taking injections. After two months, my own personal doctor scared me into quitting. I had lost 32 pounds. Again, at 190 pounds, I began to panic. I tried all of the liquid diets, candy pills, health clubs, exercise clubs and any diet that I heard about from national magazines and newspapers.

I tried diets of protein only, low-carbohydrate diets, and various "guaranteed-to-lose" diets. I tried one that instructed me to eat nothing but grapefruit and eggs until I achieved my weight goal.

During this time of trying to control my weight and not being very successful, I worked as a secretary at the Calvary Evangelistic Temple, a church in Forth Worth, Texas. My husband was employed as a deputy sheriff in our city. Part of my job was counseling people. I was great on the phone because I knew they couldn't see me. But at the same time, I felt guilty. I was helping others with their problems, while I couldn't even help myself. I had dieted myself "up and down" and still weighed 240 pounds. I lost all my self-confidence and withdrew from life socially. I made excuses to avoid going to reunions, weddings, and even funerals.

To my extreme sadness, I missed all of those joys of being a mother with boys in school, not because my sons were ashamed of me — they never once showed any sign — but because I felt ashamed for them.

Desperate people do desperate things. I announced, as I usually did to my family and friends at work, that I had finally found the answer, and I would be slim again. I had my jaws wired. But I couldn't stand the extreme hunger and weakness I experienced. Soon, the liquid I was sipping through a straw became a malt. I eventually ended up clipping the wires so I could eat a meal, and told the orthodontist that they had broken. But I knew he wasn't fooled. I was only fooling myself. I made a vow that I would never diet again. Many times, I went to sleep at night thinking about my devastating situation —hating myself for being fat. The one thing I desired most was to be thin. The answer to my prayers was soon to happen.

A friend at church told me of a new diet that was helping her. I was curious, but I didn't even want to hear about another diet. I had quit weighing myself and caring about my weight. I didn't go anywhere except to work. I had three dresses, all tent style, and that was my total wardrobe. I even quit going to most church services. For three more weeks, I observed my friend as she lost weight. I envied her enthusiasm and newfound energy. She finally coaxed me into calling Faye Craft, the counselor, at the local Diet Center.

I began the Diet Center Program on Saturday morning, August 24, 1981. My father and mother had given me enough money to sign up, but I figured that I would just return it to them. I wore my black tent dress. At 243 pounds, I felt and looked awful.

For two weeks, I followed the diet to the letter just to prove to myself that I could find the gimmick. I was an expert at all the diets, and I was searching for something fraudulent about this one.

As I succeeded on the Diet Center Program, I began to regain the hope I thought was gone forever. It wasn't easy and sometimes there were tears, but I always knew what to expect. When Faye and I saw the scale drop below 200 pounds, we both cried.

In April 1982, I reached my goal of 142 pounds. I had lost 101 pounds and 107 inches in 8½ months.

6

Dieting and Children

NOTE: The Diet Center Reducing Diet for Children is based on the Diet Center Reducing Diet for Women and your child's age, sex, maturity, and activity level. Follow the diet schedule and amounts prescribed in the Reducing Diet for Women (pages 130–135), but keep in mind that food amounts may require reduction based on your child's needs. Observe the daily weight changes carefully. Calcium supplementation must be increased to 1,200 mg. daily while on the reducing diet.

HE climbed the stairs slowly, huffing and puffing, until he finally reached the top. Spotting the sandwich his mother had so conveniently left for him, Billy took it and settled down into the sofa to watch TV until dinner. Another day at school — thank goodness it's over! No more jokes, smothered giggles, or shame at his failures in physical education. Billy's parents call him "chubby"; the kids at school call him "fat."

Billy is not alone. Nearly one out of every seven children is overweight. In fact, childhood obesity is perhaps the greatest "nutritional danger" in our country today. In the last century, children have grown both taller and heavier. However, in the last decade, the problem of childhood obesity has increased rapidly — from a 10 percent prevalence in 1966 to a 15 percent prevalence in 1978 — a 50 percent increase in just twelve short years.

PHYSICAL EFFECTS

The physical effects of obesity in children are similar to those suffered by obese adults — a body that cannot handle extreme physical exertion without dangerously straining the heart, bones, joints, and muscles. Obesity among children has been associated with increased risk of arteriosclerosis, high blood pressure, hyperinsulemia, and carbohydrate intolerance. Obese girls not only grow faster and mature earlier than normal-weight girls, but they are also more likely to develop uterine cancer. A study of five thousand Iowa school children associated an increase in weight with an increase in coronary risk factors. Obesity at fourteen initiates the degenerative process on the coronary arteries that kills at forty-four.

The greatest tragedy is that, unless checked, overweight children become overweight adults. The odds against an overweight adolescent becoming an average-weight adult are approximately 28 to 1.

EMOTIONAL AND PSYCHOLOGICAL EFFECTS

Overweight children are labeled with a social stigma, and the effects carry over into adulthood. Stereotyped as "gluttons," lazy, and lacking in self-restraint, such children are judged harshly by siblings, peers, parents, and other adults alike. Research has shown that overweight children receive less encouragement and approval from their mothers, less acceptance from peers, and outright discrimination from adults. In fact, overweight adolescents stand a smaller chance of being accepted by colleges or for job positions than normal-weight adolescents.

Overweight children perceive themselves as unattractive and inferior. Self-confidence is eroded as they become the brunt of jokes and the object of ridicule.

I have seen these emotions in countless children who have come to Diet Center for help. I also have observed how overweight children are treated by their peers. Living in between a junior high and an elementary school for many years was very revealing to me. It seemed every age group had one overweight child who was a social outcast to the rest of his or her schoolmates. My heart always ached in sympathy for these children as I remembered my own childhood and how important it was to "belong."

Helping an overweight child gain new self-confidence and self-love through a slim, healthy, active life is the greatest reward anyone could receive. Many parents neglect their responsibility and fail to realize their own chance to help.

Other adults often have negative feelings about the *parents* of overweight children, too: the parent is seen as "coddling" the child, or worse, as indifferent to the child's plight (not only the physical problems but the psychological pressures of being overweight).

The parent who tells his or her overweight child that "it's just baby fat" or "you have other qualities that are more important" or "just ignore the taunts — 'sticks and stones can break your bones but names can never hurt you' " means well, but children know that words really *do* hurt. The promise that they'll "grow out of it" — aside from being more optimistic than realistic in many cases — is scant consolation for the pains of here and now.

Often parents will just tell the child with a weight problem to stop eating so much "junk food" and to get more exercise. Good advice — but if *adults* can't manage it without help (and many can't), how can a child? And they'll suffer from the failure at least as much as an adult.

THE DIET CENTER PROGRAM COULD BE YOUR CHILD'S BEST FRIEND

As we've discussed, being overweight not only imposes physical pressures but mental ones as well, especially for a child. Ten-year-old Daphene Bucklew knows from her own experience.

From a roly-poly baby to a chubby toddler, she was almost fifty pounds overweight by the third grade. It was very difficult for Daphene to understand the teasing she received from her classmates. It was extremely painful, and coming home from school in tears was not uncommon. She felt angry — why should being overweight exclude her from participation in games and limit her circle of friends?

Daphene's grandparents, with whom she lives, didn't realize the seriousness of her weight problem until she began complaining about chest pains. They made an appointment for Daphene with their family physician. Her grandmother explains that the doctor informed her that "Daphene was entirely too fat, and the fat was pressing against her heart." He promptly referred her to the local Diet Center.

Daphene desperately wanted to lose the unwanted weight. The teasing had left an impression on her. Daphene was extremely cooperative and concerned and did everything exactly right.

Through the duration of the diet, Daphene never put one "illegal" bit of food into her mouth. Even on her tenth birthday, which occurred in the middle of the diet, Daphene refused to cheat and have a birthday cake.

Her strict adherence to the diet paid off. As Daphene began to lose weight, her classmates began to notice, and their ridicule turned into compliments.

"They would say things like 'You look great!' or (the ultimate) 'I'm jealous of you,' " cited a pleased Daphene.

Real support and encouragement came from Daphene's grandparents too. Her grandmother stopped buying sweets and making pastries. Instead, every day her grandmother carefully packed Daphene's lunch with nutritious and filling foods. Myra Skrentny, Daphene's Diet Center Counselor, could only describe their cooperation as "absolutely magnificent."

Daphene's enthusiasm about the changes that were taking place in her life increased when she was able to participate in sports and physical education class without becoming winded. She now enjoys playing soccer, softball, kickball and baseball . . . and the television set receives less attention.

Athletic ability is not the only area in which Daphene has shown improvement. She has attained the status of an "A" student. Daphene admits that when she was overweight and not eating properly, she was often tired and experienced difficulty concentrating.

Daphene is looking forward to fall. This year is going to be the best of her life. She will be able to proudly show off her new school clothes, which are four sizes smaller than last year's wardrobe!

"Her whole personality seems to have changed. She is more sure of herself now and enjoys meeting and talking to people instead of hanging back," explained her grandmother.

"It was really worth it!" says an excited Daphene, who can now fully experience the joys of a normal childhood.

Because of her high motivation, Daphene is one of Diet Center's most successful young dieters. Whether your child is this motivated or not, similar success is possible. One of the most crucial factors to your child's success will be your understanding and support. Please remember that all overweight children experience similar feelings of hurt, rejection, and shame. Help your child by working together to set goals, weigh daily, prepare foods, and plan meals. The Diet Center Program can provide the solution, but your involvement as a parent is essential.

LEARNED EATING HABITS

Parents have the greatest effect on shaping children's perception of food. Food often becomes more than a way to nourish the body. It attains its own emotional value when offered as a reward or withheld as a punishment. A recent study of thousands of preschoolers showed that:

1. One in four mothers used food as a reward.
2. One in ten mothers used deprivation of food as a punishment.
3. One in three mothers used food as a pacifier.

Parents have a far greater effect on their children's weight than they realize. If one parent is overweight, his or her children have approximately a 40 percent chance of also becoming overweight. However, if both parents are obese, the possibility of their children being overweight increases to 80 percent!

This relationship begins early in infancy. Parents control what types of foods are purchased, in what quantities, and when and how they are consumed. Thus, the "feeding situation" in infancy evolves into "the eating situation" in childhood. The overweight six-month infant usually becomes the overweight thirty-year-old adult.

Overfeeding or incorrect feeding of an infant becomes crucial when related to the "Fat Cell Theory." This theory, which has received tentative biological support, states that the number of fat cells present in the body are determined early in life. This number is greatly increased in children who become obese in their first year of life. Later in life, these fat cells expand as the child becomes overweight. Obese adults with a greater number of fat cells have less control over weight. They can control the size of the fat cells, but never the number. It has been found that an obese adult who was an obese child can have three times the normal number of fat cells.

Additionally, the idea that children learn best by example relates directly to eating. Fat children often imitate exactly what their parents do: they eat more, eat faster, and talk less. This difference shows up as early as ages eighteen months to two years.

By the time children begin school, influences on eating have switched from parents to television and friends. A child of this age is bombarded by over five thousand television commercials each year about food. Unfortunately, these foods are generally commercial, prepackaged sugared cereals, candy, and soft drinks.

DIET

Another major factor causing obesity is the composition of the diet, more importantly in quality than quantity of food consumed. It can be hypothesized that the recent increase in childhood obesity can be directly related to an increase in the amount of "junk foods" and "fast-food meals" consumed by children. Almost half of a selected group of children chose cola as their favorite beverage and ice cream as their favorite dessert. As a result of these and other factors, diets of many children are lacking vital nutrients and fiber. Additional research shows many children dislike vegetables, do not eat breakfast, and tolerate a narrow range of foods.

Interestingly enough, when given the option, children enjoy nutritious snacks if they are offered on a tempting tray or dish.

Diet Center believes that the only effective solution to childhood obesity involves the restructuring of eating habits and attitudes toward food, both for children and parents. The first step a parent can take is to analyze (1) what the child consumes and (2) what the family consumes. Remove the high-calorie foods, which are usually high in refined sugar and fat. Repalce candy and cookies with fresh fruits and raw vegetables. In most cases, the child will lose unwanted pounds without even being conscious that you are helping to do so. Do not make an issue of dieting.

Start by checking your pantry, refrigerator, and freezer to see what foods are there. Examine the labels to see what ingredients these foods really contain.

Next, carefully plan your grocery list. Diet Center emphasizes the importance of "staying power" provided by foods that are digested more slowly and satisfy the body's need for energy over a longer period of time. Foods purchased in "Nature's own wrapper" contain greater quantities of fiber and naturally occurring nutrients.

Breakfast

Breakfast usually falls victim to time. You can easily prepare foods (e.g., making sure you have fresh fruit on hand, measuring out cereal, cooking cracked wheat) the night before. All non-food preparations, such as table setting, can also be done. Prepare extra servings of foods (such as bran muffins [see page 314] or wheat waffles [see page 339]) and store them in the freezer until needed. Remember to focus on foods with "staying power." Shredded Wheat, Grape Nuts, Corn Flakes, and Cheerios are next best for convenience foods. Remove all sugar-laden cereals. Sweeten cereals with fresh berries. Use whole-wheat breads for toast. Watch the jam. Serve whole fruit rather than juice. Boiled, fried, or scrambled eggs only take a moment, but remember, use no grease. An eggnog is a great hurry-up meal with toast and fruit. These foods will last all morning, giving the child good energy and allowing him better concentration.

Lunch

Remember, what goes in the lunch bag is usually what the child eats. It is important to discover what foods your child (or yourself) likes! Whole-wheat breads have longer staying power, but you may need to start with cracked wheat until the child gets used to eating them. Pita shells also provide a good base for a sandwich. Use tuna, lean beef, turkey, or eggs, with sprouts and vegetables for added crunch! Always include a piece of fruit and some raw vegetables.

Check out the hot lunch program provided by the school cafeteria. Recent efforts by parents and food-service directors have resulted in changing traditional, tasteless lunches to nutritious, appealing alternatives. Parents have also been influential in replacing candy with fruits in vending machines.

Snacking

Snacking is a way of life for teenagers and children. The rule of thumb is to "substitute." Do you have a bowl of fresh fruit or raw vegetable strips available? If given the opportunity, many children will choose a nutritious snack over a non-nutritious one.

"BUT, MOM, THE COMMERCIAL SAID . . ."

Parents should learn for themselves the nutritional importance of foods and how they affect the body, then pass this knowledge on to their children. Careful attention must be paid to the child's diet. Parents must take the time and give the extra effort to ensure that the child receives adequate "macronutrients" (protein, carbohydrates, and fat) and "micronutrients" (vitamins and minerals). Once the principles of sound nutrition are learned, parents and children can make intelligent choices concerning the foods they eat. Children, grades 5 and up, are very interested in learning to read labels. Take time to teach them. Teens are most concerned about their hair, complexion, and waistline. They want to know about chemicals and additives.

Instilling the principles of sound nutrition requires more than just a change in eating habits. It requires an accompanying change in attitude. Teens are bombarded by thousands of fast-food temptations — double cheeseburgers, malts, pizza, Mexican foods, candy, cake, and hordes of other rich, oily, and sugary foods. Small children see TV commercials hidden with sales gimmicks especially designed to appeal to children. Take the time to explain basic nutrition! They are never too young to learn the basic principles of good nutrition.

IT'S NEVER TOO EARLY

Most new mothers worry that their infants are not being fed enough. They are pleased when they have a fat baby with a big appetite. While you must be very careful to ensure that a baby gets all of the required nourishment, keep in mind that you can overfeed an infant and cause health problems too.

Focus on mealtime as a relaxing experience, not a stress-filled situation or a sparring ground for arguments. If you have young children at home during the day, you may be tempted to use food as a reward or withhold it as punishment. At times, you may resort to using food as a pacifier to give you time to regroup your nerves. Be very careful not to attach food to emotional events, as this teaches a child that food can be a comfort or a crutch.

At Diet Center, we recommend the take-away system to help young children acquire a taste for wholesome foods. We have the parent put a variety of fresh fruits and vegetables in a bowl and tell the child it is for the parent's diet. We tell the parent to give the youngster a taste and then say, "That's all for now. No more." We even encourage parents to put the bowl away, just as we did for candy and cookies. "Save it for later" or "We will eat it after a while," or "That's for me" really works. NEVER use "Eat this, it's good for you!" Soon, your children will be begging for fresh fruits and vegetables, just as they did for candy and other sweets, but with an important difference. Healthy, natural foods will fill and satisfy the child for longer periods of time. They will actually eat less food and get better nutrients from the food they eat. The child will not crave the sugar-filled, refined food, and you will notice a calming effect on the child's personality. You may even notice a great improvement in the child's overall emotional and physical health. If you control what your youngster eats at this age, there won't be a weight problem later. Taste for food is acquired and developed over the years, so the younger your child when you start, the better.

Use the same good eating habits with your school-age children. After they leave the house for school, they become subject to the eating habits of their peers. Most school lunch programs will work against you at this time. TV commercials concerning food begin to have more influence on your child. Unfortunately, the majority of these commercials deal with sugared cereals, candy, and soft drinks. Your work is really cut out for you if you haven't done a good job of training your child up to this point. Do not panic, however, if you are not prepared for this phase of your child's life. Children are often smarter than many adults realize. With just a little direction, you can make any child curious about foods and how they af-

DIET CENTER
Weight Chart for Children

Average Weight Chart for Boys

(A variable of five pounds should be allowed)   (weight without shoes)

Age (yr) Height (inches)	5	6	7	8	9	10	11	12	13	14	15	16	17
38	34	34											
39	35	35											
40	36	36											
41	38	38	38										
42	39	39	39	39									
43	41	41	41	41									
44	44	44	44	44									
45	46	46	46	46	46								
46	47	48	48	48	48								
47	49	50	50	50	50	50							
48		52	53	53	53	53							
49		55	55	55	55	55	55						
50		57	58	58	58	58	58	58					
51		61	61	61	61	61	61						
52		63	64	64	64	64	64	64					
53		66	67	67	67	67	68	68					
54			70	70	70	70	71	71	72				
55			72	72	73	73	74	74	74				
56			75	76	77	77	77	78	78	80			
57				79	80	81	81	82	83	83			
58				83	84	84	85	85	86	87			
59					87	88	89	89	90	90	90		
60					91	92	92	93	94	95	96		
61							95	96	97	99	100	103	106
62							100	101	102	103	104	107	111
63							105	106	107	108	110	113	118
64								109	111	113	115	117	121
65								114	117	118	120	122	127
66									119	122	125	128	132
67									124	128	130	134	136
68										134	134	137	141
69										137	139	143	146
70										143	144	145	148
71										148	150	151	152
72											153	155	156
73											157	160	162
74											160	164	168

DIET CENTER
Weight Chart for Children

Average Weight Chart for Girls

(A variable of five pounds should be allowed)   (weight without shoes)

Age (yr)	5	6	7	8	9	10	11	12	13	14	15	16	17
(Height inches)													
38	33	33											
39	34	34											
40	36	36	36										
41	37	37	37										
42	39	39	39										
43	41	41	41	41									
44	42	42	42	42									
45	45	45	45	45	45								
46	47	47	47	48	48								
47	49	50	50	50	50	50							
48		52	52	52	52	53	53						
49			54	55	55	56	56						
50			56	57	58	59	61	62					
51			59	60	61	61	63	65					
52			63	64	64	64	65	67					
53			66	67	67	68	68	69	71				
54				69	70	70	71	71	73				
55				72	74	74	74	75	77	78			
56					76	78	78	79	81	83			
57					80	82	82	82	84	88	92		
58						84	85	86	88	93	96	101	
59						87	90	90	92	96	100	103	104
60						91	95	95	97	101	105	108	109
61							99	100	101	105	108	112	113
62							104	105	106	109	113	115	117
63								110	110	112	116	117	119
64								114	115	117	119	120	122
65								118	120	121	122	123	125
66									124	124	125	128	129
67									128	130	131	133	133
68									131	133	135	136	138
69										135	137	138	140
70										136	138	140	142
71										138	140	142	144

*Prepared by Bird T. Baldwin, Ph.D., and Thomas D. Wood, M.D. Published originally by American Child Health Association. Adapted for Diet Center.

fect the body. Many times, once children learn about the harmful effects of certain foods, they cannot even be forced to eat them. In a controlled study, when a group of children was informed of the negative effects of cola drinks, their intake dropped immediately.

No change in diet will be successful unless the entire family alters its eating habits. Parents can encourage controlled eating patterns and regular exercise habits. A deemphasis must be put on the emotional value of food.

Parents should learn for themselves the nutritional importance of foods and how foods affect the body, then pass this knowledge on to their children.

WHAT IF MY CHILD IS ALREADY OVERWEIGHT?

Is your child overweight? Use the Diet Center Average Weight charts for children to find out. Be sure to take maturity, frame size, etc., into consideration.

Being overweight not only imposes physical pressures, but mental ones as well, especially for a child. (You might consider the help of a Diet Center Counselor if you haven't prepared yourself with enough knowledge or if the problem is getting to be a serious one.) Often, one of the big reasons for overeating is little self-esteem in the home. In this case, the parent is ineffective in helping the child to lose weight. Don't hesitate to seek professional help for a problem of childhood obesity.

Weight reduction and control is never easy, especially for children. It requires not only the cooperation of the entire family, but also the willingness to change harmful eating habits and diet. However, this effort seems minute when compared to a life filled with physical and emotional pain.

7

Dieting and Men

NOTE: The Diet Center Reducing Diet for Men is altered from the Diet Center Reducing Diet for Women to include a total of 9 ounces of protein servings per day: added protein choices of lean beef, tuna, turkey, cottage cheese; and added vegetables (both a raw vegetable and a cooked vegetable are allowed each meal). If men are hungry on this diet, larger quantities of vegetables are allowed as are more eggs and cottage cheese. Be sure to drink the water; as with the women's plan, the schedule is as important as the food — eat on time, on a schedule, and be prepared.

IN the past, most men regarded dieting as an activity "for women only," until a severe heart attack or serious illness scared them into trying to diet. Today, however, men are increasingly aware of the importance of good nutrition and the severe consequences of obesity.

Typically, a man can gain additional pounds through the years without the emotional problems that are so apparent to an overweight woman. During the teen years, he is called "husky" or "strong," instead of "fat" or "obese." Unless he is tremendously overweight, it is just too easy to ignore those additional pounds. In many cases, a man is fifteen to twenty pounds overweight, yet feels he is in good health. Poor eating habits are reinforced, and soon his health begins a downhill slide. His job exerts extra pressure and his doctor starts prescribing high blood pressure medicine and warning him to lose weight. He begins to become self-conscious about his weight, noticing, perhaps for the first time, the glances and comments of people around him. Few men are versed in nutrition or don't know "how" to lose weight. Skipping meals and fad diets result in even more weight and increased feelings of frustration, embarrassment, and failure. Just like any woman, he falls into the trap of "yo-yo-ing," which continues until a heart attack or stroke occurs, sometimes fatally.

John Von Rueden of Bismarck, North Dakota, experienced many of these same feelings and difficulties before learning to control his weight permanently at Diet Center. John had yo-yo'd for years, trying a variety of diets ranging from liquid protein to diet pills. John's wife, Joan, first introduced him to the Diet Center Program where she had lost fifteen pounds. John then began the program himself and lost eighty pounds. Today John no longer needs his daily blood pressure pills or medicine for gout. "I've never felt better," says John. "I'm no longer fatigued by the end of the day, and my energy level is high. My wife and I actually went to a late movie last week."

While you may be conscious of the health risks linked to obesity for both men and women, the detrimental effects of those extra pounds carry into every facet of life. Many men may not realize how their weight, and subsequent looks, could be jeopardizing their careers. In hiring, companies tend to by-pass the obese or heavy man, knowing that more sick days are taken and insurance claims for serious illness are more frequent.

It may be decided, behind his back, that his being overweight is too great of a risk for the company to invest a great deal of money and training for a promotion to a more important position. It may be decided in the private thoughts of the president of a company to exclude him from an important assignment because of the impression he will make on the public. The obese person may feel this is discrimination, or he may not realize the actual reason until it starts to become obvious. Because of the high cost to the employer, obesity is now a valid reason for not hiring an individual. In the military services of the United States, an overweight serviceman is graded down on his annual fitness report for being overweight. If that person fails to control his weight, he can be discharged from his job. Even overweight politicians and other public people could gain more influence and support if they were not overweight. Our society thrives on the image of a slim and healthy, energetic person — an image that cannot be achieved by someone who is overweight or obese. Overweight and obese men have an immediate disadvantage in any social or business sphere to which they belong.

CHANGING PERCEPTIONS

The fact that most men know little about nutrition and dieting requires some attitude changes before they can even begin to diet. To be successful, a man must be convinced that his extra pounds do not look good, do not make him strong, and are very harmful to his health and future. He must be convinced that dieting is not a "sign of weakness," but a "sign of intelligence."

Consequently, commitment and motivation are essential for success. A male dieter must make a commitment to reach goal weight and to not stop even one-half pound short! For many men who have "always" been ten or even twenty pounds overweight, this is a difficult concept to grasp, and even a harder challenge to accept. When some men lose to the point that they feel and look good, they will be tempted to quit dieting. If they do quit at this point, however, it will be very easy to regain the weight. But once a man finds out how much better he feels, how much more energy he has, and how much better he looks after reaching goal weight, there is nothing that will stop him.

Men tend to rationalize and tell themselves that they are not overweight: it's just their broad shoulders, or they are "husky." Possibly they hide those extra pounds under a size 44 suitcoat when, in fact, they are too heavy. Often, men insist that their wives lose weight, when they themselves need to drop twenty pounds. One man came to see us about having his wife go on the diet. I put him on the scale and *he* needed to lose twenty-five pounds. It took him twenty-five days to lose the weight and he felt great!

The reason most diets fail for men is because they fail to take into account the drastic difference a man's life-style and size has on his need for food. If a man attempts the fad diet designed for a 5'2" woman, he will never be successful and may dangerously impair his health in the meantime. A successful reducing program for men takes into account such factors as: How did he gain his weight in the first place? How active is his life-style? What type of work does he do? And what is his motivation for wanting to lose weight?

In order for a man to diet himself, he must understand the need to completely modify his thinking about what foods he can eat, how the food is prepared, and when the food is eaten. In fact, he must learn about nutrition in order to be in control of what he eats and to maintain his weight after it is lost. He may even need to teach his wife the importance of natural foods.

Many men are overweight simply because they eat too much of the wrong types of food. Often, eating junk foods, working long hours, and grabbing only a candy bar leaves dieters wanting more junk food (low blood sugar levels).

The life-style of a man often will determine how his body handles foods. Usually, construction workers and men who work out-of-doors are able actively to work off the food they consume. Short and small men, or men who lead inactive lives, will have trouble with eating too much food. Sometimes, a shorter man will have to use the woman's diet, and not vary from it, in order to be successful. For most men, however, an entirely different diet is required, including larger quantities of vegetables, fruits, and protein to satisfy them.

If a man is involved in heavy labor, or is working two jobs, an adjustment can be made to the foods on the list. Diet Center's Diet for Men is based on the average man with the average life-style. This diet must meet the health needs of the individual, so a supplement may be needed for extra energy if the man does daily physical labor. He must eat breakfast, and he must increase his protein consumption. Diet Center recommends mixing protein powder into a thermos to be drunk throughout the day.

For the man working two jobs, it would be well to take a fruit break at about 8 P.M., and again at 10 P.M. to eat a vegetable snack or a salad. This will control hunger and maintain good health and strength.

Men are able to handle more and different types of food than women. They have larger frames and a higher metabolic rate, and as a result they lose weight so easily that they put it off and don't take it seriously.

The Diet Center Recipes section features two sets of recipes for men. Since men can eat all the foods on the Women's Reducing Diet, any of the recipes in "Diet Center's Reducing Recipes for Women and Men" are allowed. However, because most men can consume additional quantities and types of food, men are allowed to choose any selections from "Diet Center's Men's Reducing and Women's Stabilization Recipes." For these substitutions, men should follow the recommended portion size indicated in the "Men's Reducing Recipes" section at the end of the book.

EATING IN RESTAURANTS*

For the male dieter who must eat in restaurants, dieting is very easy. Most restaurants have salad bars with a wide variety of approved foods. (Some fast-food places have a salad bar for quick snacks.) Check the menu for the "dieter's special." It will usually be a broiled chopped steak or broiled ground

* These suggestions on menu selection apply specifically to men. Women who travel or dine frequently in restaurants should see the "restaurant" section on pages 238–240.

round with cottage cheese and a fruit. It may be a fish serving, and this is good also. You might ask for a serving of cottage cheese and a well-done hamburger if you do not see it on the menu. Watch out for very greasy food. If your hamburger patty is greasy, soak away the excess with a napkin before eating.

Most restaurants offer half a grapefruit, fresh strawberries (in season), honeydew and fresh lime, or cantaloupe. It is very easy to stop for a fruit break, and very refreshing and satisfying.

Do not overlook an omelet on a restaurant menu. A large, three-egg omelet, or one with mushrooms, peppers, onions, etc., is a good meal any time. (Remember to avoid the cheese, however, while reducing.)

For breakfast, you might try poached eggs, omelets, or grilled fish. Do not forget steak (well-done) and eggs for extra protein if you need it.

If you are dining out in the evening, you will have to be a bit more crafty in your choice of foods from the menu. When ordering, you must specify how you want the food prepared. You may be surprised at the way a fish entrée, for example, is cooked and served, unless you specify when ordering. If you are in a situation where you do not want to make a fuss, you could order shrimp in the shell or lobster. Diet Center recommends that you simply tell the waitress that due to a health problem, you cannot have any special sauces, added salt, foods smothered in butter or gravy. Stay away from prime-rib dinners, because they contain too much fat!

On business trips, it is good to carry apples with you in your suitcase for emergencies. If your business meetings become so involved that you are unable to get away, you can eat an apple before a meeting or before you retire, and you will feel great! Be sure to drink your required water, and try to get some exercise during the day.

If you are driving on a trip, take a thermos of ice water to drink along the way. Take fresh fruits and vegetables for snacks, and plan your meal stops so that you eat on schedule. Stay in control of your diet, plan ahead, be prepared, and commit yourself to diet.

The Diet Center Reducing Diet was specifically designed to deal with each problem a male dieter encounters: how he lives and works, his special problems and individual tasks. Men like the nutritional information and motivation. You will lose weight easily, quickly, and with no hunger. You will rarely experience plateaus, and will continue a one-pound-a-day weight loss if the diet is followed exactly.

The challenge is to fit the diet to each individual dieter by taking into account the man's size and the type of work he does. Then, a weight goal is determined, and measurements need to be taken for neck, waist, chest, and wrists (see pages 19–20). Most men are surprised by how little food it takes to be healthy, if the right foods are eaten. They lose only adipose tissue, not muscle. You will maintain your new weight goals because, as with any woman dieter, you've learned the basics of nutritious living.

SCHEDULE YOUR MEALS

A *schedule* is just as important for male dieters. While reducing, you should aways plan several meals and in-between-meal snacks at the same times each day. If you are tall or have a large frame size, are employed in a job requiring heavy labor, or are very active physically, it is recommended that you eat breakfast, lunch, and dinner, with mid-morning, mid-afternoon, and early evening snacks, Your meals should consist of a protein selection, cooked vegetables serving, salad, and bread serving. Snacks can be additional protein, fruit, and vegetables as needed. If your height is below 5'7" or your frame size is smaller, you are occupied in a sedentary job or are less physically active, you may need to reduce the amounts suggested above.

The following is an example of a one-day menu planner for a typical male dieter — moderately active, average height and frame size. It is adapted from the Women's Seven-Day Reducing Menu Planner (pages 130–135). Additional menu planning can be adapted in the same way. You may need to adjust this schedule to suit your personal life-style.

Remember:

- Eat on time, on a schedule.
- Be prepared with foods.
- Eat two fruits each day, one of which must be an apple.
- Drink eight 8-ounce glasses of water each day.
- Eat a large salad and cooked vegetable with each meal.
- Eat two bread servings per day.
- Eat nine ounces of protein each day and up to 1 cup cottage cheese.

SUGGESTED TIMES AND FOOD FOR THE REDUCING PHASE OF THE PROGRAM

7:30 A.M.	1 (500 mg. time-release) vitamin C 750 mg. calcium tablet(s) Hot lemonade (2 Tbsp. pure lemon juice in 8 oz. hot water)
8:00 A.M.	1 scrambled egg (use no oil, fry in no-stick pan) 1 Wasa Brod (Lite Rye), toasted 1 Tbsp. Wildberry Jam (page 313) 1 glass (8 oz.) water
10:00 A.M.	½ large orange ½ cup cottage cheese 1 glass (8 oz.) water
12:00 noon	Lean ground beef patty (3½ oz.; blot off any excess fat) 1 cup Stir-Fry Vegetables (page 331) 1 cup cottage cheese and 1 sliced tomato arranged on leafy greens 1 Diet Center Custard (page 317) 1 glass (8 oz.) water
2:30 P.M.	½ large orange ½ cup cottage cheese 3 Diet Center Thins or 1 Wasa Brod (Lite Rye) 1 glass (8 oz.) water
6:00 P.M.	Turkey Soup (page 336) 2 Melba rounds Sliced cucumbers, cauliflowerettes, sliced zucchini and green pepper strips with Cottage Cheese Vegetable Dip (page 334) 1 glass (8 oz.) water
7:30 P.M.	1 (500 mg. time-release) vitamin C 1 glass (8 oz.) water
8:00 P.M.	1 Baked Apple (page 315)

REMEMBER: These guidelines are based on recommendations for a typical dieter. Your individual needs increase or decrease the amounts of types of foods listed above. Don't forget to weigh daily, chart your progress, and adjust the diet to suit your particular situation.

8

His-'n-Her Dieting

In today's world, two seems to be the magic number, especially if one of the two is male and the other female.

Challenges that are difficult when tackled alone become much easier when mutually confronted and shared with another person. The his-'n-her aspect can turn drudgery into enjoyment.

For instance, Diet Center feels weight loss can be made fun and effective by trying his-'n-her dieting. By working together toward a common goal, you can improve your waistline and have fun doing it.

LOOK BEFORE YOU LEAP

Before you begin dieting, you both should consult a physician. He can assure you that you are in good physical condition to proceed with a diet. He can also explain what a resting pulse is and how to read it and apply it to your dieting and exercise program.

Afterwards, sit down together and discuss your individual and mutual goals in detail. Decide how you are going to conduct your program. Write down your goals and then set up a timetable. This action will reinforce your decisions and lessen chances of giving up before you attain your goal. Diet Center recognizes the importance of goal setting, and encourages its dieters to write their goals down and put them in a highly visible place. You are then constantly aware of your goal and can review it several times a day.

THE WRITTEN EVIDENCE

Diet Center stresses the need for the frequent recording of weight and measurements. This allows you to realistically observe the effects and progress of your dieting efforts. These recordings may also indicate the need to modify your diet program.

Before begining your diet program, carefully weigh each other. Choose a time that will always be convenient and make it a point to weigh at that same time daily. Yes, DAILY! Diet Center has found that its dieters are more likely to stay on the program if they know there will be a confrontation with the scale every morning. Also, if you set a realistic goal (one-quarter pound per day, for example), you will be more encouraged by your daily progress.

The measurements play an extremely vital role in dieting. Almost every dieter will experience plateaus when losing weight. These times can quickly promote discouragement. Diet Center teaches its dieters that even though they are not losing pounds, they are losing inches (if they are not cheating). Although the discouragement may still exist, the inch loss compensates and keeps dieters from giving up in despair.

Starting with day one, write down your height, weight, and measurements. Remember, weigh daily and measure every two weeks.

THE THRILL OF THE RACE

If you are a competitive couple, you may wish to conduct a contest to initiate incentive. If you do choose this course, ladies beware! However unfair, it is a fact that men lose weight faster than women while being able to eat more (women should lose half a pound to men's one pound).

Because men have lower amounts of body fat in proportion to muscle tissue (about 4 percent less at ideal weight), they lose weight at a much faster rate than women. Also, many men are more active than their counterparts and burn up more calories.

You may also want to take into consideration that there will be some days you will lose more weight than others. Some people lose very well over the weekends; but for others, it is the most difficult time. By daily weighing, you will be able to pinpoint your weight-loss pattern.

THE POWER OF SUGGESTION

An important part of his-'n-her dieting is becoming attuned to the other person's needs and feelings. It is easy for discouragement to set in when dieting. If you are aware of your partner's moods, you can be each other's greatest asset.

Discouragement should not be the only time to compliment the other person. Offer positive feedback daily, and you will discover that verbalization is the world's most powerful reinforcer. Don't assume your partner knows that he/she is showing the effects of dieting. For some unknown reason, people tend to be critical of themselves and have a hard time distinguishing their own weight loss. So, TELL THEM HOW GREAT THEY LOOK!

DOUBLE THE FUN

There are several things you can do together that will cinch your diet's success.

It is extremely valuable if you are able to isolate the factors that contribute to your weight problem. Possibly, something as simple as watching TV is responsible. Many times, evening snacking in front of the TV is the main culprit.

After you have discovered these harmful habits, eliminate them from your life. Replace them with constructive, new habits that you both can enjoy.

Select some type of exercise you can do together. Tennis or racquetball are both activities that are a lot of fun and, at the same time, high-energy burners. This physical exertion will not only help your waistline, but will increase the strength of your heart as well.

You will be able to monitor the improvement of your heart by comparing your resting pulse with your pulse following strenuous activity. As the amount of time it takes for your heart to return to its resting pulse decreases, you can be assured that your heart's health is improving.

Make out your shopping list and go to the grocery store together. This way, you will be less likely to succumb to temptation if you are both there to help the other resist. Remember, if you don't buy it, you can't eat it.

Of course, you can't and shouldn't spend every waking moment together. Take some time to be alone and just deeply relax. Diet Center offers these helpful suggestions.

1. You need a private, quiet, dark place away from the hustle and bustle of everyday life. Sit in a comfortable chair (don't lie down); remove your shoes and wiggle your toes (or if

conditions don't permit, just close your eyes and proceed). Plant your feet flat on the floor; get comfortable and BEGIN!

2. Progressively tense and relax all your muscles, starting with the feet and working up. Tighten the muscles in your feet so you can recognize how your body feels when it is under stress. Then, let the tension slowly drain out; work up through the legs, stomach, chest, hands, arms, neck, and face. Totally relax.

3. Breathe deeply through your nose. Concentrate on a breathing pattern. Inhale, count to three, then exhale. Repeat.

4. Empty your mind of any problems or thoughts and continue breathing deeply, letting the oxygen flow to all parts of your body. Visualize yourelf in peaceful surroundings (by a lake, in a meadow, etc.).

5. Write the word *RELAX* on a card and keep it in a visible place, possibly next to your goal card. Every time you see the card, it will remind you to relax.

You may not notice a considerable difference at first; but with continued practice, you can attain a state of relaxation that can help change your life. Remember, you need to be good to your mind and body if you want them to be good to you.

VARIETY — THE SPICE OF LIFE

Many times, diets are abandoned for no other reason than the fact that the person becomes tired of the regimen. If you find your diet becoming boring or tedious, experiment with some of the fun and creative Diet Center recipes, or be imaginative and try some ideas of your own.

A perfect picnic suggestion for those who love the outdoors:

> Diet Center Deviled Eggs
> Rolled Breaded Chicken Breasts
> Cole Slaw
> Stuffed Celery Sticks
> Fresh Fruit Salad
> Lime-Fizz Fruit Punch

Or may we suggest a romantic "diet" candlelight dinner for two:

> Spinach-Tossed Salad and Vinaigrette Dressing
> Mushroom-Stuffed Chicken with Sauce
> Fruit Ambrosia
> Diet Center Mock Cold Duck

(You will find the recipes for all the above suggestions in the Diet Center Recipes section.)

Many husband-wife duos have achieved success together on the Diet Center Program. One couple relates:

Until now, we never realized how those extra pounds affected our physical and mental well-being. Now, people tell us how different we look, but that's only half the story. We both feel good about ourselves and what we have accomplished! Together we lost 192 pounds and gained a whole new way of life.

Dennis and Sue Spomer
Grand Island, Nebraska.

VI

LEARNING
TO APPLY THE TOTAL
DIET CENTER
PROGRAM TO YOUR
LIFE — PHASE FIVE

1

Modifying Your Attitudes and Behavior

THIS section of the Diet Center Program is just as important as any of the material previously presented. Dieters CANNOT permanently control their weight by just following a "diet." Once the weight is lost, the poor eating habits and non-nutritional life-style will take over once again. The weight that has just been lost will be quickly regained! Permanent weight control requires a total restructuring of the way we think, and act about, food.

This section outlines those changes you'll have to make to lose the extra weight successfully and maintain your new weight forever. Losing weight requires a personal commitment derived from the willpower associated with a positive self-image. The skills of visualization and relaxation are also vital to successfully accomplish any goal. These same skills will help you cope effectively with the stresses of everyday life — the stresses that have contributed to obesity.

The final portion of this section treats what happens when you successfully attain your weight goal and must deal with both a new body and a multitude of emotions. This part of the Program, from establishing a positive self-image to handling a multitude of compliments, is just as vital to your success as any diet!

PERSONAL COMMITMENT AND GOAL-SETTING

How important is your attitude in losing weight? Read this dieter's account. Does it sound familiar?

Diet Center made its greatest contribution for me on the inside. By the time I met Diet Center, I had been a glutton for at least 25 years. Although I managed somehow to keep my weight to less than 40 pounds overweight by strenuous physical exercise and crash diets, I was hungry all the time and preoccupied with food. In fact, food was one of the most important things in my life. I binged frequently, stopping the binge only when nausea, a stomachache or sores in my mouth made it impossible to eat anymore. I hid snacks under the bed, in the laundry hamper, in the car and at the office. I even ate what food had been thrown away in the garbage. I ruined my body chemistry.

On the Diet Center Program, I lost 20 pounds in six weeks, then 10 more. Little by little, my health has been returning. My blood pressure has dropped to normal. My migraines are almost gone. Last week, I forgot to put sweetener on my bran and fruit. The physical cravings for sweets and salts are gone.

Not only has my health been returning and my taste buds changing, but my attitudes toward food are changing too. Sometimes the memories of a two-decade love affair with certain foods stir up old cravings, but Diet Center gives me the way and the Lord gives me discipline. I know that I am healthy; I am helping others; and I can resist those temptations. I have said goodbye to my gluttonous spirit forever. And, it is that inner healing which has changed my life.

Martha Hargadine
Monroe, Louisiana

You must have a firm commitment to losing and permanently controlling weight if you want to be successful. Commitment is that passionate belief that *nothing* will stop you. It is the knowledge that you are successful! You can achieve! You can be slender and healthy! You are a beautiful, wonderful person!

Commitment requires the realization that there is a problem, a "plan" to overcome it, and the action to solve it. Commitment is actualized through goal-setting. Creating goals is simply the process of putting your commitment into words.

How do you gain a commitment to losing weight, or any other goal for that matter? Commitment requires some insight into knowing your "inner self." Once you truly know what you want, you can make your own decisions and assume full personal responsibility for their outcome. You need to cultivate a positive self-image in order to gain the insight and personal responsibility needed for total commitment.

THE ART OF GAINING A POSITIVE SELF-IMAGE

How much do you like yourself? Although this is a relatively simple question, it is one that is rarely answered.

The way you feel about yourself, your self-esteem or self-assurance, affects your life more than you know. Often you may treat a partner, a child, or co-worker badly simply because you do not feel good about yourself. It is a simple psychological fact that you cannot love anyone unless you first love yourself. This may sound self-indulgent, but it isn't. Self-esteem leads to a better life for you and everyone with whom you come in contact.

Are you able to love yourself? Do you have a healthy regard for yourself? To find out, just answer the questions on page 196. Remember, there are no right or wrong answers, only answers that will help you lead a much more rewarding life. Each question can be answered with the word never, seldom, occasionally, frequently, or always. Select your answer, then write down the number that corresponds to the word you have chosen. Total up your answers for all 30 questions. Then, check the following table to see how you rate.

How much self-esteem you possess can determine the course your life may take. Remember, you are what you think you are! If you are internally motivated, your own values will decide your course. If you develop and exercise high standards, if you accept yourself as you are right now — but are willing to change when change is necessary — you can achieve whatever you truly desire to achieve. There is no magic formula for such success.

If you do not submit to fear and anxiety, you can then realize that loving yourself and feeling great about yourself is not egotistical. You know that, more than any other positive trait, your self-image holds the door open to your happiness and high achievement. You are a winner!

One of the most difficult hurdles for an overweight individual to overcome is a negative self-image. Overweight people often feel shunned and withdrawn. One look in a mirror and the mirror-image becomes their inner perception of who and what they are. Because of this negative self-image, an overweight individual often develops external shields — a jovial disposition, or perhaps shyness — while internally he or she is crying for help.

More often than not, an overweight person turns to food for solace and contentment, failing to acknowledge that food is not only the major contributor to his or her overweight condition, but also a dominant factor in a negative self-image. The

NEVER (1)   SELDOM (2)   OCCASIONALLY (3)   FREQUENTLY (4)   ALWAYS (5)

1. If someone hurts my feelings, I tell them so.
2. People value my opinion.
3. I feel intelligent.
4. Nothing is too good for me.
5. With few exceptions, I'm satisfied with myself the way I am.
6. I consider comparing myself with other people to see if I rate higher than them a waste of time.
7. I enjoy meeting and talking with new people.
8. I feel at ease at parties.
9. I'm happy being me and, with few exceptions, wouldn't want to change places with anyone.
10. I don't want to be somewhere else, doing something else.
11. I'm content with the way I live my life.
12. I like the place where I live.
13. I enjoy my work.
14. People generally admire me.
15. I'm a kind person.
16. I enjoy getting up in the morning.
17. I can take care of myself.
18. Other people need me.
19. I enjoy watching what I eat, getting proper nutrition.
20. I try to make sure I lead a balanced life — enough sleep, enough work, enough play.
21. I don't mind being alone.
22. I enjoy my time alone.
23. I like myself.
24. I respect myself.
25. I value myself.
26. I see myself as a good-looking person.
27. I see myself as a sexual person.
28. I see myself as a loving person.
29. I see myself as a sharing person.
30. I see myself as a confident person.

150–129 points:	Your self-esteem is in the high/normal range. You can take people and situations in stride. You also have enough confidence to improve if you need to.
128–90 points:	You are in the low/normal range. Try to raise your self-esteem — you have the confidence to do it yourself.
89–60 points:	Your self-esteem is low. You can build it up yourself, if you are willing to work hard.
59–30 points:	You may need professional help to raise your self-confidence level. If your score does not improve, you may need a psychologist or a psychiatrist to help you.
Below 30:	Professional help is strongly indicated. You will be amazed how such help will change your life.

type of food ingested under such circumstances is typically low in nutritional value and high in refined sugar. Foods high in refined sugars can cause instability in the blood sugar level, often leading to intermittent periods of depression. The more frequent these periods of depression, the more prone an overweight person is to overindulgence. The cycle will continue until the overweight person gets help.

Help can come in a variety of ways. The only successful method of helping an individual overcome a negative self-image is through behavior modification and proper nutrition.

Think back to your quiz score. Were you satisfied with the results? Would you like to increase your level of self-esteem? If so, locate the areas in which you need help. Look back at the quiz and recheck those questions you answered "never" or "rarely." Is your answer fair or are you being too hard on yourself? Most people who lack self-esteem do so because they are too hard on themselves. Try this exercise: Stand before a full-length mirror. Look at the person you see there. Say: "You are a very special person who deserves the best break possible." Every chance you get, take advantage of your good nature and treat yourself better. Give yourself credit when things go right. Remember, you have the power to see the positive as well as the negative. You can see the good as well as the bad. You have the power to treat yourself like a leader or a slave. It's all up to you.

Here are some other Diet Center suggestions that will help you toward a positive self-image:

- Practice using your imagination. Recall your favorite experience in vivid detail. Concentrate on only the positive aspects. The human mind is a remarkable biocomputer capable of marvelous action. For example, the subconscious level of your mind cannot distinguish between real and imagined behavior. If you vividly imagine an action in your conscious mind, your subconscious mind treats that action as if it really occurred, triggering your behavior toward achievement of that action. Open your mind to clear, positive thoughts.
- Learn to listen. We always learn more about ourselves and our environment when we're listening. We are equipped with two ears and only one mouth. We should listen twice as much as we talk.
- Limit your TV viewing time. Invest more time in reading, writing, visiting, and giving some service to others.
- Write a short résumé (no more than two pages) of your professional and personal assets. Concentrate this résumé on present activities and future potential (e.g., current job, future

career goals). Read it every week, and visualize yourself exercising those positive traits. You should continually upgrade and revise the résumé.

- Eliminate the clutter in your life.
- Concentrate your thoughts on what a great person you are. You are special. You are unique. You are the best there is at being you.
- Always project a positive attitude toward your family, friends, and co-workers. Positive actions, combined with positive attitudes, create success and happiness. Always be enthusiastic — it's contagious.
- Align your thinking and actions with others who have the same feeling of positive action.
- There will aways be times when you let down and feel depressed. All winners experience it. But a winner won't stay down. A winner will be right back on top. A winner remains optimistic and always has a strong sense of self-worth.
- Always assume total responsibility for your actions. You are what you are.
- Unless prescribed by a physician, avoid depressants or stimulants.
- Show your spouse or loved ones that you care about them. Say, "I love you" — even to yourself.
- Be glad you are alive and enjoy good health. DO NOT, AT ANY TIME, FEEL SORRY FOR YOURSELF.
- Apply all of these suggestions to your life. Choose to be a winner and DO IT NOW!

HOW TO HAVE THE WILLPOWER TO MAKE YOUR OWN DECISIONS!

Everyone has willpower. Even people who say, "I have no willpower" have willpower. They just don't have as much as they want or they don't know how to use what they already have.

Willpower is not something that is discovered. It is neither a secret formula nor a magic process. Willpower is developed through practice and hard work.

Do you get out of bed each morning? Do you bathe and brush your teeth regularly? Do you show up for work or other commitments? If you do these activities, you have willpower. If you had no willpower, you could never do any of these things. As a matter of fact, if you had no willpower you couldn't do anything at all. Even to raise your arm or turn your head requires willpower, because your brain tells your muscles what to do. Willpower is simply your brain making up its mind to give the instructions.

At times, it is easier to believe what others say than to stick to our own beliefs. We let others convince us that the "reason" we are overweight is because we are over forty, work, don't work, eat out a lot, cook for the family, have children at home, don't have children at home, and on it goes . . . All these factors have an impact on our eating habits, but they are not the reasons we are overweight. When you believe that outside circumstances have control over your body, you cannot realistically deal with a weight problem.

At other times, it is as if your brain actually has a will of its own. Despite many good intentions, the mind sometimes seems to do as it wishes. There is some truth to this belief in that the subconscious mind does act independently of the conscious mind to some extent. Some of our ideas, feelings, memories, and fears come to us unbidden. We don't have to summon these thoughts, they just come to us from the "tapes" of our subconscious mind. Most of this information was developed in our early childhood. But the subconscious mind can be retrained by giving it repeated instructions from the conscious mind.

In order to develop willpower, you must

1. stop telling yourself that you don't have it;
2. start noticing that you do have it already; and
3. get at the hard work of developing greater willpower.

Begin developing this willpower by:

1. realizing that your subconscious mind is, in the long run, under the control of your conscious mind;
2. reprogramming your subconscious mind toward greater willpower, in general, by pointing out ways in which you already have willpower; and
3. reprogramming it in relation to specific tasks by pointing out that you can do it and how you can do it. In developing willpower to lose weight, you could say to yourself, (1) "I am in control here. I refuse to let my eating habits control me. I will control them." (2) "I do control my temper and my alcohol intake [or other behavior you have control over] already, so I can control my eating." (3) "I can control my eating by adopting a nutritionally well-balanced eating program and planning my meals ahead so I won't get into a food situation I can't control."

Once you have the positive self-image to perceive your true worth and the willpower to act, make a specific personal decision. This decision must be yours alone. You alone will receive credit for success or responsibility for failure. Assuming personal responsibility is indicative that you are a mature individual in control of your actions.

Making the decision to lose weight must be yours alone. Ask yourself exactly WHY you want to lose weight. Be honest in your assessment. Are you doing it because a husband or boyfriend insists? Is it because a total stranger made a cutting remark? Is it because all your friends are trying a new diet? While these reasons will not prevent weight loss, they will block your chance of permanent success. No one "forced" you to become overweight in the first place. You alone were responsible. Your decision to act must follow this realization. Lose weight because you truly want to become slim and healthy! You will succeed because every ounce of your determination will be behind this personal decision.

One Diet Center dieter sees this decision as the key to her success. Having been overweight since childhood, she recalls trying every diet that came along, never losing much weight and always gaining it back — plus more. "Finally," she says,

something clicked. Whether it was total disgust, desperation, boredom or just the thought of not being able to buy cute, summer clothes again another year, I decided to give Diet Center a try. Once I got started, it was easy. I wasn't tempted to eat off the program.

The most important thing Diet Center did for me was to teach me that I am responsible for myself. I learned that people make their own choices; and because of my actions, through my own choosing, I had chosen to be fat. Now, I have chosen to be thin, healthy and happy for the rest of my life. And I know I can, because I am in control.

Lisa Edelstein
Danvers, Massachusetts

2

Setting Your Personal Goals

ARMED with a positive self-image and the willpower to make your own decisions, you have achieved total commitment to permanent weight control.

The next step is to transfer this feeling of personal commitment to action by setting your goals. There are several basic rules to remember when creating a personal goal.

FIRST, DO IT! Don't delay once you have made a firm decision to make goals. Goals commit you to immediate action. A decision to lose weight means little if you don't start dieting!

SECOND, BE REALISTIC. How many pounds should you lose to achieve goal weight? (Consult the Diet Center Ideal Weight Chart.)

THIRD, WRITE IT DOWN. Be as specific as you can. "I will lose _____ pounds," not just "I will lose weight." A goal to lose weight doesn't necessarily have to be measured in pounds. You may want to say "I will lose weight and inches until I fit into my new size 10 pants."

FOURTH, SET A TIME SCHEDULE. Ensure that your goal will require working at it to succeed. Losing ten pounds by the following year allows too many other problems to interfere.

On the Diet Center Program, dieters are encouraged to focus on the end result. Instead of stating "I will" or "I want," state firmly, "I am."

Try this technique:

I AM SLENDER

1. Select your weight goal.
2. Write that weight on a 3 x 5 card.
3. Repeat: I am a slender _____ pounds (40–50 times daily).

4. Do this for at least twenty-one consecutive days.
5. Do this when tempted to eat off the diet.

This technique has been used successfully by millions of Diet Center dieters. As Phyllis Courtney of Idabel, Oklahoma, describes: "I made it! I set a goal that I had been trying to reach for eight years and could never get anywhere near. With the help of Diet Center, I made it." These words describe the importance of setting the "right" goal and achieving it for one young mother of three children. Three pregnancies had resulted in sixty overweight pounds and still gaining. She tried every diet imaginable. "I'd lose eighteen pounds, then go on an eating binge and gain back what I had lost, plus three or four more pounds." After hearing about Diet Center, she decided to give dieting "one last try." She wasn't sure that she could lose weight, much less reach the goal she had in mind. "After I looked at a picture of myself and stepped on the scale, I couldn't believe it! That was someone else, not me! But, then I realized it WAS me and something had to be done." During the twenty-four weeks on the diet, she never had a morsel of anything that was not allowed. "I never thought of going off the diet. Now, I'm a different person, not only physically, but mentally too."

Set daily, weekly, monthly and even yearly goals. DON'T LIMIT YOURSELF TO JUST ONE SPECIFIC GOAL FOR LOSING WEIGHT. EXPAND YOUR LIST OF GOALS TO INCLUDE MANY OF THE ACTIONS YOU CAN TAKE TO CREATE A NUTRITIONALLY SOUND LIFE-STYLE.

The following are suggested goals:

- I will exercise.
- I will visualize.
- I will drink my water.
- I will prepare my foods ahead of time.
- I will follow the diet exactly.
- I will cut back on salt.
- I will get adequate sleep each night.
- I will not get angry.

MAINTAIN A POSITIVE APPROACH

Remember that you, and you alone, have absolute control over your attitudes. Combining attitude with determination equals success.

Develop enthusiasm for your goals. Remember these points in maintaining a positive attitude toward your goals:

- All emotions are within you.
- You love or hate life as much as you love or hate yourself.
- Replace a negative thought with a positive thought.
- Learn how to handle disagreements and putdowns; don't strike back.
- Don't put yourself down.

Periodically, review your goals to see if they are still realistic. Can you set your sights higher, or do you need to lower your expectations?

PICTURE YOUR GOAL

In addition to visualization, picture your goal visually by designing a poster! Cut out photos, words, labels, or anything that will inspire you to achieve that goal. Hang this poster in a place where you will be able to see it each day.

3

When Stress Gets Your Best — Burn-out: Are You Experiencing It?

IN the morning, it is hard to get up. You find yourself working later into the evenings. Tears come easily to your eyes; you are bone tired, listless, depressed, and irritable. You find it hard to face work in the morning. How could this possibly happen to you when you love your job, your activities, your family, and your home?

What is wrong? You should be happy and excited about life. How can you have these feelings when you are "successful"? A newly coined term that has taken the modern world by storm is *burn-out*.

If you recognize yourself as having some of these feelings, you may possibly be experiencing one of the many stages of "burn-out," a condition often very hard to recognize, and even harder to cope with.

Just what is "burn-out"? Burn-out is the end product of stress. It begins with overwork and unrealistic expectations of yourself. Finally, an individual may find it difficult to cope both personally and professionally.

What are the symptoms? Check out the following list. You may find that you have some or all of these symptoms. Generally, the farther down the list you go, the closer to burn-out you are!

1. Easily fatigued.
2. Bored with work.
3. Angered easily.
4. Restrain emotions by separating home, social, and professional lives, and refuse to discuss one while in any of the other settings.

5. Depersonalization of others.
6. Loss of concern for others — attitudes begin to shift toward cynicism, hostility, and apathy.
7. Begin to have trouble seeing others' problems and concerns.
8. Withdrawal from others — both physical (smile or a hug) and psychologically (few compliments or less encouragement).
9. Become rigid and inflexible.
10. Become ineffective and inefficient. It becomes harder to think clearly, to make a decision, to accomplish even routine tasks.
11. Feelings of resignation and futility.
12. Deep tiredness, regardless of how much sleep.

Do any of these symptoms sound familiar? If so, it may be that you are beginning to feel the effects of the stressful situation in which you work or live.

There are two major causes for burn-out — work and you. Heavy demands, long hours, high public visibility and expectations are all work-oriented stresses. Most important, it is our reactions to these problems, and others, that can create or prevent burn-out. Many dieters are unsuccessful because they feel that their situation is so hopeless. You may want to take a few minutes to sit down and ask yourself these questions.

1. Are your goals realistic? (What good will it do you to work twelve hours a day if you are tired and frustrated, your spouse is unhappy, and your children never see you?)
2. Are you taking everyone's problems on your shoulders? You need to walk a tightrope that is balanced between not caring enough and caring too much.
3. Are your expectations of yourself realistic? Too often, people become frustrated because they feel they are doing an inadequate job. Three vital points to remember:
   A. You cannot help everyone.
   B. Not all things can be changed.
   C. Not everyone is going to love you.
4. Did you know that success often breeds burn-out, because it creates greater expectations? If you look at any profession in which people are highly successful (e.g., builders, counselors, teachers, lawyers, doctors), you will find people who have burn-out. The greater the successes, the greater the self-expectations. A vicious cycle can develop between greater success and greater demands, culminating in burn-out.

What can you do if you see yourself slipping into burn-out? First of all, recognize that you have it. This is not as easy as it sounds. People who tend to burn-out also tend to be characteristically charismatic, energetic, impatient, given to high standards. They thrive on intensity. "Failure" just is not in their vocabularies!

Failure, however, does occur — in meeting goals, handling stress, and satisfying job expectations. To admit burn-out seems like just one additional failure. Subsequently, a typical "cure" is to work harder, spending more time at the office and creating higher goals. All that this accomplishes is to intensify stress and speed up the burn-out process. In admitting you are having problems with stress and burn-out, you have reached the first point in defeating it.

The next step is to recognize what causes your stress. Is it any of these factors?

1. The way you are organized.
2. Your workload.
3. Your self-expectations.
4. Too many additional demands.
5. Communicating with others.
6. Limited range of interests.

Take a quick survey of what you spend your time doing. Work? Household chores? Recreational activities? Escapes? Next, evaluate the frequency and length of each of these activities. Where does your time go? Where would you like it to go?

Once you have realized the need to reorganize your life, do it in these ways:

1. Reevaluate your job situation. Can you let up a little and still do an excellent job? Can you better delegate your responsibilities?
2. Reevaluate your home situation. Are you at home enough to satisfy the needs of your spouse and children? Do you spend quality time with the important people in your life? Make sure you do not just allow a rushed hour between other responsibilities or the small remainder of an evening when you are exhausted. Take the time to communicate!
3. Reevaluate your life-style. Are you eating incorrectly? Are you overweight? Do you avoid exercising on a regular basis? If you answer all these questions with "yes," you are headed for ruined health. Reread the sections in this book explaining how to put a nutritionally sound life-style to work for you!
4. Take time, when needed, for simple relaxation. Relax? How? Remember those relaxation and visualization skills? Are you scheduling relaxation and visualization into your

day? Remember, you need to relax and unwind just as much as anyone else.

Do you have your own personal escape? Are you taking that time to play tennis, paint, sail, or whatever hobbies you do for relaxation? All work and no play creates burn-out!

5. Recognize the symptoms of stress early before you burn-out. Realize that stress is inherent in any profession. While there are many rewards, the pressures are constant — the perfect conditions for burn-out. You must deal with stress on an on-going basis. Do not let it pile up! Reevaluate your goals continually; save some time for your needs and keep an eye out for the early symptoms of burn-out.

Take care of yourself first, then your husband or wife, your family, then your business — in that order — and you will be successful.

VII

EXERCISE: ANOTHER KEY TO DIETING SUCCESS!

START YOUR OWN DAILY EXERCISE PROGRAM

Being physically active on a regular basis can have immediate benefits! These include:

1. SUPPRESSED APPETITE: Contrary to what some people may think, exercise does not increase appetite. Actually it does just the opposite and acts as an appetite suppressant.

2. BETTER DIGESTION: Exercise encourages food to pass through the intestinal tract much faster. The faster the food goes through, the less is absorbed to become excess weight. You can understand why it becomes so important to have regular bowel movements to show a good weight loss. Active athletes can pass a meal through their system in as little as four to six hours. The transit time for most people is usually twenty-four to twenty-six hours. One theory used to explain this increased intestinal activity (peristalsis) is that exercise causes the body to release more magnesium into the intestinal tract. Magnesium works as a laxative.

3. MORE CALORIES BURNED: Your body continues to burn calories after you have finished your exercise session. Once your body's metabolism is speeded up, it takes a while to slow down. Dr. Herbert de Vries has shown that the increased metabolic rate that occurs after exercise in an average person can result in a five-pound weight loss in one year.

4. BETTER MENTAL HEALTH: Exercise helps ward off depression. Many overweight people eat in response to feeling blue. Because exercise improves mood, it can be helpful in solving two problems: depression and eating.

5. BETTER MUSCLE TONE: Exercise is especially important for

dieters. A regular program of light exercise will help firm and retone muscles as you lose excess adipose tissue. Brief sessions of exercise every day will aid good muscle tone, good stamina, and, most importantly, good health.

Exercise is important for everyone. However, it is especially important for two types of dieters. *Short* dieters (generally women under 5′2″ and men under 5′5″) need to expend more energy. The Diet Center Program recommends a minimum of thirty minutes of exercise every day for short dieters. The second type, *pear-shaped* dieters, carry the majority of excess adipose tissue in the hip area. Diet Center also recommends a minimum of thirty minutes of exercise every day.

Gradually build physical activity into your schedule until it becomes a part of your life on a regular basis. The first step in increasing your activity is to look at your daily routine. See what can easily be incorporated to increase activity. Some examples are:

1. Walking to work or walking at least part of the distance.
2. Using stairs instead of the elevator.
3. Parking at the far end of parking lots.
4. Getting off the bus two stops earlier.
5. Avoiding purchase of convenience items that eliminate steps (riding mowers, remote-control televisions and garage doors, and extension telephones).

Because these seemingly small amounts of exercise do add up, rather small changes in our daily habits can have a profound effect on weight control.

No exercise program can be effective unless adjusted to personal life-style. Consider your available time, degree of physical fitness, skill level, and personal likes and dislikes in designing your own exercise programs.

You may also want to consider these:

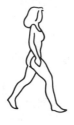

WALKING: A good brisk walk can tone up the muscles and get the blood circulating throughout the body and brain as well as, or better than, any sporadic exercise. Everyone can walk; you will need no special facilities or equipment. You must walk briskly, breathe deeply — a golfing pace will not do. Time yourself, starting out slowly at first if you must, but working up to 3½ to 4 miles an hour. You will feel great! Walking for thirty-six hours will burn one pound of fat. Someone looking at this statement might think that it would be impossible for him to walk this much; therefore, exercise would have a minimal effect. One should remember that his

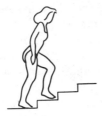

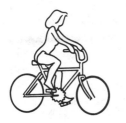

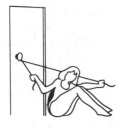

thirty-six hours of walking does not have to be at the same time. Walking one hour a day will give you thirty to thirty-one hours a month, which will be almost one pound burned. In a year, that will add up to approximately ten pounds.

STEPPING: It is great! Stepping can be done anywhere in any home. Step 25 stairs up or down per minute and time yourself. Start out slowly at first then go faster as your weight comes off and you begin to tone up your muscles.

BICYCLING: Of course, this is seasonal but very enjoyable. Bicycling allows you to enjoy the countryside. Pedal fast and breathe deeply. A good stationary bicycle is a fine method of exercising. When buying a bicycle, be sure it has gears, a timer, and a mileage indicator on it.

SWIMMING: This is an excellent method for keeping your body in good physical condition. If you are an average swimmer, you use every muscle in your body painlessly. One hour

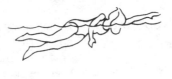

of swimming is approximately 670 calories of energy expended. This means that five hours of swimming equals one pound. On a regular basis, this can contribute significantly to your energy output.

JOGGING: This may be too strenuous for some of you, and we suggest that you alternate jogging with walking — five minutes of jogging and five minutes of walking.

DOORKNOB EXERCISE: This is done by connecting a stretch rope (which can be bought commercially) to the doorknob and to the part of your body you wish to exercise. This exercise is recommended by the Diet Center because it lets you exercise at your own rate. You can increase the exercise as you build up your muscles.

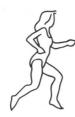

BOUNCE YOUR WAY TO BETTER HEALTH!

Do you enjoy a good massage to perk you up after a hard day or after strenuous exercise? The mini-trampoline will accomplish the same results . . . and while you are exercising. A massage will manipulate the muscles in such a way as to force the cells together and work the waste from around them and back to the lymphatic system. This causes your muscles to

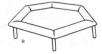

mini-trampoline

tingle and feel relaxed. This is where the massage ends but rebound exercise continues to work.

The effect of acceleration, deceleration, and gravity when you bounce on the mini-trampoline also stimulates circulation in the lymphatic system. The lymphatic system, also known as the immune or auxiliary circulatory system, has more liquid volume than the blood circulatory system. However, it has no pump and must rely on muscular activity, changes in atmospheric pressure, and gravitational pull to circulate its fluid. If the circulation of the immune system is not working properly, a person is more likely to become ill. When exercising on a mini-trampoline, the lymphatic fluid is forced through its network of tubes and one-way valves to its own cleansing organs, the lymph nodes and the spleen. The fluid, loaded with cellular waste, is cleansed of impurities; and you will feel great, look like you feel, and act like you look.

What Is Rebound Exercise?

Rebounding is a new and exciting form of exercise, and its popularity is just beginning to emerge. It is simply bouncing on a mini-trampoline. The idea is so simple that some people become skeptical of its value as an exercise program. Yet it has been said to be the most effective form of exercise ever devised by man.

What Rebound Exercise Can Do for You

The mini-trampoline permits the body, through muscular contractions and bouncing motion, to experience the forces of gravity, acceleration, and deceleration simultaneously. Because the cells in the body cannot distinguish among these three forces, they identify all three as increased gravitational pull. Each cell works to adjust to these environmental pressure changes and automatically strengthens its walls by a buildup of cellular protein. Because this combination of forces is being applied to every cell in the body at once, each cell individually becomes stronger and, therefore, the entire body is strengthened.

When exercising on a mini-trampoline, every cell in your body is being forced to oppose gravity — even without allowing your feet to leave the mat. This includes the muscles, the internal organs, the eyes, and even the bones of the skeletal system. (To feel the effects of rebound exercise, position your hands directly above both thighs. By bouncing lightly, you can feel the gravitational pull on your abdominal muscles.)

An Exercise Program for Everyone

By exercising on a mini-trampoline, participants of sports can increase their endurance as well as improve their balance. For the healthy athletic types who desire a hard workout, the mini-trampoline can increase their strength and endurance dramatically. There are exercises for improving tennis skills, skiing muscles, coordination, and other specific disciplines.

It is amazing that a person of little strength can benefit greatly by using a simple, gentle bounce. Positive effects can be gained just by sitting in the middle of a mini-trampoline while someone standing behind provides the bounce. People confined to wheelchairs can exercise their legs by having someone bounce while they rest their legs on a mini-trampoline. Elderly people are able to exercise regularly by placing the mini-trampoline near a wall or by holding on to a stationary object for balance while gently bouncing.

By using a very gentle motion (never lifting the feet off the mat) for a few counts several times a day, the ill person or people with an arthritic condition, lower back pain, or knee problems have been able to improve their overall health. Just the effect of the gentle motion increases circulation and nutrient flow to the body.

Many businessmen and women who spend long hours behind a desk are finding a tremendous benefit by taking short breaks throughout the day and exercising on the mini-trampoline. They do not have to change clothes, leave the office, or even work up a sweat. Most have found that by exercising this way (at mid-morning, after lunch, mid-afternoon, and just before leaving the office), for three or four minutes each time, their total health has improved; and they are amazed at the results.

One Diet Center dieter who is also an avid big-game hunter confirms that the mini-trampoline* makes a difference.

Ever since my father took me duck hunting at the age of four, I've been hooked on hunting of all kinds. Big game hunting has been my real interest which has provided me with many trips all over the U.S., including Alaska, and Canada.

Unfortunately, as we start pushing 40, our hunting trips become farther apart, as do the notches on our belts. The one short trip isn't fun anymore because what you seem to remember most is the aches and pains and the continual struggle to cover half the ground you did 10

---

* Mini-trampolines are available at sporting goods stores. The Diet Center has also developed one especially for dieters — the DCX X-Er-Sizer — available at your local Diet Center.

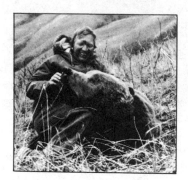

Stephen Bing not only lost 59 pounds with the Diet Center Program, but through rebound exercise, regained the necessary stamina to resume big game hunting.

years before. I had resigned myself to the fact that my trophy room would never have the greatest trophy in North America among its collection, a Kodiak Brown Bear. These bears inhabit an island off the coast of Alaska, bathed in rain or snow almost daily the year around. A hunter has to not only put up with the weather conditions, but has to continually wear hip boots and climb the volcanic mountains daily, covering several miles a day — definitely, not the place for a soft 40-year-old.

One day, I learned that a hunting buddy of mine was about to leave for Kodiak Island. I didn't know if I could lose the weight I had to and get back to good physical condition, but I was going to try. I had heard some good things about Diet Center's Program; one that I could live with, but did it work? I am happy to say in three rather short months I lost 59 pounds.

I then began to exercise on the mini-trampoline and go for long walks in the mountains. Following a year of this program, I can assure you that I was in better shape then when I was in college some 20 years ago. With the loss of weight, my pulse and blood pressure, even under stress, is that of a trained athlete.

Oh yes, I went on that bear hunt and was lucky enough to have taken the largest bear to have come off Kodiak Island in many years.

Stephen Bing
Fort Morgan, Colorado

... Safe and Convenient

The mini-trampolines are small and take up no more space than a living-room chair. They can be tucked under the bed or stood in a corner, out of the way, when not in use. They weigh only a few pounds, and some models fold into a small case that can be taken on trips or carried to and from the office.

The mini-trampoline is constructed of a mat, made of strong material, attached to a steel frame by a unique triangulation of springs, which allows a person to bounce up and down without bottoming out on a hard surface.

Locate the mini-trampoline in a place where it is convenient and accessible. Use it for short periods of time throughout the day, every day. Working people can best benefit from its use by locating it in the bedroom for a quick exercise program before getting ready for work. At night, it can be used during the commercials while watching TV. For more strenuous exercise, a mini-trampoline is excellent for running in place. It is not so jolting to the skeletal system as running. Some joggers prefer to jog on it to rest their bruised feet or a shin splint while still staying in shape.

Diet Center recommends rebounding as one of the finest exercises known to man. Try it!

BEFORE YOU BEGIN

Be sure to get your doctor's advice before you begin any form of exercise. Start out slowly and increase your endurance as your body gains strength. If a mini-trampoline sounds too good to be true, try it for yourself and see why thousands of people are bouncing their way to better health.

MINI-TRAMPOLINE EXERCISES

1. BOUNCE — Gently bounce to warm up, keeping toes forward. Do not bounce too long or too high.
2. PIGEON TOED — Repeat "Bounce" with toes pointed inward.
3. SPREAD FEET BOUNCE — Repeat "Bounce" with toes pointed outward and feet slightly spread.
4. EXTENDED ARMS BOUNCE — Repeat "Bounce" with arms extended (palms upward).

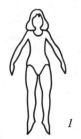 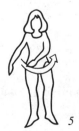 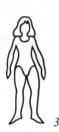 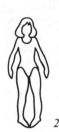

5. TWISTING BOUNCE — Repeat "Bounce" and alternate twisting either direction. Twist only at the waist.
6. EXTENDED ARMS BOUNCE (REVERSE) — Repeat "Bounce" with extended arms, with palms facing down instead of up.
7. BACK BOUNCE — Repeat "Bounce" with arms extended behind your back. Allow your arms to raise and drop as you bounce.
8. RELAX! — Take three minutes to return pulse rate to normal.
9. BOTTOM BOUNCE — Sit on the mini-trampoline and grip sides with your hands. Gently bounce up and down, twisting at waist if desired.

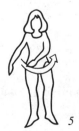 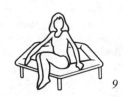 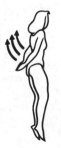 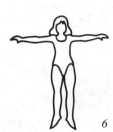

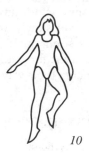

10

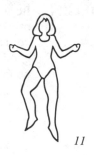

11

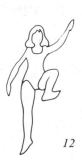

12

10. ONE-FOOT BOUNCE — Repeat "Bounce" on one foot alternating from left to right (two bounces per foot).
11. JOG BOUNCE — Jog in place in the middle of the mini-trampoline, lifting knees to chest.
12. KICK BOUNCE — Repeat "Bounce" thrusting alternate legs forward in a kicking action.

SUGGESTED METHOD: Start slowly, devoting an equal amount of time to each exercise. Then slowly build up speed and duration. For total workout, spend 2½ minutes per each exercise. For additional information on "rebounding" or the DCX mini-trampoline, contact your local Diet Center.

STRETCHING EXERCISES FOR BEGINNERS

Let your arms hang loosely at the side of your body as you stand, or as you sit in a straight-back chair. Now shake your wrists. The easiest way is to rotate the forearms quickly back and forth. Try other side-to-side or back-and-forth shaking motions too.

Raise your knees to a position that is comfortable. Now roll slightly from side to side.

Lie on your back in bed, pointing toes upward. It takes effort, although very slight, to keep them pointing up. Relax this effort. Let them fall to a natural, outward position. Bring them back to a vertical position and let them fall outward again. Keep doing this for two or three minutes, perfecting your ability to let go. Have them fall outward without any help from you.

While lying on the bed on your back, raise your knees against your chest as far as you can without producing pain. Fold your arms across your knees and rock your knees back and forth with the power of your arms pulling on them. Relax, pull, relax, pull . . . you will enjoy this beneficial routine.

Continue this for two or three minutes. Each week, gradually increase this routine until you are doing it steadily for ten minutes. Enjoy this rocking motion every night and every morning.

Sit on a table or other object high enough to permit your feet to hang loosely without touching the floor. Stretch one leg forward. Then let go and let it swing back and forth like a pendulum until it comes to rest. Try not to control the motion. Let it happen. Now do the same with the other leg. Keep doing this for two minutes every hour, increasing to three minutes as improvement is noticed.

A PHYSICAL FITNESS STRETCHING PROGRAM

For those of you who wish to have a regular outline of exercises, this exercise plan contains a chart of ten exercises arranged in progressive order of difficulty. The chart is divided into fifteen sets, numbered from 1 (the least difficult) to 15 (the most difficult). You are to do all ten exercises each day. The number of times you do each exercise increases as you advance to higher sets. Do not skip sets as you progress. You should probably spend at least two days at each set. Move to a new set when you can perform the routine without undue strain. When you have reached your maximum level of performance, about three exercise periods a week should be adequate to maintain this level.

DIET CENTER EXERCISE TABLE

EXERCISE	Set 1	Set 2	Set 3	Set 4	Set 5	Set 6	Set 7	Set 8	Set 9	Set 10	Set 11	Set 12	Set 13	Set 14	Set 15
1. Waist Whittler	5	7	9	9	10	10	11	12	13	14	15	16	17	18	20
2. Bend and Stretch	8	9	10	11	12	13	13	14	15	17	19	21	23	24	25
3. Arm Circles	16	17	18	20	22	24	25	26	27	29	30	31	33	34	35
4. Bent Knee Sit-ups	9	12	15	18	21	24	27	30	32	34	37	40	42	44	46
5. Knee-to-Nose Touch	10	12	14	16	18	21	23	25	27	30	32	34	36	38	40
6. Side Leg Raise	25	28	31	34	37	40	43	46	49	52	53	55	57	59	60
7. Leg Splits	25	27	30	33	35	37	40	43	46	48	51	52	53	54	55
8. Leg Lifts	10	12	13	15	16	17	19	21	23	24	26	27	28	29	30
9. Knee Push-ups	5	8	11	14	17	20	22	24	26	29	31	34	36	38	40
10. Run and Hop	160	170	180	190	200	210	220	230	240	250	260	270	280	290	300

The exercises are illustrated on the following pages.

1. WAIST WHITTLER
   Position: Stand with legs about 4″ apart, raise right arm, left hand on hip.
   Count 1: Bend to the left side, slide left hand down leg as far as possible. Raise body until standing straight again. Bend to the left side.

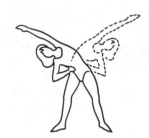

2. BEND AND STRETCH
   (increases flexibility)
   Position: Stand erect, with feet 12″ apart, arm overhead.
   Count 1: Bend trunk forward and down, keeping knees straight. Stretch gently in an attempt to touch your right hand to your left foot then your left hand to your right foot. Return to starting position.

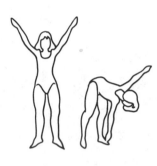

3. ARM CIRCLES
   (firms upper arms and bust)
   Position: Stand with feet about 12 inches apart and arms outstretched.
   Count: Rotate arms in circles, backwards.

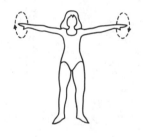

4. BENT KNEE SIT-UPS
   (strengthens abdominal muscles)
   Position: Lie on back with knees bent, hands clasped behind neck.
   Count 1: Sit up; touch right elbow to left knee. Next time touch left elbow to right knee. Return to starting position.

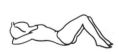

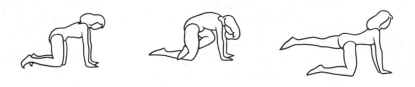

5. KNEE-TO-NOSE TOUCH
   (stretches lower back, strengthens upper back and hip muscles)
   Position: Hands and knees on the floor.
   Count 1: Try to touch nose and knee then extend leg backward parallel with floor while raising head. Do not arch back. Do half of recommended number with each leg.

6. SIDE LEG RAISE
   (strengthens muscles on side of hip and thigh)
   Position: Lying on side.
   Count 1: Raise and lower upper leg as high as you can. Do half of repetitions with left leg; half with right.

7. LEG SPLITS
   (strengthens muscles on insides of thighs)
   Position: Lying on back, raise knees to chest, extend legs until perpendicular to floor.
   Count 1: Slowly lower legs to the sides, raise legs until together again.

8. LEG LIFT
   (strengthens muscles on front of thighs)
   Position: Lying back down, arms at side.
   Count 1: Raise alternate lege perpendicular to floor, left plus right is one count.

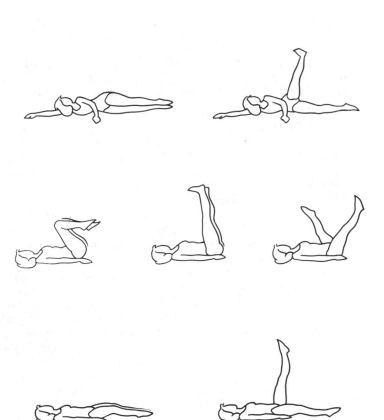

9. KNEE PUSH-UPS
(strengthens arms, shoulders
and chest muscles)
Position: Lie on floor, face
down, legs together; hands
on floor under shoulders,
palms down.
Count 1: Push upper body
off floor until arms are fully
extended and body is in
straight line from head to
knees. Lower until chest
touches the floor.

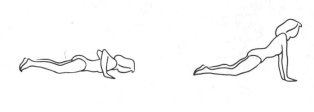

EXERCISE TIPS

Choosing an exercise program is a very personal decision. There is a wide range of options to select from and one will be just right for you and your individual needs. It is something you should plan on doing for the rest of your life, so make sure it is an exercise you can enjoy.

1. Make sure your exercise is an exercise and not just a leisure activity. Be sure you are exercising the major muscles. It is also a good idea to learn exactly what your particular exercise does for your body.
2. It is prudent to have a doctor's approval before embarking an any exercise program.
3. Begin by exercising three times a week and build up your endurance for daily exercise. The actual exercise itself should last about 10 to 15 minutes. Do not worry about the element of time until you have mastered frequency.
4. Plan on exercising at the same time of day every time. If you know that at that specific time you are to exercise, it will be easier to form the habit. As to time of day, the choice is yours. Use morning exercise as a stimulant or evening exercise as a relaxant. Both times work great!
5. Set up some type of record to show your progress. You may even want to attempt keeping a journal of the thoughts you have while exercising. It is a free time to contemplate issues you otherwise do not take time for.
6. Make sure you have the proper equipment and apparel. Your clothing should be loose and comfortable. And because your feet take a lot of abuse in any activity, invest in a good pair of shoes.
7. Never start exercising until you have warmed up your muscles. This is one advantage of exercising at night: your muscles have been partially warmed up from the day's activities. Warming up, if only for a few minutes, will save you from a lot of injuries.
8. To prevent soreness and stiffness, make it a point to do a few minutes of cool-down exercises. However, if either soreness or stiffness does occur, continue to exercise on schedule. Exercise is the best way to loosen those tight and aching muscles.
9. Although it is important to be enthusiastic about your program, *start slowly*. Be aware of your breathing pattern. If you are not able to carry on a conversation while exercising, you are pushing yourself. Never exercise to the point of total breathlessness for the first few weeks.
10. Good posture should always be considered in an exercise program. If you demonstrate correct posture, your body will perform more naturally. Concentrate on slow, smooth movements instead of fast and jerky actions.

10. RUN AND HOP
    (cardiovascular endurance; strengthen heart muscles, legs and hips)
    Position: Standing.
    Count 1: Run in place, lift feet 4″ high, left plus right is one count, after each 50 counts jump up and down 10 times lifting feet 4″ off floor.

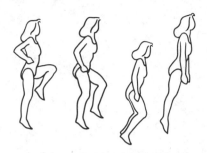

11. Whatever the exercise, stay with others of your same level of ability. This action will prevent you from overdoing or underachieving your capabilities. It will also decrease discouragement.

12. Do not exclude daily opportunities for exercise. Climb the stairs instead of using the elevator, or park the car several blocks from the shopping center. These activities burn up more calories than you might think.

13. Continue your exercise program during your vacation. A rest from work should not result in a break in your exercise program. Impress upon yourself that exercising is one of your daily highlights.

14. Realize that an exercise program is *NOT* an excuse to eat more. Exercising alone is a very ineffective way to lose weight. It does, however, tighten up those sagging muscles while simultaneously helping to control your appetite and occupy your thoughts.

15. Many nutrients may be lost through increased perspiration. Prior to exercise, supply your body with the extra fluid it will need. However, do not overdo it. Large amounts of water can flush vitamins and minerals out of your body, leaving it depleted.

16. Do not worry about increasing your salt intake. True, you are losing more water through perspiration, but unless you have dramatically increased your water intake you will obtain adequate salt from your normal diet.

17. Be sure to keep your body warm after exercise until it returns to normal temperature. Even though it is warm outside, rapid cooling of your body can result in summer colds.

18. Take special precautions with your skin. As your pores open to perspire, your skin becomes a prime candidate for sunburn, dryness, and chapping. Sunscreens and a good moisturizing lotion are a must for your summer exercise kit.

19. Summer activities leave little time for normal meals, but now is when good nutrition is vital. Strenuous exercise and long hours require that the body have a generous supply of essential nutrients.

20. Make it a point to get enough rest. Sleep is the time when your body makes its repairs and readies itself for the next day. Illnesses will be more of a problem if you allow your body to become worn down. And you have got better things to do with your summer than be sick!

21. When you reach a goal in your exercise program, reward yourself. Buy a record album or a new blouse. Never use food as a reward — it is only a temporary reward while other things can be long-lasting.

22. The most helpful tool you have in your exercise program to guide you is your body. Listen to it and learn what it is telling you. Your body is quite accurate in making its needs known. You must appreciate it enough to know how to read the signs.

VIII

MORE STEPS FOR DIETING SUCCESS

By now, you should be able to understand the basic nutritional principles that can aid weight loss while maintaining good health. You should understand the importance of maintaining a stable blood sugar level, eating foods with "staying power," and counting nutrients, not calories. You should also be mentally geared for success after learning the skills of relaxation and visualization. You should be confident that you can succeed and have the skills to do it.

What happens, however, when you run up against a special occasion or special temptation? This section is designed to assist you in overcoming special-problem situations dieters often encounter when traveling, entertaining, and snacking. Some fun ideas are also suggested for cool summer meals and his-'n-her dieting. Once you have learned the basics of dieting, these ideas are easy and fun to try.

1

Low-Fat, Low-Sugar, Low-Cost Entertaining

ENTERTAINING can be exhilarating. Entertaining does not have to be time-consuming, expensive, or fattening. In fact, just the opposite is true! Even with a demanding schedule, you can simplify food preparation so that you can spend quality time with your guests. You should keep one goal in mind for a successful dinner party, buffet, or casual get-together — guests must feel at ease. To achieve this, offer a variety of foods in a relaxed atmosphere. A variety of foods does not have to cost a lot either; you can provide a generous buffet even with a limited budget.

Many guests have specific needs. Some people have health problems that require restrictive diets; some are dieting, others may not be. Offering a variety of foods so your guests can make choices is the secret to successful entertaining. You'll be the "Hostess with the Mostess" when you entertain with the guests in mind.

For example, offer two bowls of punch that are the same color. One punch bowl can be filled with a delicious, festive Diet Center drink made without sugar, and the other one with a beautiful, festive holiday punch. Garnishes, such as fresh strawberries and lime slices, can adorn both bowls. Inform your guests of the difference; but because the punches are the same color, your guests can freely indulge in either without explanation or apology. Both your dieters and many guests who have such health problems as diabetes, hypoglycemia, and heart conditions will appreciate this consideration from any hostess.

Most winter-holiday tables are usually dominated by glazed

hams. Other meat entrées along with ham, such as chicken or fish, could also be served. Offer your guests several choices so those who wish to eat lean meats may do so without drawing attention to themselves. Fish and chicken are both excellent lean meats. Both can be prepared in a variety of ways. Herbs can be used generously as seasonings. Avoid using excess salt in preparation.

Idaho baked potatoes are perennial favorites and very low in calories. While they are very filling, they are truly time-savers, meal-appeasers, and appetite-pleasers! Some guests prefer to saturate their potatoes with the usual sour cream and butter. That is fine; but also offer an alternative of puréed cottage cheese sprinkled with chives and a tiny bit of pepper and Diet Center "Buttery Flavor Salt." It is delicious and you cannot tell the difference! However, rich butters and cream should be avoided. Local corn-on-the-cob is served in season, but so are fresh green beans and spinach from the garden as an alternative for guests on restricted-food diets. A large, crisp five- to seven-vegetable salad is always welcomed by everyone.

Parties, receptions, and even sit-down dinners invariably have beautiful trays of fresh fruits and raw vegetables with low-fat dips. The vegetables are readily eaten in the form of celery fans, radish roses, and cauliflowerettes. These trays, not surprisingly, are the foods that have to be replenished continuously throughout the course of the evening, which is the most sincere sign of appreciation from guests.

For dessert, a tray of fresh fruits, such as red-ripe strawberries, bite-size cantaloupe squares, honeydew melon balls, and small clusters of grapes will suit some guests, while others may want the rich cheese cake to go with it. What makes guests comfortable, however, is having a choice.

In order to maintain a desired weight, or even achieve that weight, you have to be consciously aware of foods without making an issue of it. (In fact, wise dieters never draw attention to the fact that they are dieting.) For example, suppose you are to entertain guests at your home on the lake or when traveling in your recreational vehicle for the weekend. Breakfast is often one of the main meals of the day; however, only serve juice, and, instead, plan on brunch.

I have found that my guests enjoy two meals each day — a brunch at 11 A.M. and a dinner at 7 P.M. For the brunch, serve a selection of breakfast foods, including baked or broiled trout, ham or bacon, scrambled eggs, waffles with a nice selection of fresh raspberries, honeydew melon with lime, cantaloupe, and bananas in sections. In offering a brunch, always make sure there are numerous low-fat, low-sugar choices. Dieters can avoid the ham, bacon, and waffles served with butter and syrup. Instead, they can choose trout, scrambled eggs, and fresh fruit — a wonderful meal, diet or not! Your dieting guest will never feel guilty because every person's plates will look so appetizing!

Another secret of effective entertaining is to never let it become a hassle. Even a large party, social gathering, or dinner does not have to overwhelm you. Time is important to everyone, so use it wisely! Not only does preparing beforehand make the actual event more relaxed and enjoyable for the hostess, but trying to do everything on the day of the party sets up tempting situations: skipping scheduled eating because you haven't got the time, then snacking and "test-tasting" . . . Here are some hints that make the difference in entertaining:

- Shop two days before the party.
- Prepare as many foods as possible ahead of time. Clean fruits and vegetables. Put them in air-tight plastic bags or containers a day or two before the party, so they will be crisp and ready at a moment's notice.
- The day before your party, prepare the main course so it is ready to go into the oven or on the grill. Favorites at most gatherings, such as baked beans, potato salads, or casseroles, are much better if allowed to refrigerate for twenty-four hours to allow flavors to permeate. The same holds true for a drink base.
- Be sure to plan a beautiful seven-variety vegetable salad, fresh and crisp, to be served along with a beautiful big tray of freshly cleaned vegetables.
- Set tables or the buffet serving area with glasses, silverware, and napkins the day before the party if small children (or pets) are not a problem. Remember, *always* "deep clean" at least two days before you are to entertain. A week before your party, begin to "deep clean" one room every day (an effective way to keep your house clean even if not entertaining!); and the task becomes fun, challenging, and satisfying. Make it easy on yourself. Do not tire yourself the day of the party. Remain rested so you can enjoy every moment with your guests.
- Do not entertain merely to impress people or because it is your turn. Entertain to spend some quality time with your family, friends, and associates. DO IT RIGHT! Doing it right does not require a lot of time or money. Just remember, doing it wrong requires the same effort.

• Fats, sugar, and salt are the major culprits in obesity and undermining health. Cut them out of your dishes so your guests may eat without guilt. Fats and salts can be slashed from foods in numerous ways. It is also prudent to cut out sugar whenever possible. However, some guests may want rich desserts to finish a meal, so again, provide choices.

Holiday time brings an overabundance of rich foods. Holiday candies, fruitcakes, and plum puddings usually adorn every holiday table — and still can appear on yours. Just offer numerous, delicious low-fat, low-sugar choices, so everyone, regardless of diet, will be able to eat and fully enjoy themselves.

Entertaining can also be very costly, an important consideration if you are on a limited budget; but there are numerous ways to cut expenses. Chicken is a low-cost meat that can be prepared simply or "deluxed." Boneless chicken breasts are one of the best meat buys and are a favorite because they have ample low-fat meat. Whole chickens can cost just as much as breasts because, with whole chickens, you pay for the bones and refuse. Chicken breasts can be broiled, stuffed, baked, or slow-cooked.

Egg dishes, such as quiches, omelets, and soufflés, are also low-cost favorites. Crepes are another egg speciality: they're simple to prepare and yet just cost pennies to serve. Crepe fillings can be anything in the meat, fruit, or vegetable department. You can add expensive or inexpensive fillers, from crab to strawberries to cole slaw, and still come out a winner. Crepes can also be served as a main course, salad addition, or luscious dessert. Crepes are a marvelous, versatile food.

Salad buffets are also good choices, for very little meat is required; and because meat can consume most of your entertaining budget, costs are minimal. Chicken or shrimp salads work well for meat additions; then potato salads, tossed salads, or cole slaw can be added. Good desserts are fresh fruits and molded gelatins. Whole-grain crackers and bran muffins are perfect additions. The result? Good entertaining with a minimum of cost!

There are some households where cost factors are not a consideration. However, keep in mind that most expensive foods are also usually loaded with excessive fats and sugars. Entertaining, regardless of how extravagant, should leave guests satisfied rather than uncomfortable. High-fat, high-sugared foods can leave you with indigestion, headaches, and a lethargic feeling. Variety, again, is the key, so learn to cut unnecessary fats and sugars out of foods whenever possible and also to offer alternate low-fat, low-sugar choices.

Good substitutes for fats and refined sugars are a little honey or crushed fruit with no-calorie sweetener in place of

TIPS FOR DIETING WHILE ENTERTAINING (OR BEING ENTERTAINED)

1. Remember that you and only you are in control of your life. Make a commitment before going to the party. Each time you successfully deal with a difficult eating situation, you gain more willpower, feel more confident, and become more self-assured.
2. Never go to a dinner party on an empty stomach. One-half hour before leaving, eat a large apple and drink a glass of water. You will not be ravenous, and you will be in control of the situation.
3. When invited to a home, you may want to call ahead and explain your situation. Ask if you can bring a large shrimp salad. Not only will you be able to eat without guilt, but other guests can too!
4. If a hostess puts pressure on you to eat her specialty, stand your ground with a compliment: "Not even your good cooking, June, can tempt me off my diet."
5. People seldom notice what you are eating (or not eating) if you do not draw attention to the fact that you are dieting.
6. We hope most holiday entertainers will offer a selection of foods that a dieter can have. KEEP IN MIND THAT THE PURPOSE OF GETTING TOGETHER WITH FRIENDS AND FAMILY IS TO ENJOY ONE ANOTHER'S COMPANY AND HAVE A GOOD TIME. EATING DOES NOT HAVE TO BE THE MAIN EVENT.
7. If high-fat foods are served, such as fried chicken, choose a breast. Lift up the skin and eat only the white meat.
8. If the foods in the meal are rich and full of sugars or creams, take a small portion and leave it on your plate. NO ONE WILL NOTICE. (If you ate an apple before coming, you will feel satisfied, and not crave sweets. You will not feel sorry for yourself for missing rich desserts!)
9. Remember, every day you stay on your diet brings you closer to good health and your weight goal.
10. Eating a balance of foods (lean meats with raw fruits and vegetables) will satisfy you longer because they digest more slowly.
11. If you are at a cocktail party, drink water or ice water with a twist of lime. Alcohol can set a dieter back three days. DO NOT DRINK ALCOHOL WHEN SERIOUSLY DIETING! If you do drink alcohol while on maintenance, do so in moderation.
12. Do not eat a food just because it is on your plate. If it is not on your diet, *do not eat it!* Let your hostess (or waitress) take away your plate. If necessary, explain you have a medical problem and just "cannot seem to eat a thing."
13. When eating out at a restaurant, always order the food exactly as you wish it to be prepared. Order all dressings on the side — use only one teaspoonful. (Allow a taste.) Order dressings of sour cream and butter for your Idaho potato on the side, not on top!
14. Act happy. Do not act as if resisting all the temptations is killing you.
15. Never finish a meal in less than twenty minutes.
16. Many hostesses who are famous for their cooking are overweight. Keep that in mind if they try to tempt you — it will help you stay on your diet.
17. If you are eating a seafood buffet and you are going to splurge, indulge yourself with crab, shrimp, and lobster; avoid the clam chowders, Newburg dishes, and others with rich sauces.
18. At a seafood buffet, squeeze lemon juice over your seafood. If you must have a sauce or dip, choose cocktail sauce, which is usually ketchup and horseradish, rather than the rich mayonnaise dips. Diet

sugar (sucrose). Tofu, skim milk, yogurt, and blended low-fat cottage cheese or buttermilk can replace rich creams in dressings and dips for fresh fruits and vegetables.

Entertaining should be relaxing and satisfying. Entertaining can be fun if you go about it with the right approach. Try

Center "buttery flavor salt" mixed with oil (polyunsaturated) is delicious on crab, lobster, shrimp, and fish.

19. Relax before the party — take a rest! It will fortify your self-control. When people are nervous, tired, and uptight, they feel as if they are hungry.

20. If you hear negative voices (imagined or real) telling you that an extra piece will not hurt, do not believe them. You, and you alone, are responsible for your own health.

21. Do not starve all day to indulge at night; most dieters do. If no food has been eaten, the blood sugar level drops, you crave sweets and completely lose control.

22. If pressed, let people know you have made a commitment to diet.

23. Eat slowly. Set down your knife, fork, and spoon frequently. Relax. Have a good time!

24. Cut your food in tiny bite-size pieces and chew it thoroughly.

25. Avoid excessive amounts of caffeine-filled beverages. They lift and then drop your blood sugar, invariably making your nervous, thus causing hunger.

26. Remember that most foods are tasted for only *three seconds,* then swallowed and are gone. Remember to choose foods with "staying power" so you will be satisfied.

27. Do not salt foods. Salt is an acquired taste. The more salt you eat, the more you want! Be aware that an additional ¼ teaspoon of salt equals ½ pound of water being retained by the body.

28. "Nibble" at your food and "linger" with your drink.

29. Avoid foods with sauces. Sauces are often rich in butter, sugar, and flour.

30. During the course of the evening, sip on ice water. No one will care, and you will be in control.

31. Remember that success comes when you can look beyond food.

32. Mentally prepare yourself before the party through relaxation and visualization. Visualize yourself in control. Your attitude makes all the difference. Be determined and confident when you say, "No, thank you."

33. Remember that the first, illegal bite can lead to dieting failure.

34. Carry a low-cal drink as a means of refusing food. "I have something, thank you."

35. If snack plates are served while you are standing, just nibble on a crisp vegetable. Avoid dips. Select a cracker. (Remember, no more than two!) You are the only one who knows how many you have had. Be responsible to yourself. Do not make a meal of crackers.

36. When going out, never use the word "try." *Try* implies failure. Use "will" instead: "I will stay on my diet. I will be thin and attractive."

37. When assisting with food preparation, chew sugarless gum through the entire preparation so tasting will not tempt you.

38. "Apple pie is just not one of my weaknesses" can easily turn an insistent hostess away without offense. A hostess will rarely force a food on you that you dislike.

39. Bring some "legal" nibbles with you, in case none are available. Do not mention them, just eat them if necessary.

40. If you feel that your diet will be sabotaged, call the hostess in advance and tell her that for health reasons (obesity threatens health), you must adhere to your diet.

41. Remember, a wise hostess will not be offended if you graciously decline foods.

it often. Be sure, however, to take the time and hassle out of entertaining and just enjoy! Be prepared.

Ready for a quiz? Try these situations and learn even more about dieting!

The First Eating-Out Area: At a Friend's Home

A home-cooked meal at a friend's home is the very hardest type of food to resist. Did you skip breakfast and lunch so when you ate the meal you could eat and not gain weight? How did you feel when you reached the table? Were you ravenously hungry? Did you eat all you wanted, thinking you had nobly skipped food all day so you could enjoy this beautiful dinner?

How many of you have had this experience?

Now that you have learned Diet Center's Nutrition/Behavior Modification principles and have learned about the body and how it functions, what do you think you should do to prepare for a home-cooked dinner party?

Answer: Eat all of your meals as you normally would on a schedule.

Q. The dinner is for 8:30, later than you usually eat, and you may not actually eat until 9:30.

A. Just before you leave your home, eat an apple and have an eight-ounce drink.

Q. Why would you eat normally during the day and have an apple just before you leave home?

A. You eat on schedule to keep the blood sugar at a normal level. If the body has had no nourishment, you crave goodies and you become ravenous. You eat everything and cannot resist a thing! You are literally out of control!

Q. Why would you eat an apple?

A. The apple has good bulk and fills you comfortably. When dinner is served, you can resist anything you wish and enjoy small portions of the dinner. You no longer feel persecuted. You can eat sensibly and usually you will not gain. Now, you are in total control.

Q. What do you do if you do gain weight the next morning?

A. Continue to weigh each day. If you are up in your weight, take it off immediately.

The Second Eating-Out Area: Home Card Parties

Q. You are invited to a friend's for an evening of cards. You know there will be candy, nuts, drinks, and desserts served. How are you going to handle this situation?

A. Call in advance and ask the hostess if you can bring a plate of deviled eggs, stuffed celery, carrot strips, onions, peppers, pickles, and a six-pack of diet drinks. Any hostess will be glad to have you bring the offering.

The Third Eating-Out Area: Holidays

Q. You always put on five pounds during the holidays. How can you handle it this year?

A. Eat on schedule. While preparing food, eat an apple and have a large drink of water. Now, I know what you are thinking — *"unheard of!"* — but, haven't you said to your children, "Don't eat before dinner; it will spoil your appetite"? Well, you were right. You will enjoy your meal, but *you* are in control, not your stomach. This year, you won't gain those five pounds, and it won't take you weeks to lose them.

How to Enjoy Your Vacation Without Forgetting Your Diet!

VACATIONS and trips usually spell disaster for anyone on a diet. Greasy fried foods, sugary snacks, and inactivity can all combine to threaten your hard-earned dieting success. However, additional self-discipline, combined with conscientious planning and preparation, will make your trip a success — both travel-wise and diet-wise!

Success is a result of PLANNING. Treat your diet like your wardrobe. How many hours do you spend deciding what clothes to pack or what shoes to wear? Staying on a diet requires the same planning and effort that packing your clothes does. You need to follow the same steps: deciding where to go, what you will need, making a list, purchasing necessary items, packing carefully, and checking everything over before you leave.

MOTIVATIONS

Diet Center recommends that you follow this same strategy when it comes to dieting while traveling. First, you need to set your expectations. For most overweight people, it is a lucky experience not to return from a vacation ten pounds heavier. Once you have made the decision to enjoy your vacation to the fullest and have combined this decision with the knowledge of how to diet, you need never gain weight on a vacation again. Whether it be the romance of a cruise ship or exotic Hawaii, you can enjoy the finest cuisine and never gain an ounce! It does take planning and self-discipline, but the secret again is preparation and eating on time. Remember, you are in control.

The first step is to set a goal. Follow these suggestions:

1. Set your goal. Yes, you can go for two full weeks and absolutely maintain your beautiful new weight or successful weight loss. Remember, you are slender, slim, and beautiful. You will stay that way!
2. Print your goal — "I will weigh _____ pounds when I return" — across the middle of several index cards.
3. Put these index cards in highly visible spots where you will see them several times a day. (Try your makeup mirror, car visor, or shampoo bottle. Slip one in your wallet. Put one in your pocket so each time you touch the card, you will remember.)
4. Each morning when you get up, stand in front of the mirror and repeat your goal, out loud, *ten* times.
5. Whenever tempted by foods not on your diet, touch your goal card in your pocket. Repeat your goal to yourself ten times to build up incentive!

Now that your motivation is geared high, work on those details: How long will you be gone? How are you going to travel? Will there be a selection of foods you need? What do you have to bring along?

You will also need to visualize yourself. See your new slender body. See yourself at the pool in your swimsuit. Watch yourself dance in a lovely new dress. Feel it cling to your body. Enjoy the thrill and excitement of what you are and the new freedom you are experiencing. Visualize yourself in every detail. Know that health and happiness are of utmost importance in your life. You are in control. You are truly beautiful.

EXERCISE

Second, take a look at your activity level. Hopefully, *by now* you have developed your own exercise program to go along with your diet (see pages 209–223). What happens, though, when you sit for six hours in a car or airplane? By the time you reach your destination, you hardly feel like swimming laps or jogging a mile. This is the time, however, when your body needs exercise the most. A lack of exercise, combined with insufficient water, will make your entire body feel sluggish and heavy, and cause constipation.

When driving, Diet Center suggests you stop as often as possible to stretch and move around. Pull over at waysides or scenic views to take a brisk, five-minute walk. Take along a jump rope to use each night (five minutes of jumping is equivalent to one mile of jogging).

Do not forget those basic rules to get more exercise in your life every day! Do not allow your vacation to become an excuse for not exercising. Use your extra time to the fullest!

TRAVELING BY CAR

If you plan to travel by car, your first battle will be to fight off the "car munchies." Eating is one of the easiest solutions to the boredom of traveling. Have you ever stopped to consider the number of calories you consume while sitting in a car? There are plenty of foods that can satisfy both the "munchies" and the "crunchies," while keeping you slim and trim. At all costs, keep those salty, sugary, fried foods out of the car! "Out of sight" really does mean "out of mind"! However, even if others in the car are eating "junk foods," be sure you have your own fruit and diet drinks. You will feel satisfied and not deprived.

Diet Center recommends you snack on foods with "staying power." Recommended snacks include hard-boiled eggs, apples, oranges, grapefruits, celery and cauliflowerettes, and whole-grain crackers. You can even bring baked chicken breast.

Be sure to refrigerate all perishable foods in a cooler to prevent spoilage. Also, make sure you bring along plenty of extras. Everyone in the car will want to have some of these delicious snacks.

RESTAURANTS

Eating out? That's no excuse to abandon your diet. Build that resolve. Make a specific goal just for that night! Promise yourself a reward (perfume or a scarf — not food) if you accomplish it!

Follow these eleven Diet Center suggestions for dieting while dining out.

1. PREPARATION IS THE KEY . . . Whether you will be dining out your entire vacation or for just one night, you will need to prepare. The worst thing you can do is to skip meals or not eat until dinner. By the time you get to the restaurant, you will either be faint with hunger or so ravenous you will eat anything and everything!

If you plan to eat at a much later hour than usual, nibble on a large apple and sip a glass of water shortly before leaving for the restaurant. The fiber and fructose in the apple will fire up your willpower and the water will prevent a famished, empty feeling.

2. COCKTAILS ANYONE? Your first hurdle may be resisting predinner cocktails and the hors d'oeuvres. Alcohol is a disaster to your diet — it is full of empty calories that will neither satisfy nor provide nutritional benefits. Liquor goes right into the bloodstream. People gain weight when they drink. Order a glass of ice water with a slice of lemon or sugar-free tonic water. Or try a diet soda. Sip these drinks slowly. No one will feel uncomfortable because you are not drinking.

Stay as far away from the hors d'oeuvres plate and dishes of candy and nuts as you can! If fresh vegetables are available, snack on them. Otherwise, just TALK.

3. YOUR BEST BET ... Do you get to make the choice of where to go? Steak houses are generally the easiest places to find the foods you want. Most restaurants have a salad bar. Beware of places that serve only ethnic foods (e.g., Italian, Mexican, Greek, or German), for their selection often is not extensive. The food is usually rich in sauces, gravies, pastas, or is fried, making it very difficult to maintain weight and impossible to stay with your diet.

Select a restaurant that offers you the options of a salad bar, fresh fish, seafood, chicken, or steak.

4. "I WOULD LIKE" ... You cannot eat what you do not order. Concentrate on fresh crab, shrimp, or lobster salads prepared to your specifications. Any fresh fish is perfect. Order only lean meats that have been baked, broiled, steamed, or grilled. NEVER EAT DEEP-FAT FRIED FOODS OR FOODS WITH SAUCES! If ordering beef, make sure that it is well done. Always order a dinner salad or the salad bar.

Quickly glance at the menu. It helps if you decide ahead of time what you would like. The less you look, the fewer the temptations. Also, jump in and order first. It will be almost impossible to order fresh fish after everyone else has ordered lasagna.

5. "MAY I HAVE" ... Be assertive when you order. Ask for fish broiled in lemon without butter. Make sure your omelets are prepared without butter or milk. Request that croutons and rich dressings be omitted from your dinner salad.

6. SALAD BARS ... While these offer a good selection of vegetables, too much comes much too easily! Stay away from

prepared salads with macaroni, or whipped cream. Avoid vegetables that have been marinated in both vinegar and sugar. Many vegetables prepared in restaurants have sugar added. Avoid sauces.

7. SALAD DRESSINGS . . . Blue Cheese and Thousand Island can be especially deceiving. They are full of sugar. You may end up with more calories from the dressing than the entire meal others are eating. Oil and vinegar is your best bet.

8. For a vegetable alternative, order an Idaho baked potato. They are very filling. If you are maintaining your weight, you may use ½ pat of butter and 1 teaspoonful of sour cream. You will not gain, but you will feel very full.

9. AND FOR DESSERT . . . Do not destroy all your work with a rich dessert. Your dessert does not have to be filled with sugar, cream, and butter to be good. A bowl of fresh fruit is just as satisfying, both to your palate and waistline.

10. WHEN DINING OUT . . . Just simply state: "I have a health problem, and it is necessary for me to eat this." When the issue is health, people become amazingly sympathetic.

Try not to draw too much attention to what you are eating. Praise yourself mentally. Do not think of having to resist temptation throughout the meal. It is amazing but true, that when you think of your new body and unbelievable happiness, you will not feel persecuted while resisting foods. Eventually, you will actually prefer salads and chicken rather than rich foods drenched in sauces.

11. TALK, TALK, TALK . . . We have all been told not to talk with a full mouth, so instead of eating, TALK! Switch the focus of the dinner from eating to socializing. You will be surprised at how much gets left on your plate. Don't feel guilty if you leave some of your food on the plate. Don't worry about wasting food — at least it won't be wasted on your own waist!

TRAVELING BY PLANE

Most airlines will now serve you a high-protein, low-fat meal upon request. (These meals are often better than the usual fare.) Be sure, however, when making your reservation that you find out exactly when your request is due. Some airlines need it immediately; others, only twenty-four hours before flight time.

All airlines now furnish diet sodas and juices as well as

sodas with sugar or alcoholic beverages. Take along an apple or some celery sticks to munch on instead of nuts or candy.

VACATIONERS ON *STABILIZATION* DIET: SUGGESTED MENU FOR RESTAURANT DINING

Eat all of the eggs, lean meat and cottage cheese that you want. Do not go hungry. Do not stuff. (For additional information, see the Diet Center Stabilization Diet, on pages 139–149.)

BREAKFAST

Choice of eggs:
  2 scrambled
  2 poached
  2-egg omelet
Choice of:
  ½ cantaloupe
  ½ grapefruit
  1 bowl strawberries
Water

LUNCH

Try to eat fish meal at noon
  Crab salad
  Tuna salad
  Shrimp salad
  Poached fish (any type — no sauce)
Chef salad (oil and vinegar dressing)
Dinner salad and choice of: Green beans, carrots, tomatoes, broccoli or brussels sprouts (no sauce)
Water

DINNER

Lean beef, any type (well-done)
Chicken (no sauce)
Fish
Cottage cheese
Baked potato
Any Reducing or Stabilization vegetable (no sauce or butter)
Dinner salad
Water

ADDITIONAL FOODS
One fruit a day allowed, such as: fresh strawberries, cantaloupe, honeydew, apple, orange, or ½ grapefruit. You may also have cottage cheese, a small salad, boiled egg and a moderate amount of raw, fresh vegetables as a snack. Eight glasses of water is a must.

TRAVELING BY CRUISE SHIP

A cruise on a luxury liner is the ultimate vacation. The dream of all dreams. Unfortunately, it can be a disaster for anyone who is trying to control his or her weight. It took me three cruises finally to learn how to eat and not gain weight while vacationing on a cruise ship. When I finally learned, I was thrilled. You can enjoy the finer things in life — romance, exotic moonlight, sun, clothes, and food. You do not have to gain weight. Do not plan to diet while on this type of vacation, but do plan on maintaining the same weight at which you started. True, it is a time to dance, stay up late and party, eat, drink, and play, love and laugh, and not a time to think about dieting. It is a rare person who can come back at the same weight as when he left, because cruises are designed for the enjoyment of everything, especially food. They offer five-course breakfasts, three-course lunches, and seven-course dinners. They have a midnight snack of French pastry and delicious desserts. Every few hours, you can find the most delicious, full-course meals that you have ever been served.

The secret to maintaining your weight on a cruise ship is keeping your blood sugar level stable by eating on time. Eat the correct foods and you will stay in control and not become hungry.

Do not forget to visualize how much better you will feel if you do not gain additional weight during this trip!

Plan ahead. Set a schedule such as the one I tried. It worked well for me!

1. Ask for fresh fruits to be sent to your cabin. You will usually receive a basket with apples, oranges, pears, and bananas.
2. Plan to suntan at the pool in the mornings. Eat your fruit and drink water before you leave your room. You may also want to take several pieces of fruit with you.
3. All ships set up a beautiful salad bar with cold cuts at the poolside. It is a lovely cold buffet where people can build their own sandwiches and salads. It is truly made for dieters! Make a large salad with thin slices of beef, boiled eggs, fresh fruits. Have a large glass of tomato juice with a twist of lemon.
4. In the afternoon, have a large, cool diet drink.
5. As evening meals are set up for a specific time, try to get the early dinner schedule. You will not be as hungry and can remain in control. If you cannot, eat an apple about half an hour before you are scheduled to dine. Drink a glass of water before you go to eat.
6. Waiters on cruise ships are taught to feed you well. They expect you to eat and eat and eat. (I am sure they wonder

where people put it all!) It is important that you enjoy this trip of a lifetime, but do so carefully. Eat slowly and enjoy the conversation. Eat only until satisfied. Let the rest of the food stay on your plate. Taste the dessert, but stay in control; leave most of it on your plate. Dance until dawn, sleep as late as you wish, pamper yourself by wearing your new clothes, learn how to dance the latest steps, relax in the sun, but VISUALIZE! Think about your new body, enjoy the freedom of your new slimness, love yourself!

Don't make food your vacation. Manage your life. Eat to live. Don't live to eat.

DIETING AND TRAVEL CAN BE DONE TOGETHER! You can do it by setting your mind to it. Do not allow traveling to destroy your diet.

Think positively by setting a goal and devising a plan. THEN FOLLOW IT! Your self-esteem will rise with every small success, while the number on the bathroom scale falls!

HINTS FOR TRAVELING AND EATING OUT

- Do plan ahead when eating out.
- Do eat an apple before leaving the house.
- When traveling, take a bag of fruit with you.
- Do eat on a schedule.
- Do order salad and diet soda or water at quick-order places when others order high-caloric snacks.
- Do take a plate of snack foods that you can eat to a party.
- Take a tape measure on your trip.
- Do exercise on your trip.
- Do drink your water.
- Do eat wisely on a vacation.
- Do put on your own salad dressings when eating at restaurants.
- Do be on a good nutrition program for the rest of your life.
- Do eat an apple and have an eight-ounce diet drink before you go out to eat; don't go to the restaurant ravenous.
- Do not skip breakfast or lunch. Eat fruit in the morning, as well as for snacks.
- Do not have drinks with sugar.
- Do eat only what is good for you.
- Do not let yourself get too hungry.
- Do not "let yourself go" on vacation. Be in total control.
- Do not overeat two days in a row.

3

Cool Summer Meals

SUMMER means a whole new way of living! Whether it is walking, swimming, biking, tennis, fishing, hiking, golfing, boating, baseball, or tennis, you're on the go! It also means tanning, reading, and just being lazy, if you wish. Meals are not always on schedule and are often eaten on the run.

While all this activity is great, it plays havoc in obtaining the proper nutrients for your body. Snacks and meals-on-the-go often mean quick trips to fast-food restaurants or stops at the nearest vending machine.

OUT OF THE KITCHEN!

Trying to provide nutritious meals for yourself or for your family can be a very frustrating experience — especially if it means preparing a lot of meals at different times. Organize your time in the kitchen so that you allow convenience for your family and some spare time for yourself. The key is organization. When you prepare salads, fresh vegetables and fruits ahead of time, it takes away much of the hassle.

Summer meals should be light and refreshing, yet easy to prepare. Broiled meats, colorful salads, and fresh fruits combine for a fully satisfying meal.

SALADS — LET THEM WORK FOR YOU!

A salad can be the most versatile part of any meal. Used as either a main course or as an accompaniment, salads are always in demand.

Salads are easily prepared and stored ahead of time. Fresh produce should always be kept in the refrigerator. You can cut nutrient loss in half by storing produce in a refrigerator crisper that is 20 to 30 degrees below room temperature.

Remember, the fresher a fruit or vegetable, the more nutrients it contains. Be careful in handling and storage, as exposure to air or high heat can drastically reduce the nutritional levels.

While putting away groceries on shopping day, follow these hints for creating "instant salads."

1. Tear up a head of lettuce and store in a large, zip-lock storage bag. Use several types of lettuce (e.g., bib, Boston, leaf, or endive) for different flavors and texture. Add shredded red cabbage for additional color and zest!

2. Shop your produce section carefully for good fruit and vegetable buys (see "Produce Hints," pages 70, 72). Slice cucumbers, celery, zucchini, okra, mushrooms, cauliflower, radishes, green peppers and onions. Store each vegetable in a small, air-tight zip-lock bag to prevent certain vegetables from overpowering the others. Make especially sure that the onion and green pepper slices are in air-tight bags.

3. Keep the rinds or skins on produce whenever possible. The nutrients collect next to the skin or rind and cutting off these parts usually means eliminating them.

4. Sprouts of any variety produce a crunchy topping to any salad. Either keep a supply in the refrigerator or grow your own!

5. Dice chicken breasts, hard-boiled eggs, or tofu. Keep cans of crabmeat or shrimp on hand for the best sources of protein for your salads.

6. Diced fruits provide an extra sweetness and added "crunch" to your fruit salad. Try apple, peach, or honeydew melon cubes. Fruits generally do not last as long as vegetables, so you may want to prepare smaller amounts. Squeeze lemon juice over fruits to prevent browning. Let the natural fruit juices serve as their own dressing. It is delicious and refreshing.

7. Mix up several types of the Diet Center low-calorie dressings. Keep them on hand! (See pages 329–330.)

Presto! A nutritious make-your-own salad bar no farther than your refrigerator door, designed to keep you slim and trim. You should note that all the vegetables are fresh and filling. All the hidden fat-laden, salt-laden, and sugar-laden extras have been omitted! If commercial dressing is used on the Maintenance Diet, just use enough to taste (2 teaspoonfuls). If you are dieting, remember: the simpler, the better!

Do not destroy the potential of a slimming salad with rich dressings! You can actually do more damage with a ladle full of rich dressing than all the vegetables it covers.

Make up several types of dressings in large quantities. Keep them on hand in the refrigerator for dressings or dips.

Diet Center suggests these recipes for low-sugar, low-fat dressings — a perfect complement to your salad — Diet Center French Dressing and Tofu Dressing and Vegetable Dip (both recipes are in the recipe section at the end of this book).

Not only will your fresh veggies be popular "salad fixin's," but they are handy snacks to anyone on the go! Make a large tray, using a wide variety of fruits and vegetables. For nondieters, use pickles, cheese and crackers. Use the Diet Center Dip recipe (page 330). Everyone will enjoy it.

"MEATING THE PROTEINS"

Summer meals easily become dieting meals when you carefully watch protein sources (meat) and how you prepare them. It is important to remember that meat doesn't mean just "beef," but includes chicken, eggs, fish, and shellfish.

Many proteins are much lower in fats and calories than you may think. The difference comes in how you prepare and serve them! Take advantage of the airy, carefree feeling of summer and enjoy eating out-of-doors. Use your barbecue or oven broiler. In the hot weather, you will enjoy light meals.

Use chicken, fish, eggs, and tofu as protein sources for dieters. Nondieters may enjoy barbecued beef or ribs. Shop your local market for specials on chicken and fresh fish. Make up extra portions and store in the refrigerator or freezer. Extra cooked fish flaked into salads provides a "seafood" flavor!

Simmer meats in their own juices or use fat-free sauces, such as a combination of lemon juice, water, and herbs. Marinate chicken or fish overnight in soy sauce (low-salt) or apple cider vinegar for a zesty new taste!

1. Use your outdoor barbecue to "grill" down that waistline. Try fish or chicken. Broiled meats are delicious, low-calorie, and trouble-free. Everything is juicy and very good. At the last minute, try broiling zucchini cut up in length-wise strips until tender. For nondieters, wrap up the French bread in foil and put it in the broiler.
2. Broiling is another calorie-cutting cooking method. If foods appear to lack moisture, brush with soy sauce, lemon, or orange juice while cooking.

3. Instead of frying fish in oil, try poaching in a small amount of water. Fish is done when it flakes. (Chicken is done when it loses its translucency.) Use the remaining liquids when done as a sauce for your vegetables.

4. A good substitute for hamburger is beef heart. Not only is it more economical, but when ground, it tastes even better! Your local butcher or meat department at the grocery store will trim and grind a beef heart for your diet. Just mix ground beef heart, an egg, soy sauce, and some crushed whole-grain crackers. Form into patties for a real tasty treat! Your entire family will enjoy this inexpensive cut of meat.

FORTIFY YOUR DIET WITH FRUIT!

Fruits are a delicious source of vitamins, minerals, and fiber. Easy to obtain and found in a wide variety, fruits may offer a solution to that unconquerable sweet tooth.

Fruits help your diet in a number of ways, some of which you are probably not even aware! First, citrus fruits are excellent sources of vitamins C and A. Second, the sugar in fruits (known as "fructose") can satisfy even the most insistent sweet tooth. In fact, fructose is actually more sweetening (drop per drop) than table sugar. Third, fruits have "staying power" because of their ample fiber content. The fiber in an apple takes many times longer to digest than the instantly dissolved sugars in a candy bar. It is wonderful to realize that when fruit is eaten, you don't feel persecuted. While on the Reducing Diet, eat only two fruits. When you reach weight goal, you can eat three to five fruits, if you desire, and will still maintain your weight.

If all these reasons aren't incentive enough for including fresh fruits in your diet, how about the fact that fruits can improve your overall health. Daily intake of fresh fruits will help your digestion and elimination system run more smoothly; your jaws will stay healthy from all the chewing; your skin will remain clearer; and you will get fewer cavities!

- Choose firm fruits — neither underripe nor overripe. Overripe fruits become too high in natural sugars.
- Take advantage of specials at your grocery store. Or for some added fun, choose your own produce from truck farmers or a local farmers' market.
- You can save money from your grocery budget by switching from sodas, candy, and snacks to fresh fruit and fresh fruit juices.

- Wash your fruits quickly to remove dirt and chemicals. Never soak fruits in water; it removes vital nutrients. Leave the skins (or if you must remove, pare as thinly as possible) to receive all the nutrients fruit can offer.
- Never thaw frozen vegetables and fruits before cooking.
- Buy real fruit juices or squeeze your own from fresh fruit. Check the labels of many frozen juices, and you will find that the main ingredients are often water and sugar. There is no better "saving" than improving your health.
- Try different varieties of familiar fruits (like yellow instead of red tomatoes) or fruits you may have never tried before (pomegranates).
- When preparing your fruits, cut them into small slices or sections. The more, the better! Arrange them attractively on a small plate. YOUR MIND WILL SEE A LARGER AMOUNT THAN IT WOULD IF YOU JUST BIT INTO A WHOLE APPLE.
- Chew slowly. Take time between slices. Eat half at one sitting and finish the rest later when you want a quick energy boost. An apple should take up to twenty minutes to eat. This allows time for you to digest the food and time to satisfy your hunger.
- Do not just use fruits as snacks. A plate of sliced fruits makes an attractive dessert. Fruit combined with chicken or shrimp makes an unusual, but delicious, main course. Do not forget, you can cook your fruits as well as eat them raw. When barbecuing on the grill, wrap apples in tin foil and let them bake slowly over the coals.
- No other food is so easily prepared and so refreshing as fruit. Use fruit to its fullest this summer!

- PREPARATION is the key to losing weight.
- Do not let yourself become frustrated.
- Plan and prepare foods ahead of time.
- Organize the makings for a salad, prepare meats for broilers, and keep extra fruit on hand. There is no need to resort to anything other than what your diet requires when it is no farther away then your refrigerator!
- Make up your mind to do it. Plan out what you need. Shop for the best buys.
- Make sure that you have fresh fruits and vegetables on hand at all times.
- Prepare your foods in the most nutritious way possible and PRESTO! You will reach your weight-loss goal with a minimum amount of effort and time.

For Exciting Cool Summer meal recipes from Diet Center, see the Diet Center Recipes. We especially recommend trying:

Seafood Salad (page 328)
Shrimp and Egg Salad (page 329)
Shrimp and Egg Salad Dressing (page 329)

4

Snack Your Way to Better Health!

THE end of the schoolday brings home an onslaught of activity, a raid on the refrigerator, and the inevitable question, "Mom, what is there to eat?" Snacking is an important habit for growing children. Caloric and nutritive demands cannot be met with three basic meals. In fact, it has been estimated that 25 percent of daily caloric intake for most children comes from snacking.

Snacking is also a very important part of eating. With our hectic life-styles, meals are often skipped, and we rely on snacks to provide the nutrients and energy we need.

It is a common misconception that all between-meal snacking is bad for you. As a child, you were warned that it would "spoil your appetite" and "ruin your dinner." As an adult, you are cautioned that eating between meals will result in excess weight. In truth, it is not the snacking itself that causes the problem, but the kinds of foods that are most often selected for those between-meal treats.

When most of us think of a snack, we picture candies, cookies, chips, pretzels or other processed foods high in salt or sugar content. We feel a craving for these additives because we have acquired a taste for them, and they are usually readily available. It should be emphasized that this is an acquired taste and one that can be eliminated. In fact, we may actually be unknowingly killing our families with kindness. Instead of the kinds of snack foods listed above, consider substituting fresh fruits, vegetables, nuts, and dairy products. Eat these foods in a form as close as possible to the way they naturally occur. Choosing the right snacks will vary with an individual's age, life-style, activity level, and personal taste.

SCHEDULING YOUR SNACKS

Planning your snacks, as well as your meals, will enable you to maintain control of your total food consumption. By taking a high-energy snack break during the mid-morning and afternoon, you will be less hungry at mealtime; and you will maintain a more constant blood sugar level throughout the day. This is the real key to avoiding binges and overconsumption of food. Use common sense. Eat when you are hungry, but select foods that will supplement a nutritious diet.

SNACKING CAN BE FUN

Design "veggie faces" from sliced celery sticks, radishes, cauliflower or green pepper strips. Create "fruit kabobs" from slices of apples, oranges, strawberries, and melon balls. Combine these with whole-grain crackers and a light, low-calorie dip — the perfect answer for those after-school cravings!

IX

HELPING YOUR FAMILY ACHIEVE A MORE NUTRITIOUS LIFE-STYLE

Controlling obesity and maintaining good health are top priorities for everyone, regardless of age. Most of us, unfortunately, are ill-equipped for putting sound nutrition to use in our daily lives. I hope this book has provided a base of knowledge from which you can continually grow and learn. The practical examples within this book are ones that can be used immediately to generate great changes in your life.

If you are a parent, or any person with a responsibility to others, this information becomes even more important. By the example of changing your own life, you can change the lives of others around you.

1

Learn the Nutritional Difference

The end of the summer approached and Charlotte, like many other young, working mothers, welcomed the relief that the routine of the school year brings.

One morning, Charlotte paused between the last-minute rush of packing sandwiches, chips, candy bars and cookies to ponder over the conduct of her nine-year-old son Ricky. Last semester, Ricky's alternating surliness and listlessness kept him in constant trouble with his teachers at school. Sighing, Charlotte wondered just how many trips to the principal's office she would have to make this year. . . .

Can you spot a possible solution to Ricky's problem in the above story? Such a solution could be as simple as one word — food!

How about you? Are you a victim of the 10 A.M. doughnut break? The three o'clock slump? The after-work munchout?

YOU ARE WHAT YOU EAT!

The average American family ingests 50 percent of all calories from refined or processed foods, almost 126 pounds of sugars and sweeteners a year.

This diet, combined with a sedentary life-style, should be labeled with a warning reading: CAUTION, DO YOU REALIZE YOU ARE SLOWLY KILLING YOURSELF? Today, scientific research has linked diet to such killers as cancer, diabetes, coronary heart disease, obesity, malnutrition, dental disease, gout, and peptic-ulcer disease.

THE YOUNGEST VICTIMS MAY EXPERIENCE THE MOST SEVERE CONSEQUENCES

Nowhere is good nutrition more essential than for adolescents and children. A child's nutritive needs, per pound of body weight, are often greater than an adult's.

Caloric and nutritive needs remain elevated through adolescence, when 15 percent of adult height and 50 percent of adult weight are gained. While some teenagers may need up to 4,000 calories a day just to maintain weight, they generally eat smaller amounts of food than an adult. Consequently, children and teenagers need *more* nutrients from *less* food than adults.

Diets of many teenagers fall far below recommended levels of calcium, iron, thiamin, folicin, and vitamins A and D. These deficiencies are present in all age groups, but are most severe with girls (often due to fad dieting), the poor, and minority groups.

Improper eating contributes to overweight — a condition experienced by 10 percent of all elementary school children and 20 to 30 percent of all high-schoolers. Research has also linked diet to previously untouched areas, such as performance in school, hyperactivity, learning disabilities, and crime. According to Alexander Schauss, director of the American Institute for Biosocial Research, until "thirty-five years ago, hyperactive children were a rarity. Today, the incidence of hyperactivity and learning disability is higher in the United States than in any other country in the world." A pioneer in the field, the late Dr. Ben Feingold, hypothesized that a diet high in additives, artificial colorings, artificial flavorings, chemicals, etc., produced symptomatic reactions, such as hyperactivity.

TAKE TIME FOR BREAKFAST

Some of the most noticeable effects of a poor diet on children and teenagers can be measured by school performance. A common complaint from both students and teachers is fatigue, sluggishness, boredom, and lack of concentration occurring mid-morning and mid-afternoon. This lack of productivity can be directly traced to what was (or wasn't) eaten just a few hours before.

This happens not only with breakfast, but also with lunch. Remember the lunch that Charlotte was preparing for her son Ricky? White bread, potato chips, chocolate-chip cookies and a candy bar. Hidden in these innocent-appearing items are twenty-five teaspoons of sugar! No wonder many children remain so "overactive" for a short period following lunch and then lapse into nonproductivity. Do you notice these same effects in your life?

YOU CAN MAKE THE SWITCH

Are you interested in giving yourself and your children a fighting chance? If so, you must work on restructuring both EATING HABITS AND EATING ATTITUDES.

Remember that you, as a parent, may have the greatest influence over whether or not your child becomes obese. We learn the what, where, when and whys of eating as children, and carry these habits into adulthood.

Parents can help their children develop good eating habits by using nutritionally sound judgment. What your children should eat depends upon their size and how quickly they put on weight.

Help your child get the most out of the schooldays with foods that produce constant energy levels. Diet Center recommends you plan a nutritious lunch box with such foods as a thermos of chicken soup, a tuna-salad sandwich, whole-grain crackers, vegetable sticks or a piece of fruit.

Control between-meal snacks by providing milk, juices, fresh fruits, and raw vegetables instead of refined sweets. You decide "what"—let them decide how much. Make meals a special time where the whole family can sit down, relax, and share the day's events. Eat only at the table, not in front of the television. Make eating fun and easy with nutritious finger foods (an assortment of crisp vegetables and a tofu dip).

Remember a sound nutritional life-style equals good health. Make sure you and your family eat plenty of leafy, green vegetables and citrus fruits to obtain vital vitamins and fiber. Eat those meats high in protein but low in fats. And, don't forget to drink plenty of water.

2

Becoming Your Own Nutritionist

NUTRITIOUS food, like gas in a car, keeps your body running in good condition. (Your body can adapt to a poor diet, but it will not be healthy. It will eventually stop working, and the result will be illness.)

Your nutritional requirements will vary according to age, sex, weight, and physical activity. If you are skipping meals and missing adequate amounts of nutrients, you can become undernourished. People often believe they are eating well, but are actually deficient in one or more nutrients. Fatigue, irritability, or depression are all possible signs of an improper diet.

Good nutrition does not just happen. It requires awareness, knowledge, and planning. How well do you know the basics?

This chapter is designed to assist you in making sound nutritional decisions through nutritional concepts, practical examples, and immediate application. Do you realize you can count "nutrients," not calories? Or, that the information you need to make nutrition decisions is on that prepackaged food you buy? Do you realize just how little actual "food" you may be eating? And do you realize the large role food manufacturers and processors, plus the federal government, have in determining what appears on your table?

The answers to these questions are all contained within this section. Read it carefully, not just for information, but the knowledge to apply these examples to your own life!

HOW TO COUNT NUTRIENTS

"Nutrition" can be defined simply as a process by which you can permanently control your weight and maintain your good health through proper eating. What you eat for breakfast has an immediate effect on how your body functions, how you feel emotionally, and how you react mentally. Your eating patterns over a lifetime help determine your health, and even your life span! By controlling what foods you do eat and when you eat them, you can have better control over your health!

This control comes from a simple understanding of the

A BRIEF REVIEW OF THE INGREDIENTS CRUCIAL TO YOUR GOOD HEALTH!

PROTEIN: Protein is the life substance of the body. It is called the "Building Blocks of Life." It is the only substance capable of building and repairing the cells and tissues of the body. Protein is the major building material for muscles, blood, skin, nails, and internal organs, including the heart and brain. Next to water, it is the most abundant substance in the body. Protein is the second major nutrient to be digested. As it is digested, it produces sustained energy.

CARBOHYDRATES: Carbohydrates are the body's main energy supplier. The brain relies almost exclusively on the carbohydrate glucose to provide it with fuel to operate. Carbohydrates also assist in bodily functions, digestion, and muscle exertion, while helping a person to think more clearly and to maintain a good energy level. It is important to consume the right kind of unrefined, complex carbohydrates to maintain a stable blood sugar level and keep you from constant snacking. Carbohydrates are the first major nutrient to be digested and provide an "instant burst" of energy.

FATS: Fats, also called lipids, are essential to the diet. They are the most concentrated form of energy and furnish nine calories per gram (more than twice as many calories as either proteins or carbohydrates). The body uses fats to hold food in the stomach for longer periods of time, thus generating "staying power," to keep the skin soft and supple, to contribute to healthy hair, to act as a reserve source of fuel and energy, to act as a lubricant and assist in elimination, and to help in the utilization of fat-soluble vitamins.

WATER: Water is the most important nutrient for the body. It accounts for 50 to 55 percent of our body weight. Most individuals would die within a week if deprived of water. The body relies on water to supply and carry nutrients, dispose of wastes, act as a medium for the majority of chemical reactions, act as a means of transportation, and help control body temperature.

VITAMINS: The human body requires about twenty substances for proper growth and good health. Since the body is not capable of synthesizing these organic compounds, they must be obtained from the diet or through a dietary supplement. Vitamins can be found in various plant and animal products. They are divided into two categories: water-soluble (vitamin B-complex, vitamin C, and bioflavonoids) interacting with water and fat-soluble (vitamins A, D, E, and K) interacting with fats.

MINERALS: Approximately 4 percent of our bodies are composed of minerals. We require fourteen known minerals and have a possible need for at least three more. Unlike vitamins, which are compounds (combinations), minerals are elements (found singly). Minerals include: calcium, phosphorus, sodium, chlorine, potassium, magnesium, and sulfur. Trace minerals (minerals found in your body in only small amounts) include: iron, iodine, manganese, copper, zinc, cobalt, fluorine and selenium.

FIBER AND BULK: Fiber and bulk are essential for healthy bowels. They move waste products through the intestines and slow digestion, allowing a more consistent and gradual absorption of nutrients. Fiber and bulk are essential for "staying power" and can be found in fresh fruits, vegetables, whole grains, etc.

basic nutrients — proteins, carbohydrates, fats, water, fiber and bulk, vitamins and minerals. This understanding becomes a "nutritional consciousness" that you should put to use every day!

HOW NUTRITIOUSLY DO YOU EAT?

What foods are you now eating and when? Do you know what nutrients these foods provide? The American diet has steadily grown worse, from a nutritional standpoint, over the last sixty-five years. In just the last century, there has been a drastic increase in fat consumption, an overall decrease in complex carbohydrate consumption (from fresh fruits, vegetables, and whole grains) and an incredible increase in sugar consumption. The average American eats too much saturated fat, cholesterol, protein, sugar, and just TOO MUCH FOOD!

Remember that a healthy balance is the key. While keeping your protein, carbohydrate, and fat intake in a healthy range, make certain you select those foods highest in vitamins, minerals, and fiber for better health.

Your best choices are:

PROTEINS: Stick to lean meats, such as chicken and fish. (Well-trimmed, cooked beef may be used on occasion. Pork and lamb are rich in fat.) Eggs can be included but limit to no more than five per week. Prepare these foods through methods that will maintain high nutrient content without adding extra fats and calories. Try legumes (beans, etc.) as an alternative protein source.

CARBOHYDRATES: Choose "natural" complex carbohydrates from fruits, vegetables and whole grains. Eat at least three to five fruits per day. Have a large variety of vegetables, with half of this amount raw. Eat a salad and cooked vegetable every day, but prepare those foods properly as well to keep their highest nutritional potential. Choose whole grains in breads, crackers, and cereals; avoid highly refined or facsimile whole wheat. Use honey as a sweetener rather than refined white or brown sugars.

FATS: Avoid foods extremely high in fat content, but low in nutrients. Use unsaturated fats as much as possible, mixed with a little unsaturated oil.

For specific suggestions on foods high in these nutrients, see "Vital Nutrients and the Diet Center Program" (pages

78–100). An in-depth analysis of all nutrients in each food found in this section is available in the Appendix.

The basic nutrients should be as familiar to you as types of breakfast cereals. The rest of this section is devoted to showing you ways to apply this knowledge to cooking, shopping, and even proper eating! Calories may be important, but nutrients make the difference when it comes to good health!

Digestion and Enzymes — A Key to Better Eating

BY now, you know the best foods from which to gain the basic nutrients. A brief explanation of digestion can be helpful to learning the difference between just eating and eating "right."

DIGESTION . . . A BIOLOGICAL MIRACLE

Ask any scientist and he will tell you that the digestion system is impossible to duplicate scientifically. The efficiency of digestion is an inspiring miracle.

Digestion is a process of the autonomic nervous system. It is accomplished without being consciously commanded, leaving our minds free to concentrate on other matters.

Our state of mind and our emotions affect the entire digestive system. For example, stress and negative behavior in people influence the speed by which food moves down the digestive tract. If people are upset or under undue stress, their food may not be in contact with the intestinal lining long enough for nutrients to be properly absorbed. The senses of sight, smell, and taste also seem to activate or slow down the digestive juices. If a person on a diet is not hungry, has no appetite, or if the food does not taste good, the digestive juices will not flow properly; and the food will be poorly digested. Many nutritional and emotional factors influence digestion.

DIGESTION . . . A TWENTY-SIX-FOOT JOURNEY

The digestive tract is a continuous tube running from the mouth to the anus. The digestive process begins in the mouth then continues with its twenty-six-foot journey. Individual enzymes have to be available to digest each different group of foods (proteins, carbohydrates, and fats). Enzymes are what make digestion happen. Without them, digestion would be impossible and the foods we eat would merely sit in our stomachs and stagnate.

Chewing and saliva moisten and break down the food. Chewing food thoroughly is important because larger pieces of food are not completely digested, and some of the valuable nutrients are lost.

FOODS DIGEST AT DIFFERENT SPEEDS

Incredible as it may seem, food accumulates in layers corresponding to the order in which it was eaten, despite the stomach's vigorous churning. Also, different types of food are digested at different speeds. If foods are not combined, they will digest in the following order:

1. Simple liquids (take the least amount of time to digest)
2. Fruits
3. Vegetables
4. Starches
5. Proteins
6. Fats and oils (take the longest to digest)

Knowledge of digestion is limited when digestion involves complex mixtures of food. It is known that whenever fats are added to a meal (for example, oil dressing on a salad), the digestion process is slowed down, resulting in a longer period of satiation. Coffee, tea, spices, and other stimulants can accelerate digestion, but these along with salt are also irritants to the stomach lining.

DIGESTION TAKES FROM TWENTY-FOUR TO TWENTY-SIX HOURS

The entire digestive process reaches completion in approximately twenty-four to twenty-six hours and is simplified by eating a wholesome diet of lean meats, fresh fruits and vegetables, and whole grains. Greasy, rich foods overtax the entire digestive process, and in doing so contribute to ill health.

Since the small intestine is where nutrient and water absorption take place, it must have a large exposed area. And it does! The surface area of the small intestine is about two thousand feet, or equivalent to the main floor area of a large eight-room home. The long narrow tubes are coiled in a series, in the abdominal cavity, in folds with uncountable villi (little hairlike fingers), reacting like a turkish towel, absorbing nutrients and water.

By the time the digestive contents reach the end of the small intestine, digestion and nutrient absorption are virtually completed. What remains is water (that is, if you drink an average of eight glasses of water per day; if not, at this point, constipation can become a problem because the waste doesn't have enough moisture for the muscles to excrete it, so it hardens and sits). Also in the remains, besides water, are some dissolved salts, some body secretions, and the indigestible fibrous material. This waste is moved into the colon (the large intestine) and moved along basically for excretion.

The digestive system is such a magnificent happening, with thousands of intricate functions, that it seems almost sacrilegious to simplify it to the point of basic understanding. It must be done, however, because few people are scholars of chemistry, and the chemical makeup of the body must be shown simply so everyone can understand it and apply that knowledge to their lives.

4

Food — A Big Business!

WHAT happens when you sit down to dinner? Do you ever stop to think just exactly where your food came from? How it was processed into what appears on your plate? While gourmet cooking may be an art, food manufacturing and processing is a highly technical science. A science that often appears hard to understand and of little concern.

Is that cheese you crumbled on your salad "real" cheese or is it "fake" cheese? Yes, "fake" cheese does exist as a combination of restructured fatty acids, chemically modified starch, chemical emulsifiers, artificial colors, and fake cheese flavor! Or, how about last night's shrimp cocktail? Are you certain it really was shrimp and sauce or could it have been shrimplike pieces faked from soybeans covered with a sauce containing artificial thickeners, artificial color, artificial flavoring, and a heavy dose of salt?

It is easy to keep that preconceived idea that green beans are green beans, cake is dessert, and food is just to be eaten. It is not a very appetizing picture to think that your favorite candy bar is loaded with artificial sweeteners, flavorings, colorings, and preservatives that are not chocolate at all! However, by understanding the way in which food is altered through processing and preparation, you can gain new insights into putting "nutrition" back into your life.

Modern man's digestive system is very much the same as his forefathers'. Primitive man was a hunter and gatherer. He ate most of his food raw. Cooking came later, but it was a cultural event, not a biological necessity. (To this day, we are able to digest vegetables, seeds, and meat raw.) The advent of food processing, however, resulted in a whole new "type" of food — foods that could be prepared thousands of miles away and months before eating. This preservation involved a new set of processes and new additives. An excellent example is what has to be done to create that loaf of white bread sitting on the grocery shelf.

First, a fracturing process takes place that breaks the original grain into several components. Some of the components are used; the rest are thrown away. The wheat germ and the bran are separated from the starchy inner part called the endosperm. The bran and wheat germ are loaded with thiamine, plus many other vitamins and minerals. They are fed to the chickens and hogs. The endosperm, which is relatively worthless in food value, is made into white bread, pasta, cereals, etc.

The next step in the process is to modify the selected components by chemical treatment, e.g., bleaching the wheat to make it white. These products, together with a large dose of chemicals, are worked into artificial and simulated ingredients.

The last step is to combine these ingredients into a product that looks and tastes natural, but is far from the original.

To make up for nutritional deficits produced by food processing, food fortification was added. Foods have been fortified since the 1920s. Originally, nutrients were added to correct deficiency diseases, such as goiter and rickets. The trend in food processing greatly increased during World War II. For example, manufacturers began adding synthetically made vitamins and minerals to these foods to replace some of the natural nutrients lost in processing. The label on the side of a cereal box often indicates that a multitude of vitamins and minerals have been added. But these additives do not ensure good health. In many cases, the original grains that were the base of this cereal contained *higher* amounts of nutrients, fiber, and bulk than present now. Another concern is that *all* the nutrients removed during processing are not necessarily replaced, or aren't replaced in the *amounts* originally present. Unless legally mandated, manufacturers have the option to "fortify" with just those nutrients they choose, in the amounts they desire.

Fortifying foods has, in many cases, resulted in a large increase in per-item cost. Consumers are led to believe that they can receive all essential nutrient requirements for the day just through several servings of cereal!

5

Food Additives

DID you know that over twenty-eight hundred substances are added to different foods — on purpose? And that over ten thousand other chemical combinations can inadvertently be added through processing, packaging, and storage? For example, vitamins are often added to "fortify" foods. To ensure these vitamins last through the manufacturing process, however, vitamin preparations are often coated with gelatin, starch, or shellac. Your label reveals the added vitamins, but not their coatings!

A food additive is a substance or mixture of substances, other than a basic food stuff, which is present in a food as a result of any aspect of production, processing, storage, or packaging. This covers a wide variety of items. Herbs and spices and even salt are food additives.

Additives are incorporated into foods for four basic reasons:

1. Nutrient maintenance or fortification;
2. Preservatives for added shelf life, flavor, color, and to prevent oils from turning rancid;
3. Coloring and flavoring;
4. Body and texture.

GRAS LIST

According to law, chemicals that were used in food prior to January 1, 1958, could be deemed *G*enerally *R*ecognized *A*s *S*afe (GRAS) without scientific testing. Chemicals introduced to the food supply after that date may not be declared GRAS unless scientific tests indicate safety. GRAS chemicals are assumed to be safe because they have been used in food for many years or because they have undergone a certain amount of testing. Most GRAS chemicals have been used for so many years in foods that they are undoubtedly safe. However, being on the GRAS list certainly does not guarantee safety, because many GRAS chemicals have been inadequately tested. Cyclamate was on the list in 1969 when it was found to be carcinogenic (cancer-causing). Because of problems of this type, the FDA announced in 1971 that it would reexamine the toxicity of all GRAS compounds and conduct tests on many of them. There is also no limit on the levels at which most GRAS substances may be added to the food; the FDA did, however, place limits on most other food additives, both as to concentration and as to the foods in which they may be used.

INTERIM LIST

Another grouping of additives is included on the Interim List. Food additives on this list can continue to be used at present levels, but cannot be expanded to further uses until more testing is done on them.

FINAL GROUPING

This final grouping of food additives can only be used in certain concentrations and only in specific foods.

How does a new food additive get onto one of these lists so that it can be used in food? A company that wants to use a new additive must supply proof of its safety. The company is responsible for all testing, after which the FDA examines the results of the tests and rules on the safety of the additive. Only at this time can the food additive be used commercially. It must be used only in accordance with the terms of the regulation. Testing is usually quite long, from two to seven years, and also quite expensive.

TOXICITY TESTS

Toxicity tests are done to see if the chemical produces any injury to the test animal. Acute toxicity tests show the effects produced by the compound when a single dose is administered to a variety of laboratory animals.

Short-term toxicity studies (about ninety days in length) usually involve feeding several different groups of rats or other laboratory animals foods with different concentrations of the chemical. The test animals are observed for general appearance, behavior, growth, mortality, blood changes, condition of organs, and other biological and pathological effects.

Long-term toxicity studies (two years or more) are also made so that researchers may study the effects of lifetime ingestion of the compound. The same observations are made as in the case of short-term toxicity studies. In many cases, investigators also examine the effects of the compound on fertility, reproduction, and lactation. Analysis may also be made to determine how a compound is broken down or changed by the animal body before being stored or eliminated.

You must realize, however, that no matter how extensive the testing, many useful chemicals can never be proven absolutely safe. Scientists can gather good evidence that chemicals are not harmful, but proof of ABSOLUTE safety under ALL conditions for ALL people is impossible. It is important to understand that although a single product has been proven safe, we are still subjected to many varieties of prepackaged, boxed foods ladened with chemicals. During an entire day (or month or year), our bodies are not capable of utilizing many of these chemicals, additives, and preservatives. They take their toll on the body, leaving it as waste material, through the skin as blemishes, and even causing cancer. Nothing is more important than good health; nothing is more simple than returning to basic food.

GO NATURAL

Variety is very important to good nutrition. Many scientists believe we should eat diverse foods to ensure an adequate supply of all the nutrients, known and unknown. A supermarket may stock ten thousand items, but the bulk of the calories they furnish is derived from four crops: wheat, corn, soybeans, and sugar cane. These four crops, plus assorted chemical additives, can be converted into such diverse products as pizzas, fast-food "shakes," simulated bacon and sausage, and artificial cheese.

We can no longer gather berries, dig roots, and chase wild animals. We have developed many cultural patterns and food preferences. We must develop an eating regimen that takes care of our biological needs for wholesomeness and variety, and also satisfies our cultural heritage.

There are basically two types of natural foods. The first type is food as nature offers it, such as apples, carrots, grains, beans, and potatoes. This food should be eaten in its natural state or cooked minimally.

The second type includes the same fresh foods that are ingredients for minimally processed foods. This would include stone-ground wheat flour for bread, cheese prepared in the traditional manner from milk, and vegetable oil that is cold pressed from seeds.

Any kind of processing also includes preservation, but the process should not destroy the essential nutrients of the food. Freezing and drying are good methods. Canning is less desirable because of the extensive heating involved and because large quantities of sodium are also added. Remember that many fruits, vegetables, and grains have a built-in preservation system that permits long-term storage. These foods, like potatoes, winter squash, wheat and rice, are actually alive.

Some fortification is necessary and essential, such as vitamin D to milk and iodine to salt. Diet Center is concerned, though, about the abuses of vitamin and mineral fortification. Do not be misled by advertising claims. The cost is high financially and physically for these modern, chemical-wonder foods.

The information presented in this chapter provides a basic understanding of essential nutrients and their role in good health. If you are interested in more in-depth information, see the Appendix, "Diet Center's Food Composition Charts." These charts can help you determine just what nutrients are in the foods you eat every day. A breakdown of composition is also included for all foods on the Reducing Diet.

6

Sodium (Salt) and You

How much sodium do you use? Just a shake or two? Do you realize that the average American addicted to a salt shaker may consume twenty to fifty times the sodium the body actually needs? In fact, if the average person never used a salt shaker, too much salt would still likely be consumed.

Where does all this sodium come from? Let's say when you got up this morning you took two aspirin and some cough syrup for your cold, brushed your teeth with toothpaste, gargled with mouthwash, and sat down to a breakfast of eggs, bacon, toast, cereal, and orange juice. Every item mentioned contains sodium! Within just two hours you would have taken in enough sodium to satisfy your body's needs for the day. If you either need or want to reduce your sodium intake, first learn the facts and then apply them.

SODIUM — A LIFE MAINTAINER!

Few people realize that salt is actually composed of both sodium (40 percent) and chloride (60 percent). Sodium is necessary for survival as it is the major mineral component in blood and tissue fluids. Sodium enters the body through the foods you eat and is absorbed from the intestinal tract into the bloodstream. It helps regulate blood pressure and control blood volume, aids in heart and other muscle contractions, affects nerve impulses and enzyme action, and controls the fluids surrounding body cells.

TOO MUCH — A LIFE STRAINER!

Controversy rages over the question: "What happens when the body must deal with a consistently excessive intake of sodium and does this excessive intake *cause* hypertension?" While no definitive research demonstrates a direct cause and effect, the "possibility" is enough for many. Hypertension is a serious disease affecting one out of every four Americans. It is the major risk factor for stroke and one of the major risk factors for coronary heart disease.

HOW MUCH IS ENOUGH?

The average daily sodium intake of the majority of people in developed countries is far in excess of the amount needed for good health. The body's need for sodium is only 200 milligrams a day, or the equivalent of one-tenth of a teaspoon of salt. The Food and Nutrition Board suggests safe and adequate intake of 1,100 to 3,000 milligrams of sodium a day (up to 2 teaspoons of salt). Actual average consumption varies between 4,000 to 10,000 milligrams a day — twenty to fifty times what the body actually needs.

Some of the traditional justifications for such a high consumption either no longer exist or are being challenged. Originally used as a preservative in colonial America, salt is now primarily a "flavor enhancer." A recent analysis by the Center for Science in the Public Interest (CSPI) took low-sodium products and added salt "to taste." Its results demonstrated that it required only one-quarter to one-half the amount used by food manufacturers to make food tasty. Another rationale for high-iodized-salt consumption was to ensure adequate intake of iodine in iodine-depleted areas. This condition has actually reversed with FDA findings that "the typical American diet is not low, but surprisingly and even dangerously high in iodine." In fact, iodine requirements can be more than satisfied with residuals left from the iodine-containing compounds used to sterilize food-processing equipment.

Regardless of the reason, there is a growing consumer concern over salt intake; in fact, 40 percent of the population is already trying to reduce it! To a salt-conscious public, counting milligrams of sodium may soon become as popular as counting calories.

IT'S NOT JUST IN THE SHAKER!

One-fourth of all the sodium you consume comes from naturally occurring food sources. Foods originating from animal sources, such as meat, poultry, fish, milk, and cheese, are all naturally high in sodium. Sodium can be found in grains and vegetables as well. Interestingly enough, these foods can provide all the sodium your body needs.

A second source of sodium is direct use of table salt and seasonings. Salting food is an unconscious habit for most people. The quickest, although not long-term, solution for reducing sodium is simply to hide your shaker. Be cautious when seasoning foods — garlic salt, onion salt, and celery salt are simply "flavored" salts. Soy sauce, itself labeled as "liquid salt," can fulfill recommended daily sodium allowances with just one shake. Many salt substitutes simply mix potassium chloride with sodium. Even black pepper contains sodium.

The largest and most unrecognized sodium source is processed foods and products. Sodium is an essential agent in food processing and preservation. It is used to flavor and pre-

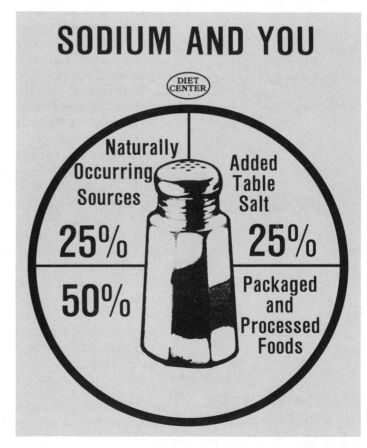

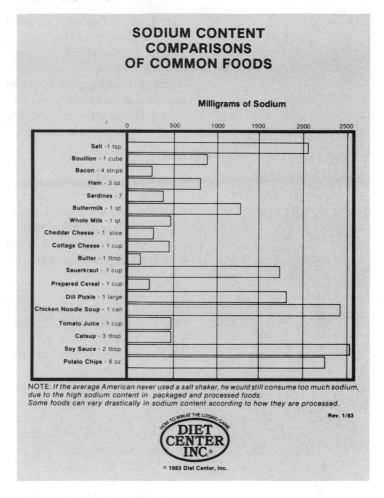

SODIUM CONTENT COMPARISONS OF COMMON FOODS

Milligrams of Sodium

NOTE: If the average American never used a salt shaker, he would still consume too much sodium, due to the high sodium content in packaged and processed foods.
Some foods can vary drastically in sodium content according to how they are processed.

Rev. 1/83

DIET CENTER INC.®

© 1983 Diet Center, Inc.

serve foods, develop color, bind types of foods together (e.g., sausage), maintain shelf life, and control fermentation in foods.

Surprising to consumers is the fact that often the foods that taste the "saltiest" are *not* the highest in sodium content. A food-analysis survey by the U.S. Department of Health and Human Services revealed that the foods highest in sodium were grain products.

The difference between natural and prepared foods could be the difference between a daily intake of under 800 milligrams of sodium and a daily intake of about 10,000 milligrams of sodium. Take the case of a relatively harmless cup of fresh green beans (it contains 5 milligrams of sodium). After being subjected to the canning process, sodium content increased 91 times (456 milligrams).

These figures may seem incredible until you examine the labels of many products. Remember, sodium can appear in countless forms, including salt, sodium, soda, sodium bicarbonate (a baking soda), sodium saccharin, sodium nitrate, sodium propanate, sodium citrate, to name just a few.

THE SODIUM CONTROVERSY

In the last five years, sodium has achieved growing consumer attention because of new emphasis and controversy in scientific, medical, and even political areas. In the absence of any other preventive measure for hypertension, *sodium restriction* emerges as a viable precaution.

SODIUM AND YOU

Diet Center recognizes the importance of sodium to maintain a properly functioning system. Excessive consumption of sodium, however, is unnecessary and can have detrimental effects on your health.

Diet Center believes that the sodium issue is one with which every concerned consumer can become involved. YOU have control over what foods you eat and how you prepare them. Adequate sodium intake can be obtained from naturally occurring food sources. YOU can conquer a "salt-dependence" by trying new ways to flavor foods.

Replace your salt shaker with lemon or herbs. Choose fresh fruits and vegetables rather than the canned or processed equivalent. Use whole grains instead of commercial cereals. Finally, eliminate or reduce salt amounts when cooking or baking.

7

Sugar, Sugar Everywhere!

You may be so familiar with sugar and salt that you do not consider them additives. However, they are used in more foods, in greater amounts, than most other additives.

Fifty years ago, if you wanted your food to taste sweet, you simply added granulated sugar to it. You controlled the amount of sugar you and your family ate. But modern food processing has drastically changed the way we consume sugar. A look at product ingredients on supermarket shelves will demonstrate how difficult it is to find any type of prepared food that does not contain sugar. It is not only used in sweet baked goods, desserts, and soft drinks but also in sauces, many baby foods, almost all fruit drinks, salad dressing, canned and dehydrated soups, pot pies, frozen vegetables, most canned and frozen fruits, fruit yogurt, and breakfast cereals. If you eat a hot dog, there is sugar in the meat, in the catsup or relish, and in the bun.

Whether in packaged salad dressing or in a packaged cupcake, sugar is the leading food additive today.

Some of the sugar in processed foods serves functions other than adding sweetness. It retains and absorbs moisture. This keeps foods from drying out too quickly. It drops the freezing point, making ice cream and other frozen desserts smoother. It can act as a preservative, and it can enhance the appearance of some foods.

Industry uses sugar for other reasons. For only a few cents per pound, sugar is a very cheap ingredient. And many people have developed a desire for a sweet taste.

Unfortunately, nutrition labeling does very little to help

promote an awareness of sugar content. The label shows only total carbohydrates and not the percentage of sugar and starch in a product. Another problem: Many different types of sugar that are not familiar to most consumers may be listed on the label. Be aware of the following forms of sugar:

1. Fructose (fruit sugar)
2. Lactose (the sugar in milk)
3. Dextrose (one of the sugars made from cornstarch)
4. Maltose (malt sugar formed from starch by the action of yeast)
5. Sucrose (cane or beet sugar)

If you are looking for the word "sugar" and find it well down the list of ingredients or not present at all, you may believe the product does not contain much sugar when, in truth, sugar may be the most prominent ingredient in the food because of all the different forms that are used.

The words "no sugar added" on a label can be misleading to anyone trying to cut down on sugar consumption. Sugar can still be present, because many foods contain natural sugars. Apple juices, for example, may have slightly more natural sugar than the sugar added to a soft drink. The difference, of course, is that fruit juice has nutrients that will not be found in a soft drink.

What happens to all this sugar in the body? It is digested very quickly and converted into glucose, the primary fuel of the body. With the help of the hormone insulin, blood glucose then enters the cells of the body and is used as an energy source. Much of the glucose that is not used for energy is metabolized in the liver into fatty substances called triglycerides, which are transported in the bloodstream to the fat deposits of the body. Because refined sugars are digested so quickly, they cause an overload on the system and most of the glucose will be converted into body fat. Fresh fruits and vegetables release their sugars slowly because they have to be chewed and digested and because they supply their own sugar buffers in the form of fiber. They provide a gradual and usuable energy boost that the modern candy bar does not.

If your diet is high in sugar, consider these points: First, did you know that what you eat directly affects your dental health? Sugary, sweet foods like cake, candy, pastry, and soda pop coat your teeth with a sticky, nearly invisible, form of bacteria called plaque. Plaque uses the sugars from these foods to form acids that attack the normal surface of your teeth within thirty minutes after eating. The end result is a cavity.

Second, it is easy to eat too many sweet, sugary foods. If you are overweight, simply avoiding sugary foods may help you lose pounds.

Third, a diet high in sugar will almost certainly be a poor diet. High-caloric, low-nutritional sugary foods replace nutritious foods.

Fourth, honey is better for you than sugar. Even though the caloric content is equal and it has no nutritive value, the body is able to digest it more efficiently.

Finally, sugar is not addictive; but because the system digests it rapidly, thus causing the blood sugar to fluctuate, then drop, the body, as a result, craves more sugar.

Diet Center recommends that you eat natural fruits and vegetables for your carbohydrate needs. They provide the body not only with energy, but with a generous supply of vitamins, a lot of important minerals, and a valuable supply of fiber. Calorie for calorie, they are a better value. A small piece of chocolate cake provides close to 300 calories and does not take long to eat. How long would it take you to eat four medium-sized apples? or eight small peaches? or a quart and a half of strawberries? Each contains the same amount of calories. (Diet Center recommends that you not consume fruits as juices. Chewing the entire food will provide bulk and "staying power.")

As a key, look for any word ending with "ose," such as maltose or dextrose. "Corn syrup" or "corn sugar" is a commonly used sucrose substitute. Ultimately, they all mean the same thing — you are buying sugar.

SUGAR

1. Sugar is the leading additive in U.S. foods.
2. There are many foods that naturally have high amounts of sugar.
3. Sugar causes an immediate rise in blood sugar, but has no "staying power."
4. Three teaspoons of sugar equal 12 grams of carbohydrates.
5. Read all labels carefully for any *"ose"* (lactose, sucrose, dextrose, maltose and fructose).

8

Read the Label

Do you know EXACTLY what is in the foods you are eating? Are canned green beans just green beans? You may be surprised at what exactly is in that tin can, under the bottle cap, and inside that prettily packaged box. Reading the label may be one of your best tools in eliminating unnecessary fillers, additives, and preservatives from your family's diet. (Did you know that preprocessed green beans usually contain salt and sugar?)

Certain foods are required to carry labeling and specific facts on that label. Other foods, such as fresh fruits and vegetables, are beginning to carry labels just because of consumer demand.

Go to your cupboard and grab a package or box. Look for the small square usually entitled "Nutrition Information." Nutrition labels generally include extra information regarding number of servings and serving size. Nutrients are generally expressed in these terms:

> Calories (a measure of the energy value of that food)
> Protein (in grams)
> Carbohydrate (in grams)
> Fat (in grams)

These are the major nutrients found in foods (often called macronutrients).

Next on a label follows a list of vitamin and minerals (called micronutrients). These nutrients are usually measured against government recommendations called RDAs or U.S. RDAs (see the next chapter for additional information on

RDAs). Any vitamin or mineral ADDED to the food *must* be listed. Naturally occurring micronutrients *may* be included if desired. This can be misleading to the consumer. For example: Many canned products, such as orange drinks, appear by the label to contain a natural source of vitamin C. While consumers may think they are buying the "real thing," in reality the drinks contain mainly chemicals and flavorings with little natural vitamin C.

Next on your label will follow a series of preservatives and additives used to create (or increase) flavor, color, texture, shape, and shelf life. The vast majority of these ingredients are chemically synthesized into the correct combinations. While some manufacturers state the purpose of specific additives, the rest leave us to wonder rather skeptically as to what we are really eating.

Ingredients are placed in descending order by weight. So, if the label states: water, sugar, oranges — you receive mainly water and sugar!

One of the major "first" ingredients in prepackaged foods is *sugar*. It would be enlightening, however, just to know how much sugar is really in that food. A candy bar, for example, lists sugar, but fails to tell you that it includes 21 TEASPOON-FULS. That can of pop you are drinking has 6 TEASPOONFULS of sugar. For those who down a six-pack of soft drinks per day, this equals 36 TEASPOONFULS.

Besides appearing as the "first" ingredient, sugar can often appear father down the line hidden by other names. Look at your label: does it include honey? molasses? fructose? sucrose? maltose? dextrose? These are all additional forms of sugar that directly affect your weight. (Or a label can say sugar-free, yet be loaded with sugars, such as maltose, dextrose, etc., which are, in fact, sugars.)

Another major ingredient to check for is flour. Did you know flour comes in a variety of types much like sugar? On labels, the word "flour" means white, processed flour, much like that you purchase at a grocery store. "Wheat flour" is nothing more than plain, white refined flour. The best flour with "staying power" is "whole-wheat flour." Do not be fooled by the name!

The next ingredient that usually dominates most labels is fat. There are several types of fats: hydrogenated, monounsaturated, polyunsaturated and saturated. Saturated fats are usually solid at room temperature, mainly of animal origin, and may raise the level of cholesterol in the blood. Polyunsaturated fats also appear in oil form, are liquid at room temperature, are derived mainly from plant sources, and may lower blood cholesterol. Monounsaturated fats are also liquid at room temperature, but appear to have no effect on cholesterol level. Hydrogenated fats (usually found in margarines and vegetable shortenings) are produced by adding hydrogen to unsaturated liquid oils (a process called hydrogenation). This process forces the oil to become more saturated.

Remember, the "best" type of fat for a balanced diet that promotes good health is polyunsaturated.

Food additives, as previously explained (see chapter 4 of this section), abound in virtually all packaged products.

Reading food labels is a must for any dieter. Cutting your total intake of foods will result in poor health if those foods contain only sugars, saturated fats, flours, sodium and preservatives. Dieters who resort to these types of foods will almost assuredly find themselves in a state of low blood sugar (constant hunger, depression and anxiety).

Even so-called diet foods often carry these same ingredients. Prepackaged foods, high in preservatives and additives, do not provide a permanent solution for dieters.

Exercise your right to know! Read the label! Food provides the nutrients we require each day to stay healthy. Diet Center knows that no single food can provide all of the necessary nutrients; you need a variety of foods every day. Food labels tell us what nutrients foods contain, and can help us select nutritious foods for a well-balanced diet.

9

Government, Food Manufacturers, and What You Eat!

CAN these three diverse subjects be related? You bet — and the connection, of which few of us are aware, has tremendous impact on what you eat every day! You have just learned what compositional changes occur when food is processed. The rules and guidelines for food processing, however, are dictated by the federal government. Regulation of new and existing food and drug products is done through the Food and Drug Administration. Besides regulation, governmental agencies and legislative committees have created guidelines concerning foods. These guidelines are designed to assist people in obtaining better health through sound nutrition.

U.S. RDA AND RDA

You see one set of these guidelines thousands of times each day. They appear on your cereal box, bread wrapper, soda can, on TV commercials and in magazines. What are they? The Recommended Dietary Allowances!

The Recommended Dietary Allowances (RDA) are exactly that — only recommendations. They are not set up for individual requirements. Their basic function is to be a measuring device for specific segments or groups. There are also standards set for infants, children, adolescents, adults, and pregnant and lactating women.

The RDA is periodically revised, usually every four to six years, by the Food and Nutrition Board of the National Academy of Science, National Research Council of the United States, to meet the changing needs of the population. The

Food and Nutrition Board is comprised of fifteen experts from academic, governmental, and industrial areas. They give advice on food and nutrition, and help promote any necessary research.

These daily allowances are set above the majority of individuals' requirements, and it is estimated that they meet or exceed the needs of 45 percent of the people. The high standards also help cover times of stress when the body needs larger doses of nutrients.

There are some nutrients for which the RDA is not known. It is presumed that eating a wide variety of foods may help cover those unknown requirements. Many foods would have to be eaten in large quantities to meet the RDA; but in that quantity, they exceed the corresponding caloric intake.

A person may not be meeting the daily allowances in all areas, and still be receiving adequate nourishment. The RDA is only a reference that serves as both a maximum and minimum guideline, and a desirable goal. An individual may not even need to receive these nutrients daily, but they cannot be consistently ignored.

In the last few years, the Food and Drug Administration has adopted the RDA for its nutrition-labeling program. They use one figure for the U.S. RDA, usually the highest RDA. The U.S. RDA will be equal to, or higher than the RDA. This system allows a comparison of the product and easy evaluation of what you are buying and the recommended amounts.

As described in chapter 8 of this section, recommendations such as these can be an invaluable tool to ensure that you, and your family, receive adequate nutrients. Most nutrition labels do all the work for you by providing the RDA. The next time you go to a grocery store, take a few minutes to check labels of the products you buy for the U.S. RDA and RDA!

U.S. DIETARY GOALS VERSUS DIETARY GUIDELINES FOR AMERICANS: CONFUSION OVER NUTRITION

Another set of guidelines created by the federal legislature has resulted in more controversy than have many tax bills. These guidelines have an interesting history that directly affects TV commercials and product ads you see today!

In 1968, the Senate Select Committee on Nutrition and Human Needs was organized to work as a mediator between food and farm interests versus health, welfare, and research interests. This committee also dealt with solutions to hunger.

Then, in 1975, the evidence linking nutrition and disease

caused the Select Committee to change its direction. They began to realize the importance of preventive medicine by maintaining good health. The United States Dietary Goals were initiated in an effort to lower rising health costs.

The Senate Select Committee on Nutrition and Human Needs is no longer in existence. However, a Subcommittee on Nutrition has been formed and placed under the Standing Committee on Agriculture, Nutrition and Forestry. This subcommittee consists only of several senators.

In February 1977, for the first time, the American public was presented with a set of dietary goals designed to improve nutritional quality and, subsequently, health. It took over two years to complete. Since that time, however, these goals have been revised, restructured, and rewritten until all that remains is a diluted version of the original outline. How and why this happened should be of vital interest to anyone concerned with nutrition.

The "Dietary Goals for the United States" were issued by the U.S. Senate Select Committee on Nutrition and Human Needs. Based on nine years of research, these goals gave specific suggestions to alter improper eating.

U.S. DIETARY GOALS

1. To avoid overweight, consume only as much energy (calories) as is expended. If overweight, decrease energy intake and increase energy expenditure.
2. Increase the consumption of complex carbohydrates and "naturally occurring" sugars from about 28 percent of energy intake to about 48 percent of energy intake.
3. Reduce the consumption of refined and processed sugars by about 45 percent to account for about 10 percent of total energy intake.
4. Reduce overall fat consumption from approximately 40 percent to about 30 percent of energy intake.
5. Reduce saturated fat consumption to account for about 10 percent of total energy intake, and balance that with polyunsaturated and monounsaturated fats, which should account for about 10 percent of energy intake each.
6. Reduce cholesterol consumption to about 300 mg. a day.
7. Limit the intake of sodium by reducing the intake of salt to about 5 grams per day.

Instead of just raising public awareness, these goals triggered an avalanche of protests from many food producers and packaging industries. Lobbyists from the meat, egg, sugar, dairy, grain, and canning industries all attempted to have the goals revoked or restated. By December of 1977, a "revised" version of the U.S. Dietary Goals were published with the following suggestions (and alterations):

The goals suggest the following changes in food selection and preparation:

1. Increase consumption of meats and vegetables and whole grains.
2. Decrease consumption of refined and other processed sugars and foods high in such sugars.
3. Decrease consumption of animal fat, and choose meats, poultry and fish, which will reduce saturated fat intake.
4. Except for young children, substitute low-fat and non-fat milk for whole milk, and low-fat dairy products for high-fat dairy products.
5. Decrease consumption of butterfat, eggs and other high cholesterol sources. Some consideration should be given to easing the cholesterol goal for premenopausal women, young children and the elderly in order to obtain the nutritional benefits of eggs in the diet.
6. Decrease consumption of salt and foods high in salt content.

Notes:

• The warning to eat less meat was modified.
• Restrictions on sodium were eased.
• The attack on sugar was limited to refined and processed.
• Lean meats were included with fish and poultry.
• Eggs were treated more favorably; their importance for the elderly, young children and women were emphasized.

The Senate Select Committee on Nutrition and Human Needs was disbanded on December 31, 1977. Control over establishing dietary standards was then removed from Congress and delegated to an administrative level.

In February of 1980, the Department of Agriculture in conjunction with the Department of Health, Education and Welfare published a twenty-page pamphlet entitled "Nutrition and Your Health; Dietary Guidelines for Americans." These guidelines were produced on the same format as the U.S. Dietary Goals. However, these guidelines are general principles with no specific suggestions.

Unfortunately, even these guidelines have not been exempt from controversy. The 1980 report by the National Science Academy suggested that not enough evidence exists to limit cholesterol consumption for normal, healthy individuals. Armed with this information, the dairy and meat industries set off new protests. The cattle industry has also questioned these guidelines and lobbied for their revocation.

DIET CENTER TOTAL PROGRAM GUIDELINES

GUIDELINE 1: Consume a wide variety of foods. Because all nutrients do not have known RDA, this practice will ensure the best possible chance that adequate amounts of all needed nutrients are obtained.

Diet Center stresses the importance of eating from all food groups to maintain good health. We also feel it is an important factor if weight is to be permanently controlled.

GUIDELINE 2: Maintain ideal weight. It is a proven fact that people who are not overweight have a better chance to live longer and experience fewer health problems than those not maintaining ideal weight.

On the Diet Center Program, dieters are taught to lose and maintain their weight while eating nutritionally balanced meals. It is for this reason that our program can be a lifetime program. It is also easier to keep off additional, undesirable pounds if the body is maintaining an ideal weight.

GUIDELINE 3: Avoid large amounts of fats, saturated fat, and cholesterol. It is felt that cholesterol may be a contributing factor in fatty deposits in arteries, increasing the risk of heart attacks. By replacing saturated fats with polyunsaturated fats, the serum cholesterol will usually be lowered. It is suggested that no more than 30 percent of calories should be obtained from fat.

We recognize that fats are essential to proper functioning of the body, and are also required for wise weight loss. However, these must be the correct type of fats, and polyunsaturated fats are recommended. All visible fats should be removed from foods. It is very important that people are conscious of invisible sources of fat.

Only lean meats, chicken, and fish should be eaten. You can also make protein choices from vegetable protein (tofu) and eggs. Eggs contain many minerals required by the body and should not be totally eliminated from the daily diet. However, Diet Center agrees with the American Heart Association in recommending a maximum of three to five eggs weekly.

GUIDELINE 4: Eat foods that contain adequate complex carbohydrates, fiber, and naturally occurring carbohydrates. Fiber gives the body its needed bulk, and may help to prevent colon cancer. Starch is an energy-giver to the body. Natural occurring carbohydrates contain many of the required vitamins and minerals while having the added advantage of "staying power."

Purchase fresh foods and prepare them at home. This practice provides for more nutritious meals that contain a minimum of empty calories. Remember, fresh is best!

GUIDELINE 5: Avoid excess refined sugar. This figure should not exceed more than 10 percent of the total carbohydrate intake. Refined sugar is of no nutritional value. It contains no essential nutrients and, therefore, is only a source of many empty calories that cause a great amount of fluctuation in blood sugar levels. Refined sugar, a simple carbohydrate, also does not give a "full feeling" that is received from complex carbohydrates, and, consequently, people tend to overindulge. Although fructose (fruit sugar) is a simple carbohydrate, the fiber in most fruits allows only small amounts of fructose to be slowly released into the system and the blood sugar level is kept within normal range. Remember the importance of blood sugar levels and how rapid fluctuations can cause hunger, cravings, and other problems.

GUIDELINE 6: Avoid large quantities of sodium. Great concern exists on the effects of salt on high blood pressure. It is felt that salt has a wide range of harmful effects. Five grams (2 teaspoonfuls) daily are usually adequate for the average individual. Actually, most foods naturally contain salt, so little or none needs to be added. Additional salt deadens the taste buds, so over a period of time, greater amounts will be required to achieve the same taste. Because salt is an acquired taste, when it is excluded from the diet, the taste buds will become more sensitive, and will be amply satisfied with the natural salt in foods. If a salty taste is preferred, use lemon.

GUIDELINE 7: If you do drink alcohol, do so in moderation. Remember that an excess of anything is not good for you. Alcohol is suspected as a contributing factor in various physical disorders. It is a great handicap to those people who desire to lose weight and, therefore, is completely restricted from the Conditioning, Reducing, and Stabilization phases.

The 1968 and 1977 editions of the Dietary Goals are now history. The U.S. Department of Agriculture ceased publication of the 1980 U.S. Dietary Guidelines in spring 1982, with availability limited to those copies already printed. The controversy, however, continues as new administrative committees reevaluate the Dietary Guidelines.

Diet Center supports the sound nutrition principles presented in the Dietary Guidelines and Goals. In fact, Diet Center followed these principles long before they were even created. Twelve years ago, the Diet Center Total Program was devised with its own set of guidelines. These guidelines have withstood twelve years of questioning and conjecture. They remain, today, the basic backbone of the Diet Center Program.

X

HANDLING THE SLIM NEW YOU

I couldn't believe my own new image because I still felt fat. Every time I walked past a mirror, I would quickly glance at myself. It was like seeing a whole new person. I had a chin and cheekbones, where I didn't before. It was so unbelievable that I could not resist touching my face. I was delighted. It was like a butterfly emerging from a cocoon. It was literally a dream. The transformation I felt was unbelievable. I wanted to tell the whole world that I was "myself" now. The change in my body was so fantastic. I found a shinbone in my leg that I never even knew existed. Oh, the joy of crossing my legs and letting the top leg hang down instead of having to stretch it straight out. In the morning, while lying in bed, I discovered my ribs and breastbone. I never even guessed there was a floating rib. I had never felt it before! Oh, the joys that were mine to finally discover the wonders of my body; feelings that never existed when I was obese.

SUDDENLY SLIM

Walking past a mirror is exhilarating! Wonderful, new thoughts race through your mind: "I am really thin! . . . This is unbelievable. I am actually beautiful!" Your mirror now reflects a new person, a human being with new hopes and even dreams! You contemplate this reflection with newfound self-confidence, now unafraid to face the world. It is a delightful, all-consuming feeling. You feel good. No . . . you feel great! It is unbelievable that this could happen to you!

For many dieters, reaching an ideal goal weight is often a far-off dream, a goal that seems at times unattainable. Once, however, you settle into the pattern of a disciplined regimen, the pounds seem to drop consistently, quarter by quarter, half by half. Suddenly, you being to notice changes . . . changes perhaps unnoticed by others, but signs of success for you. Chairs get bigger; belts unwind; dresses grow longer; suitcoats begin to sag; steering wheels get farther away; and shoes and rings no longer pinch. Incredibly, men find old neckties even become too long!

Then, others around you begin to notice your changing appearance. Friends and co-workers begin to voice their compliments and neighbors give you a second look, wondering what's different. An acquaintance you haven't seen for weeks passes you by one day on the street, not recognizing you. The more weight you lose, the bigger the change.

Then, the day arrives when you reach your ideal weight goal *permanently*. For dieters who have struggled constantly with the problem of obesity for many years, reaching goal is a complete turning point in their lives. The thrill of achieving success spreads a warm glow of self-satisfaction that reflects throughout every aspect of your life. While you are basically the same person no matter what your weight, becoming slim, healthy and self-confident results in new feelings and growth. The experience is one few dieters ever forget. As one successful Diet Center dieter describes after losing 101 pounds and 107 inches in eight and a half months: "I can't begin to tell you how I feel today. But just let me say that when I awoke this morning, I really felt as though I was Alice in Wonderland or Cinderella after she was rescued by the handsome prince. I used to read stories with happy endings, but never in all of those stories did I read about someone as thrilled as I am today . . . I was actually proud to be me!"

Some dieters have been overweight since childhood and never remember being thin. Physical changes are often overwhelming — a beautiful face emerges that was hidden before, and with it a slender body with small hands and feet, shapely legs and figure. "I'd never seen what I looked like normally, even as a kid I was overweight," recalls a now succesful 107-pound Diet Center "loser." When she flew to Florida for a family reunion, her own father didn't recognize her! "I had to walk right up to him and say, 'Hi Dad!' and then he just recognized my voice!" Even her brother agreed that the voice was familiar, "but when I look at you, I see someone else!"

Each day brings new revelations: "I can walk with energy and vigor! I am no longer tired and worn out — I now want to participate in everything. I am living! I love shopping for new clothes, bright colors, high fashion . . . slim-cut pants, tucked-in blouses, even belted styles." All this excitement is hard to imagine for the person who has never had a weight problem; but for the newly slim, these are marvelous new experiences. No longer are you afraid to go to the store, to a movie, to a play, even out on a date! Men not only notice you, but are actually flirting with you — not someone else, YOU! Your friends are full of compliments, and from some, you can even detect a note of jealousy. You are happy to be alive and proud of your accomplishment.

For men, attaining a new ideal goal weight is just as exciting. Friends admire your new physique. You no longer feel lethargic and listless, but alive and full of life. Your tasks at work seem easier to accomplish and each workday seems to fly by even faster. Incredibly, you even have energy when the day ends to go out or join a health club. After losing seventy pounds, one male dieter states, "I've never felt better, I'm no longer fatigued by the end of the day, and my energy level is high. My wife and I actually went to a late movie last week." You rejoin sports you had abandoned since high school or college. You are no longer winded and you can feel your "competitive spirit" reemerging. Women start to give you second glances. You abandon baggy shirts and worn pants to purchase shirts that tuck in (no more overhanging stomach!) and tight-fitting jeans. You no longer send a wife or friend out to buy your clothes — you do it yourself! Suddenly, you want a different hair style, perhaps some new aftershave. You are proud of who you are and how you look, and this pride is apparent in your every action.

CHANGING RELATIONSHIPS

A suddenly slim body not only produces immense physical changes, but great mental changes as well. Former insecurities and fears are much slower at retreating or changing. These changes often have a direct effect on relationships.

For many women, rekindled romance or second honeymoons often occur. As one husband expressed: "I feel as though I have a brand-new wife. I can literally wrap my arms around her now, and I love it!" Many women confide how wonderful it is to be able to undress without hiding or insisting that the lights be turned out. One woman said, "It is impossible to 'think sexy' when you ache and cry on the inside, hating your body, but then, so great to realize that you are now physically attractive to your husband!"

On the other hand, some husbands or boyfriends try to sabotage their wives' or girlfriends' attempts to lose weight. Possibly out of their own insecurity or the fear that other men will find their wives attractive, these men place both physical and psychological roadblocks in the way of their wives' success. Suddenly, cartons of ice cream and cookies, delivered pizzas, and bags of candy seem to bombard these wives. Their husbands urge them to take a second helping, try a new dessert and bring presents of candy, instead of flowers. Compliments seem to revert to negative remarks, perhaps because some husbands felt more secure with their overweight wives and want them back. Many men also feel confused by the suddenly active and enthusiastic person that is now their mate or girlfriend. She no longer seems content to stay at home, but wants to go out to movies, parties, or shopping. For a husband who is himself overweight or no longer possesses the physique he once did, a slender, healthy wife is often a threat to his own self-image.

NEW FEARS ARISE

For many men, these fears are real and well-founded. As some women lose weight, their suppressed feelings emerge. Now men begin to flirt with them, and they become flirtatious back, especially those women who have experienced little "real" attention in their lives. For the woman who has seldom experienced this attention, it may be puzzling, and even destructive. Others, having been starved for affection, may now overreact to the slightest flirtation. Many problems can result, especially if the spouse is indifferent or reacts negatively to her success. If the husband does not respond to his wife's new awareness and needs, the marriage can be seriously threatened. Some husbands turn from elation to insecurity — even to contempt. Meanwhile, the wife is experiencing a whole flood of new emotions. Can someone else be seriously interested in her? Can he actually think she is desirable? Maybe she is in love. These are new feelings. What is happening?

For people who have always been overweight, this time is particularly traumatic. Rejection, especially in relationships, has always been a common occurrence. Many have *never* experienced a close relationship with either sex. Friendship, dating, and marriage are often alien words and feelings of "love" were always more imagined than reciprocated.

Many old doubts and insecurities remain even with a new,

slender, attractive body. "How can I ask that beautiful girl out?" "I can't go out with him, I wouldn't know what to do!" "What if she says no?" "What if he doesn't like me?" For the newly slim, these fears are very real. For women, this new-found attention may make them fearful. For men, it may seem almost impossible to cross that first hurdle of asking a woman out.

DEALING WITH NEW RELATIONSHIPS AND NEW FEELINGS

So, how do you deal with these new relationships, new people, new friends, and new feelings?

As a successful dieter, you must learn to evaluate your life, your feelings, and your future. Determine what is really important to you. These are irrational times — strive for rational thinking. Give yourself time. Do not make hasty decisions. Take the new feelings and attentions in stride and enjoy the newfound you! You no longer feel sorry for yourself, so take time to consider the feelings of others. It's been so long since you've flirted or had anyone flirt with you that you will need to go way back and think of your high school or college days where you said flippant, cute things, and boys constantly made advances. You knew then that it was simply "fun and games." It's still the same today. This type of exchange has continued through each phase of life, but you have been excluded. Don't take these exchanges seriously. Have fun! Attention and compliments build your ego and help you feel desirable. But don't rush into something as serious as a divorce or permanent changes. Be sure to put things in proper perspective. Remain excited about yourself, your energy and newfound zest for life — and shower this new awareness on the ones you love. Husbands and children usually respond, and the relationships can flourish.

If you have never experienced a fun-and-games type of relationship, follow this same philosophy. However, you may want to practice. For one week, spend time observing people around you. Notice comments and actions in all types of situations. Then, go home and practice on an inanimate object. You may feel silly at first, but take time to find what techniques work best for you. Then, practice talking to everyone around you. Push yourself into socializing situations. Take the initiative! You'll feel more comfortable in any relationship or dating relationship!

The best way to deal with saboteurs is to evaluate your relationship with that person. Are your new behavior and attitudes making that person insecure? Are you directly threatening that person? When's the last time you said, "I love you"? Take time to make that person feel a wanted part of your life. If real problems do exist within your relationship, take time to sort them out. Once the differences are resolved, the pizzas and ice cream cartons have a magic way of disappearing.

THE FAT TRAP

Each dieter reacts differently to success. Periodically, the newly slim person does not feel comfortable with her more appealing figure. She doesn't know how to handle the attention, the new sensations and the new feelings. She may feel more secure being fat because she has hidden in that cocoon for as long as she can remember. People seem to expect more from thin people, and competition may become more keen. It's difficult to cope with these new pressures, so there seems to be safety in the protection of the "fat" cocoons.

For other dieters, achieving a new slim figure didn't erase other problems that in the past were easy to blame on being overweight. Being overweight may have contributed, but it was not the sole cause of problems at home, work, or with a spouse or friend. The security (and excuse) of "it's just be-

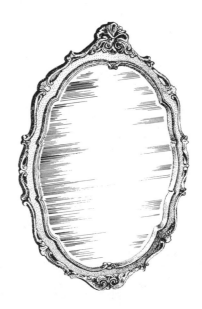

cause I'm fat" is removed. For these dieters and others, food, once again, becomes the all-consuming mentor, the mental and emotional pacifier, the insecure person's place to hide. In an attempt to regain a husband's favor, some women become even more submissive, becoming even more trapped in their own insecurities.

Don't let this happen to you. If you feel overwhelmed with problems but no solutions, don't panic. Take your time to slowly sort through new feelings and emotions. Analyze your problems to find the true cause. Work gradually on each problem or situation one at a time. Remember, this is a necessary part of rediscovering the inner you to fit the slim new you. If you are feeling these insecurities or self-doubts, go to a full-length mirror. Look at your slim, new figure. Look at the healthy glow in your cheeks. Think of how much you have accomplished. YOU ARE IN CONTROL! YOU ARE NOW IN CHARGE OF YOUR LIFE! Never look back. Instead, look ahead to your new and improved personal relationships or the new challenges you can now face with the assurance of a person who has, and will continue to succeed!

XI

IF YOU NEED FURTHER HELP, DON'T GIVE UP!

I have never forgotten what frustrations, temptations, and struggles I had to overcome while learning to eat nutritiously and permanently control my weight. Your spouse, family and friends can all be supportive, but if they have never had their own weight problem, it is very hard for them to understand how difficult it is for you. There are days when you feel great, your determination is strong, and your commitment is unchallengeable. There are other days, however, when nothing seems to go right.

During one of those difficult days, I remember turning to my husband, Roger, and saying, "If only there was someone I could go to every day, someone who could answer my questions; a special person who could give me extra encouragement and advice." I never forgot this feeling. Dieting is a difficult struggle if you do it by yourself. Skipping meals and counting calories seemed always to result with my ironclad determination of the morning dwindling to desperation. Inevitably, by late afternoon I would be starving and ready to give in and eat that leftover piece of cake. Dieters throughout America feel these same frustrations. The following story tells of one woman's struggles, not only with being overweight, but of improper dieting. Today, Arlene Jaffie's life is free from many of the problems she battled just one year ago.

A lifetime of frustration and discouragement in the battle against gaining weight came to a peak for Arlene Jaffie during the summer of 1981. As with most parents when they reach

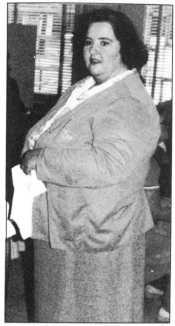

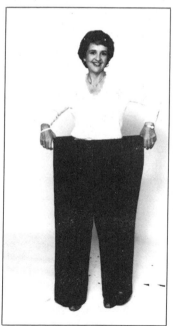

Arlene Jaffie lost 185 pounds and 149½ inches in less than fifteen months.

milestones in the progress of their lives, Arlene paused during her daughter's confirmation ceremony to reflect upon her own life. As she looked at her three children, Jeff, Susan, and Lynn, she thought to herself that they were the most beautiful sight she had ever seen. The terrible thought of not being able to finish raising them came as a chilling vision of the future, and she wept quietly as she tried to hide the agony she felt.

Arlene knew the medical histories of her parents and other relatives. Heart trouble, diabetes, and other diseases related to weight problems were prevalent, and Arlene had been over-weight all of her life. She knew her days were numbered if she didn't do something about her weight, and soon. It wasn't that Arlene had just discovered she was heavy. On the contrary, if medals were given for courage, willpower, and extreme effort in dieting, Arlene would deserve the highest that could be awarded. She had, however, through her superhuman effort at trying to control her weight, actually dieted herself to a life-time high of 326 pounds.

As for her background, Arlene was born into the perfect environment to become an overweight adult. At birth, she weighed 9 pounds, 5 ounces. Food was a big part of her early life because her family owned the best bakery in Savannah, Georgia. Her family had eight heavy, big-boned, tall brothers and sisters who were family-oriented. All holidays and Friday nights were celebrated by eating a generous meal. Good pastries and breads were always available — but her family did not care for vegetables of any kind.

After graduating from college, Arlene married Norman Jaffie, and began her nineteen-year career as a nursery school teacher. She felt she had the perfect job — she received love from the children no matter how she looked. During this period, the only time she managed to control her weight was through each of her three pregnancies. Because Arlene was vitally concerned about having healthy children and was, therefore, under the direct care of an obstetrician, she actually lost weight.

Trying desperately to lose weight, including fifteen years as a customer of a national weight-loss program, Arlene tried every diet that came along. One year before her son's Bar Mitzvah was to be held, she weighed 301 pounds. Arlene wanted to look nice for this special occasion, so she had a local doctor in Savannah wire her jaws shut. As Arlene lost weight, however, she developed serious side effects. At times, the

lower part of her body would have no feeling. Because of lost equilibrium, her balance became more and more difficult. Falling down became a major problem, and she was hospitalized twice during this time. Neurologists took numerous tests and, of course, they discovered that Arlene had a very serious vitamin deficiency. They informed her that the state of her health was similar to that of victims of the concentration camps of World War II and they were doubtful that she would be normal even after treatment.

Her doctor insisted that she have the wires removed. But Arlene was so determined to look nice for the Bar Mitzvah that she kept them on for the entire year. No one can even imagine the pain and suffering she endured that year for the sake of losing weight. The reward for her sacrifice was a hundred-pound weight loss, and an attractive appearance at her son's Bar Mitzvah. She paid the price of pain and poor health to the point of nearly causing her death — just to be presentable so her son would be proud of her. Within two months after that, she gained all hundred pounds back.

Arlene's doctor had a colleague, Dr. Lynch, whose wife had lost seventy-five pounds and, in fact, was a Counselor with Diet Center. He recommended the diet to Arlene.

Arlene's motivation to diet came during the confirmation of her daughter. She started at Diet Center the next day, June 1, 1981. At the first weigh-in, Arlene was recorded at 326 pounds. But the weight came off steadily.

Sharon, Arlene's Diet Counselor, and Arlene became very close friends. Arlene included vegetables with her meals for the very first time in her life. She enjoyed learning about foods and how to control her eating through proper nutrition. She did not realize how poorly she had felt until she began to feel so good.

On August 26, 1982, Arlene reached her goal of 141 pounds. With much determination and a lot of help from Sharon Lynch, Arlene had lost 185 pounds and 149½ inches in just fourteen months and twenty-five days. The spirit of Diet Center was passed on, and today, if you happen to enter the office of Diet Center at the Professional Plaza on Paulsen Street in Savannah, Georgia, you may see two lovely ladies counseling dieters and enjoying every minute of it. You better believe they know what they are talking about, because they have both lost weight on the Diet Center Program and have changed their entire lives. One is Sharon Lynch, a super Counselor. The other, well, is Sharon's newest Counselor and

dear friend — who looks beautiful and feels wonderful — Arlene Jaffie, a lovely lady with a bright and healthy future.

*   *   *

There are many dieters who will read and follow the diet in this book. They will succeed because this diet works. But there are many of you who, like me, need a person who can help you through very tough days. Someone who cares; someone who understands your frustrations, your hopes, fears, and desires. Someone who can help you to return to the diet when you failed miserably the day before. Someone who can give you the vision of what you can become.

For people like me it must be recognized that everything helpful about this comprehensive program simply could not be included between the covers of a book. For this is not just a "diet," but an exciting new concept — a whole new way of living.

Many of you will be interested to know how the Diet Center operates, how it differs from other organizations, and why it has been so successful. Essentially, our program is based on *service,* a service which includes daily counseling for positive reinforcement, education about the body, nutrition, emotions and stress, and information on every aspect of dieting. This service is performed by thousands of qualified Counselors throughout the United States and Canada. They know this Program works. They are "Counselors Who Care."

Our Counselors' secret for success is easy to determine. It is because they are interested in YOU. More importantly, they have struggled against this same illness and have found a permanent solution.

With your Counselor's help, you will begin to understand the serious nature of your illness. You will learn how great you can feel just by eating nutritious foods. The two of you will work together to help you stay on the Program. Soon, any challenge will become a shared laugh and the reassurance that "Yes, you can meet that challenge; yes, you are in control!"

These dedicated people provide a special reassurance. Not only because they believe in you, but because they have succeeded as well! They know that success is possible for you as it has been for the millions of Diet Center dieters across the United States and Canada who have found permanent success.

The daily weigh-in/consultation session that dieters receive is one of the key ingredients to success. Your Counselor will

meet with you *privately, each day.* To the dieter, this daily session becomes far more than just an "appointment." Such specialized attention helps to solve potential problems and difficulties often before they are even noticed. Dieters find the ten minutes they spend with their Counselor helps them to stay on the diet for the entire day. Each day is a commitment.

Most importantly, it involves people helping other people to help themselves, yet offers a high level of professional service. It is an exciting place to be. It is a place where you can gain that exhilarating feeling of, "Yes, I'm on my way to success!" Gene Fitzke found success that he never dreamed was possible.

Gene was carefully watching the progress of Marilyn, his sister-in-law. She had just started going to Diet Center and had lost 28¼ pounds in just six weeks.

Although Gene realized he desperately needed to lose weight, he just wasn't in the right frame of mind. What he needed was not a diet, but a miracle! Even though he was unusually tall (6'7") and had a large frame, his excess weight (210 pounds extra!) was a health threat. This excess weight also caused his feet to hurt until he could hardly walk. His doctor warned him continually about his high blood pressure. But that didn't hurt as much as his embarrassing, heavy breathing and the cold stares he received from strangers in public.

It was near the end of October 1979, right before Gene and his wife, Gail, were leaving for a special vacation to California, that Gene got a terrible nosebleed. It seemed as if it would never stop!

Once again, his doctor warned him of his high blood pressure and explained that the nosebleed may have been a blessing in disguise; possibly, it may have alleviated a stroke.

Gene had been looking forward to spending some leisurely time with Gail; but, once again, his weight problem hampered their trip by bringing about embarrassing situations. Not only was it difficult to fit into the airplane seat, but when the food was served, his tray could not be lowered because of his protruding stomach. He decided this was the last straw.

After coming home from their trip, Gene decided he was ready to diet. By this time, Marilyn had already lost 54 pounds and went on to lose 46 more (a total of 100 pounds). With the holidays coming up, a little added incentive would surely help. That's when Gene and his boss Jerry made a bet.

In less than one year, Gene Fitzke lost 210 pounds and learned how to maintain his ideal weight, with the Diet Center Program.

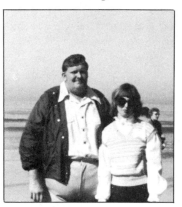

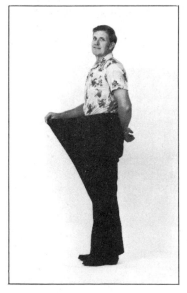

Jerry's cigarettes were as addicting as Gene's food and, certainly, as damaging. His doctors had warned him to quit smoking — or else. The bet was on; the stakes were high — one thousand dollars! In order for Gene to win, he had to lose 100 pounds in six months' time; and Jerry had to be off cigarettes for at least six weeks before Gene reached goal if it were to be a draw.

Many dieters who want to lose weight for a special function or occasion figure how long it will take them to lose if they are perfect on their Reducing Diet, then they don't start dieting until just that long before the event. This was Jerry's plan in his attempt to stop smoking. He kept an eye on Gene's progress, planning to quit just six to eight weeks before Gene's anticipated target date. As is often the case with a dieter, Jerry never quite found the "right day" to stop smoking. (He lost the bet, and Gene lost 100 pounds in just four months!)

Ah, the magic 100! This was not new to Gene; he had done it before, although not that fast. You see, he had been on many, many diets — high-protein, low-carbohydrate — even acupuncture. But this time, on the Diet Center Program, Gene didn't start gaining weight at the 100-pound mark as he had before. He went on to lose another 110 pounds in the next 7½ months, making a total weight loss of 210 pounds in just 11½ months.

When asking Gene just how he accomplished this great feat, he gave a lot of credit to his wife, Gail, who not only gave moral support, but also prepared his nutritious Diet Center meals. "I was really surprised to learn how little food my body actually requires, when it is the right type of food," reported Gene. "I was never even hungry. With the daily encouragement from my Diet Center Counselor, Gloria Pitney (the help she gave with each and every problem, and the praise with each and every pound), how could I go wrong? She knew I could make it to my goal. Her continued support and faith in me made me all the more determined to succeed. The way she guided me through each pound — I just couldn't let her down."

When speaking of the joys his weight loss has brought, Gene smiles as he talks of the things he now does with his family, his lovely wife, teenage daughter, and his six-year-old son. "All the movies, ball games, symphonies, etc. . . . I hate to think of all the things I've missed the last few years," he says.

"What a thrill it is to be able to buy a suit; it used to be quite an ordeal. The tall-man shops never had anything with a 64-

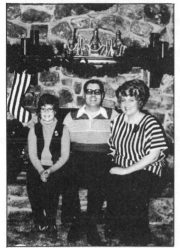

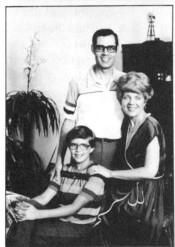

Van, Carolyn, and Kristy Osborn demonstrate the effectiveness of the Diet Center Program. Together, they lost 217 pounds and have maintained their ideal weights ever since.

inch waist, while the stout-man shops never had pants with a 38-inch inseam," he added.

Not only has it made a difference in Gene's life, but also his daughter Tami's. She, too, had had a tendency toward being overweight. But now, she has become more aware of the foods she eats and how they affect her body. Her figure isn't all that has benefited — so has her relationship with her father. She no longer needs to feel guilty that she was sometimes ashamed "to be seen with Dad." Although she always loved him deeply, she could not help but be affected by the offhand remarks made by her friends.

Gail, once again, has an escort to community and cultural affairs; Tami has a father to take her to school functions; and Jeremy, Gene's son, can run and play games with him.

Today, Gene knows the importance of eating foods high in nutritional value, eating on time, and on a schedule. He also knows that he never needs to be deprived of an active, healthy life, for he will never again be overweight.

Gene has maintained his ideal goal weight for over two years, and he realizes that if he gains a few pounds, he can call Gloria and she can immediately help him. She is his friend and will always be there to help him and Marilyn keep their weight under control.

The Diet Center Program has helped millions of individuals overcome the problem of excess weight. Entire families have also changed their lives through our nutritionally balanced Program. One such family, the Osborns of Jacksonville, Arkansas, lost a combined total of 217 pounds! For over nine years, Carolyn Osborn worked as a home economist teaching nutrition to low-income mothers, yet at the same time she was struggling with her own weight problem. Following a car accident and weighing an all-time high of nearly 300 pounds, Carolyn came to Diet Center. Her success at losing 136 pounds inspired her husband to lose 62 pounds and their daughter, Kristy, to lose 19 pounds all at Diet Center. As Carolyn describes, "I had fallen into a vat of fat and the only thing that saved me from myself was my Counselor's outstretched hand. . . . Diet Center makes getting your life back together such a joy — because you see success from the very beginning — all the way to your goal!"

I guess that's what Diet Center Spirit is all about, knowing that you can "win at the losing game" with a "Counselor Who Cares." Your Counselor has a personal and professional in-depth knowledge of the illness of obesity. He or she understands how this illness affects you physically, emotionally, and mentally and is there to help you obtain this same insight. You will learn how to "cope" with feelings and situations and you will be instructed in the basic behaviors that make dieting so much easier.

Your Counselor will also help to explain the role that stress plays in your life. The amount and types of stress often vary greatly from individual to individual. Your Counselor will help you to determine what areas of your life are stressful and could, consequently, have a direct affect on your weight loss. You will also be instructed in the skills of relaxation and visualization that will allow you to control stress and focus on success.

Counselors are professional and will work closely with your personal physician, specialist, psychiatrist, or whatever other professionals are involved in your life to help you receive the maximum benefits of this Program. We are not medical doctors. More importantly, we do not pretend to be. Counselors do not diagnose or prescribe. Instead, we believe that no one knows your health history better than you and your personal physician. Therefore, we will work closely with you and your doctor. The most important goal at Diet Center is attaining and maintaining optimum health.

Besides daily counseling at Diet Center, a dieter will also receive the Diet Center Supplement,* which was specially formulated for use in conjunction with the Diet Center Reducing Program.

The Diet Supplement is not a placebo or appetite suppressant. Its unique formulation helps the body to function in the way it was meant to. It helps with the metabolism. Dieters who use the supplement have found that they have great levels of energy, they do not crave sweets, and more importantly, they are not hungry even during the Reducing Phase of the Program. The Diet Supplement helps dieters maintain a stable blood sugar concentration, which, I believe, is the main key to effective dieting.

At each Diet Center, there is a glow of warmth and understanding, sharing and caring. It is called "The Diet Center Spirit." This spirit appears in a hundred different forms each

---

* The Diet Center Supplement is manufactured and distributed exclusively by Diet Center, Inc.

day. It is seen in the tears and smiles of a dieter as she reaches a weight she cannot remember being at since the eighth grade. The hugs and laughter of a dieter who reaches goal after losing anywhere from ten to twenty to hundreds of pounds. The recognition and admiration of fellow dieters for achieving the "Winner of the Week" award at a Nutrition/Behavior Modification Class. Or, the heartfelt congratulations of a dieter who has regained control of her life.

The Diet Center Spirit began with my first successful dieter who, in turn, endeavored to do everything she could as a Counselor helping other dieters. The chain has never stopped since that point. Our Counselors are the most unique group of professionals you will ever meet. Not only do they instruct and guide each dieter, but they provide the daily support and honest concern that is so vital to success. Each one, however, possesses the same common denominator — a love for and a belief in the Program and the genuine desire to help overweight and obese people everywhere.

It is this belief and this Spirit that I endeavor to take with me wherever I go. It is the same message I want to give you through this book. If you are overweight and are looking for a solution, don't give up! If you feel like you have tried every drug, pill, diet, book and exercise and yet have failed to accomplish your goal, don't give up! If you attempt the Diet Center Program through using this book, but you need further help, don't give up!

This Program found in the pages of this book is medically sound and will produce results. If you follow the Program, I promise you that you will lose weight. But if you do need further help, you will find at your nearest Diet Center a dedicated professional Counselor who is trained to give you just that. Each one gives all, plus more, to each and every dieter. Experience the exhilaration in your life and that of your fellow dieters as you see the tremulous smile on the face of a dieter who has successfully lost weight. Through the Diet Center Program you will again believe that there is a way to permanently control the problems of being overweight. Finally, you will know that you *can* achieve a healthful lifestyle — one where you are slim, happy, and in control.

XII

DIET CENTER RECIPES

Diet Center Reducing Recipes
for Women and Men

INTRODUCTION

These recipes were specifically designed to provide delicious alternatives while on the Reducing Diet. Some of these recipes are used in conjunction with the Women's Seven-Day Reducing Menu Planner, pages 130–135. The others can provide zest and variety to keep your dieting exciting! Never succumb to the boredom of the same chicken salad every noon or broiled fish each night. Use your imagination to create new combinations of vegetables, fruits and proteins.

Remember these important points, however, when using recipes:

1. Make sure you know the diet EXACTLY before you begin adding recipes. It is a good idea to stick to the basics — 3½ ounces of protein twice per day, 2 fruits, 1 large (5–7 vegetable) salad, 1 cooked vegetable serving and 2 bread servings — for up to two weeks before you begin combining foods.

2. Eat only while at the table! Those "tastings" and "nibblings" all count as part of your daily food intake. You may want to eat an apple and sip a glass of water while preparing meals. Save your food for the properly scheduled times!

3. Don't substitute! Follow these recipes exactly as outlined. Use only those amounts listed. Adding or subtracting even a "little" could have a negative effect on your weight loss.

4. These recipes have been specifically designed for use with Diet Center seasonings. If you wish an alternate, choose a product that does not contain sugar and is low in sodium, fats and preservatives.

5. Review the material presented in "Before Even Beginning

to Diet." Remember, *how* you prepare your foods can be just as important as the foods themselves!

The following sections are included within this chapter:

Appetizers, Condiments and dips
Breads
Desserts
Eggs
Chicken
Fish and Seafoods
Other Protein Dishes
Beverages
Salads and Salad Dressings
Vegetables

APPETIZERS, CONDIMENTS AND DIPS

CHICKEN LIVER PÂTÉ

14 oz. chicken livers
2 tsp. minced garlic
1 small onion, chopped
2 Tbsp. apple cider vinegar
½ tsp. parsley flakes
Dash salt
Dash pepper
1 hard-cooked egg

Place all ingredients (except egg) in baking dish. Stir, and microwave on high for 6 to 8 minutes, or until meat loses its pinkness. Stir at half cooking time. Drain. Place livers and egg in blender, adding cooking liquid 1 Tbsp. at a time until pâté is thick and smooth.

Spread pâté on reducing crackers (see page 127), cucumber or zucchini slices, celery sticks, or spoon into mushroom centers.

Yield: 4 servings.

DIET CENTER MAYONNAISE

1 egg
2 Tbsp. apple cider vinegar
⅛ tsp. dry mustard
½ tsp. salt
Dash pepper
Garlic powder to taste
Onion powder to taste
¾ cup corn or safflower oil

Place all ingredients (except oil) in blender. Blend on high, adding oil slowly. Mixture will become very thick. Store in refrigerator in a tightly covered jar. Mayonnaise will keep for several weeks. Stir if separation occurs.

Yield: 1 cup. Each serving (1 Tbsp.) = daily oil allowance.

WILDBERRY JAM

2 cups fruit, blackberries, blueberries, raspberries (or others)
1 tsp. no-calorie sweetener
1 tsp. lemon juice
Dash cinnamon
1 package unflavored gelatin
¾ cup water

Mash fruit in pan. Fold in remaining ingredients. Let stand 1 minute. Heat over medium heat until gelatin dissolves. Pour into container and chill until set.

Yield: 1 quart.

DIET CENTER STUFFED CELERY STICKS

8 6-inch celery stalks
1 8-oz. cake tofu
1 Tbsp. lemon juice
2 tsp. dry mustard
1 tsp basil
1 tsp. dill
Dash of salt
Dash of paprika

Clean celery stalks and cut into eight, 6-inch pieces. Blend all additional ingredients (except paprika) thoroughly. Fill celery stalks. Sprinkle with paprika. Serve.

BREADS

4 Melba rounds
2 Wasa Brod crackers (Lite
  Rye)
¼ cup (or more) water
2 tsp onion, minced
2 Tbsp. mushrooms, minced
2 Tbsp. celery, minced
Dash sage
Dash Diet Center "buttery flavored salt"*
Diet Center Poultry Seasoning*
Dash pepper

SAGE STUFFING

Crush Melba toast and crackers. Add remaining ingredients and mix well. Dressing should be reasonably moist but not sticky. Use as dressing with Stuffed Chicken Breasts (page 320) or bake for 20 minutes at 350°.

Yield: 4 servings.

APPLE-BRAN PANCAKES

2 eggs, beaten
1 Tbsp. Diet Center Protein
  Powder (vanilla)*
1 grated apple, peeled
2 Tbsp. bran
Dash cinnamon or nutmeg
⅛ tsp. vanilla

Mix all ingredients together. Drop onto hot skillet sprayed with Pam (or similar product) and "fry" as for pancakes.

Yield: 1 serving.

* Diet Center products may be purchased at your local Diet Center.

DIET CENTER'S BRAN MUFFINS

3 tablespoons water
3 Tbsp. non-fat powdered milk
1 Tbsp. no-calorie sweetener
¾ apple, cored
¼ tsp. vanilla extract
4 drops almond extract
Pinch of cinnamon
Pinch of nutmeg
4–6 Tbsp. unprocessed bran

Place all ingredients (except bran) in blender. Blend until apple is chunky. Pour into bowl and add bran. Divide batter among 4 cupcake holders and bake at 350° for 35 minutes.

Yield: 4 muffins.

LO-CAL DELICIOUS DESSERTS

APPLE COOKIES

1 egg, beaten
2 Tbsp. Diet Center Protein
  Powder*
1½ tsp. (nonfat powdered) milk
½ tsp. artificial sweetener
⅛ tsp. soda
¼ tsp. cinnamon
⅛ tsp. nutmeg
½ tsp. vanilla
1 apple, grated
2 Tbsp. unprocessed bran

Combine beaten egg, protein powder, milk, sweetener, soda, and spices with vanilla. Beat well. Add grated apple and bran. Drop by teaspoonful onto cookie sheet sprayed with Pam (or similar product). Bake at 350° for 12–15 minutes.

Yield: 1 serving.

APPLE FLUFF

6 Red Delicious apples
2 envelopes unflavored gelatin
⅓ cup water
Cinnamon to taste
Nutmeg to taste
3 egg whites
No-calorie sweetener
½ tsp. vanilla
Grated rind from 1 orange

Cut top ⅛ inch off apple. With a spoon scoop out inside, leaving a thin shell. Brush inside of shell with lemon juice so it doesn't turn brown. Cut up pulp from apple. Cook until clear. Put into blender and blend until smooth. Dissolve gelatin in water, on the stove, until mixture becomes clear. Add to blender with apples. Add cinnamon, nutmeg, and sweetener. Refrigerate until you can spoon it (partially set).

Beat egg whites until stiff, then add sweetener and vanilla. Mix together with apple mixture. Spoon back inside apple and top with orange rind. Eat just like an apple.

Yield: 6 servings.

APPLE PIE

CRUST:
½ apple
1 egg
¼ tsp. no-calorie sweetener
¼ tsp. cinnamon
¼ tsp. nutmeg
2 Tbsp. Diet Center Vanilla
  Protein Powder*
1½ tsp. vanilla
2 Tbsp. unprocessed bran

FILLING:
2 apples, shredded or ground
½ tsp. apple pie spice
No-calorie sweetener to taste
2 packages unflavored gelatin,
  dissolved in hot water
1 tsp. vanilla or butternut flavoring

To prepare crust, blend ingredients and pour into an 8-inch pie plate sprayed with Pam (or similar product). Cover side of pie pan with crust.

To prepare filling, blend until foamy. Pour into center of pie plate. Bake in preheated 350° oven for 40 minutes. Remove from oven and cool for 2 hours before serving.

Yield: 8 servings.

APRICOT FLUFF

1 can orange diet soda
1 package unflavored gelatin
2 tsp. lemon juice
Dash allspice
Dash nutmeg
1 (8-oz.) can "dietetic" apricots
  (no added sugar or syrups,
  preferably water-packed),
  chopped

Pour 1 can diet soda into small pan and sprinkle with gelatin. Let stand 5 minutes. Heat over moderate heat until gelatin is dissolved. Add ½ cup liquid from fruit, lemon juice, and spices. Mix together and chill until partially thickened. Pour apricots and gelatin mixture into blender and blend until fluffy. Pour back into pan. Chill until gelatin is set.

Yield: 2 servings.

BAKED APPLE

1 Rome apple, cut in half and
  cored
1 can black cherry or strawberry
  diet soda
Dash no-calorie sweetener
Dash cinnamon

Place apple in baking dish skin-side down. Pour soda over apple. Sprinkle with sweetener and cinnamon. Bake in preheated 350° oven for 25 to 30 minutes. (*Microwave alternative:* 2½ minutes baking time.)

Yield: 1 serving.

FRESH FRUIT CUP

1 cup sliced peaches
Lemon juice
1 cup blueberries
1 cup raspberries
1 cup strawberries
1 cup blackberries

Slice peaches into lemon juice (to avoid discoloring). Gently combine with remainder of fruit. Place 1 cup mixed fruit in 5 dessert glasses.

Yield: 5 servings.

FRUIT AMBROSIA

2 cups cantaloupe balls
1 cup blueberries
2 cups honeydew balls
2 12-oz. cans diet 7-Up (or similar soda)

Layer cantaloupe balls in the bottom of a transparent bowl. Add layer of blueberries. Top with honeydew balls and pour chilled diet 7-Up over fruit. Serve immediately.

Yield: 5 servings.

(For Fresh-Fruit Salad, see Salad Section.)

FRUITY CHEESECAKE

8 oz. tofu, pressed
1 12-oz. can diet creme soda, room temperature
No-calorie sweetener to taste
½ tsp. pure vanilla extract
2 packages gelatin (dissolved in ⅓ cup hot water)

Put in blender: Tofu, sweetener and vanilla. Blend well while slowly pouring in the creme soda. Add the gelatin-water mixture. Blend one minute. Pour into a one quart casserole sprayed with Pam. Refrigerate 2 hours or up to 3 days. If storing longer than 2 hours, cover tightly with plastic wrap.

Optional Fruit Topping: In a small saucepan combine 1 cup blueberries (or 1 fruit serving of any fruit except citrus from the reducing list) with ½ cup water and sweetener to taste. Bring fruit mixture to simmer. Meanwhile, dissolve one package gelatin in ⅓ cup hot water. Stir the gelatin into the fruit mixture after taking fruit off the stove. Refrigerate. When almost set (stir after 15 minutes), spread the fruit mixture over the cheesecake.

Yield: 4 servings.

POP SQUARES

2½ cups black cherry diet soda
4 packages unflavored gelatin

Pour diet soda into a small saucepan. Sprinkle gelatin over diet soda; let stand 3 to 4 minutes. Warm mixture over medium heat until gelatin is completely dissolved. Pour into a 9-inch square pan. Chill until firm. Cut in 1-inch squares and serve.

Yield: 81 one-inch squares.

BAKED APPLES (MICROWAVE)

4 medium apples
½ cup diet raspberry soda
Dash cinnamon

Core apples. Place in custard cups. Fill each cavity with diet soda and sprinkle with cinnamon. Cover with plastic wrap. Microwave on high 4 minutes or until tender. At half cooking time, turn a half turn. Let stand 1 or 2 minutes and serve warm.

Yield: 4 servings.

PEACH "ICE CREAM"

1 peach, peeled
6 ice cubes
1 Tbsp. nonfat powdered milk
½ tsp. vanilla
¼ tsp. almond extract
No-calorie sweetener to taste

Blend all ingredients in blender until smooth. Spoon into dish. Serve immediately.

Yield: 1 serving.

STRAWBERRY PARFAIT

1 package unflavored gelatin
¼ cup ice water
½ cup boiling water
Dash no-calorie sweetener
½ tsp. strawberry extract (optional)
1 cup fresh or frozen unsweetened strawberries, diced
3 egg whites, stiffly beaten

Soften gelatin in cold water. Add boiling water and stir until dissolved. Add (optional) strawberry extract. Add sweetener. Stir well and refrigerate until completely set. Whip lightly with whisk or electric mixer. Fold in strawberries. Fold entire mixture into stiffly beaten egg whites. Spoon into 6 stemmed goblets, custard cups, or parfait glasses.

Yield: 6 servings.

EGG DISHES

DIET CENTER CUSTARD

1½ quarts water
1 cup non-fat powdered milk
9 eggs
1 Tbsp. no-calorie sweetener
1 tsp. vanilla
Dash nutmeg

Blend all ingredients (except vanilla) in blender. Add vanilla. Pour into double boiler and sprinkle top with nutmeg. Cook until a knife inserted in the center comes out clean.

Yield: 9 servings.

MUSHROOM OMELET

5 medium mushrooms, sliced, or
1 4-oz. jar mushroom pieces,
    washed and drained
Dash Diet Center "buttery flavor
salt"*
1 egg

Sauté mushrooms in a no-stick skillet, using a small amount of "buttery flavor salt." Brown evenly. Beat egg until foamy and add to the mushrooms. Lower heat and allow egg to cook evenly but not brown. Fold over and serve immediately. Serve with Melba toast and a fresh orange.

Yield: 1 serving.

SPINACH "SOUFFLÉ"

3 egg whites (beaten until stiff)
3 egg yolks (beaten)
1 cup cooked spinach (drained)
Dash salt
Dash pepper
Dash cayenne

Beat 3 egg whites till stiff. Fold in the 3 beaten yolks, drained spinach, salt, pepper, and cayenne. Bake in a small dish at 325°–350° for approximately 45 minutes, until puffed and slightly browned. Test for doneness by inserting a table knife in the center. "Soufflé" is done when knife comes out clean.

Yield: 1 serving. Equals 1 protein portion and 1 cooked vegetable portion.

TOFU QUICHE

CRUST:
  1 egg
  6 Wasa Brod (Lite Rye)
  ¼ tsp. dillweed
  ¼ tsp. onion powder
  3 Tbsp. water

FILLING:
16 oz. tofu
  2 eggs
  1 cup spinach, cooked
Dash garlic
Dash onion powder
½ tsp. salt
Dash pepper
½ cup water
  2 thin slices onion
½ cup mushrooms

To prepare crust: Blend all ingredients in blender and let stand 5 minutes. Pour mixture into a small cake pan sprayed with Pam (or similar product).

   To prepare filling: Blend tofu, eggs, spinach, and remaining seasonings. Pour mixture into crust mixture. Crust mixture will be pushed to the edges of the pan, encircling the filling to form the crust. Place mushrooms and onions in a circle on top of filling. Bake at 350° for 1 hour.

Yield: 3 servings.

DIET CENTER DEVILED EGGS

3 hard-cooked eggs
Diet Center "the good stuff
    seasoning"* to taste
Dash of salt and pepper
⅛ tsp. prepared mustard
2 Tbsp. apple cider vinegar
Paprika

Peel and halve the hard-cooked eggs. Remove the yolks and mash with seasoning, salt, pepper, mustard, apple cider vinegar and add a few drops of water if needed. Fill egg-white halves with mixture and sprinkle with paprika.

Yield: 6 deviled eggs.

CHICKEN

CHICKEN BREASTS IN ORANGE SAUCE

4 4-oz. chicken breasts, boned
    and skinned
½ tsp. onion powder
    Dash pepper
1 orange, peeled and blended
½ tsp. Kikkoman soy sauce (or
    other low-sodium product)
1 tsp. grated orange peel
¼ tsp. coriander

Sprinkle chicken breasts with onion powder and pepper. Place in a small baking dish.

Stir remaining ingredients together and pour over breasts. Cover with wax paper. Bake at 325° for 1 hour 15 minutes or microwave for 20 minutes (or more if needed) on medium until meat loses its pinkness and is tender. Serve with sauce.

Yield: 4 servings.

CHICKEN CHOW MEIN

5 Tbsp. water
2 green onions, sliced
¼ cup green pepper, diced
¼ cup celery, chopped
¼ cup mushroom pieces
½ cup bean sprouts (preferably
    fresh)
1 cooked chicken breast, cut in
    bite-size pieces
Pinch salt
Pinch pepper

Place vegetables, water, and chicken in no-stick pan and simmer until vegetables are tender-crisp. Salt and pepper lightly.

Yield: 1 serving.

SKEWER CHICKEN (MICROWAVE)

6 6-inch wooden skewers
2 chicken breasts, boned and
    skinned, cut in 12 pieces
1 zucchini, cut in 12 pieces
1 apple, cut in 12 pieces
1 tsp. lemon juice
1 Tbsp. water
Dash Diet Center "buttery flavor
    salt"*
Pepper

On skewers, alternate chicken, zucchini, and apple, repeating once. Combine lemon juice and water. Brush on kabobs. Season lightly. Cover with wax paper. Microwave on medium heat 8 to 12 minutes or until chicken loses its pink color. At half cooking time, turn over; baste and turn rack.

Yield: 2 servings (3 skewers each).

CHICKEN KABOBS

4 oz. raw chicken (cut in 4
   pieces)
2 slices of each of the following:
   apple, cabbage, green pepper,
   mushroom, onion, zucchini
Diet Center Poultry Seasoning*
Diet Center "nice 'n spicy seasoning"* (or other seasonings
   of your choice)
Onion powder
Garlic powder
1 egg, beaten
1 Wasa Brod (Lite Rye),
   crushed
Chicken broth (from cooked
   chicken)

Alternate chicken and vegetables on a skewer and season with
spices. Dip in egg and roll in Wasa Brod. Cook in a covered
pan with ¼-inch chicken broth (if no broth, use water) for 1½
hours at 350°.

Yield: 1 serving.

CROCKPOT CHICKEN

4 chicken breasts, boned and
   skinned
2 stalks celery, chopped
½ cup onion, chopped
1 tsp. garlic powder
¼ tsp. curry powder
1 Tbsp. chopped parsley
Salt to taste

Place all ingredients in crockpot. Do not add water. Cook on
high for 2½ hours. Store leftover chicken, broth, and vegetables in individual serving packages in freezer for easy reheat-
ing.

Yield: 4 servings.

STUFFED CHICKEN BREASTS

4 skinned and boned chicken
   breasts (4-oz. each)
4 portions of Sage Stuffing (page
   313)

Pound chicken breasts until flat. Place ¼ of dressing in the
center of each breast and roll up. Wrap each breast in foil.
Bake for 40 minutes at 350°.

Yield: 4 servings.

DIET CENTER MUSHROOM-STUFFED CHICKEN WITH SAUCE

4 whole chicken breasts
4 Wasa Brod (Lite Rye), broken in small pieces
4 Tbsp. onion, minced finely
4 Tbsp. celery, minced
1½ cups cooked mushrooms, chopped
1½ tsp. sage
Dash salt and pepper
4 Tbsp. water (enough to moisten dressing)

Wash chicken thoroughly, including cavity. Mix Wasa Brod, onion, celery, mushrooms, seasonings and water. Stuff chicken. Place in an open pan and cook 30 minutes at 350°. Cover pan and cook 30 more minutes. Serve with Mushroom Sauce (below).

Yield: 4 servings.

DIET CENTER MUSHROOM SAUCE

8 oz. tofu, pressed
1 cup fresh mushrooms, diced
2 Tbsp. plus 2 tsp. water
2 Tbsp. plus 2 tsp. lemon juice
Diet Center "buttery flavor salt"*
Pepper to taste

Place all ingredients in blender. Blend and serve.

DIET CENTER ROLLED BREADED CHICKEN BREASTS

4 3½-oz. portions chicken breasts, boned, skinned and pounded to ½ original thickness
4 Ak-Mak crackers, crushed
4 Tbsp. unprocessed bran
Seasonings to taste: poultry seasoning, pepper, Diet Center "the good stuff seasoning"*
1 egg, beaten with 1 tsp. water

Mix Ak-Mak, bran, and seasonings. Dip chicken breasts in egg mixture. Roll in crumbs and place on baking sheet sprayed with Pam (or similar product). Bake in preheated 400° oven for 20 minutes. Reduce heat to 350° and cook for an additional 10 minutes. Test chicken with a fork.

Yield: 4 servings.

SWEET-AND-SOUR CHICKEN

2 Tbsp. onion, chopped
¼ cup apple cider vinegar
No-calorie sweetener to taste
1 orange, peeled
4 chicken breasts, boned and skinned
Dash garlic
Dash onion powder

Combine onion, vinegar, sweetener, and orange in blender and blend until pulpy. Sauté chicken in skillet sprayed with Pam (or similar product) until golden brown. Pour vinegar mixture over chicken. Season with garlic and onion powder and cover. Cook 30 minutes or until done. For variation, add one-half orange, peeled and diced.

Yield: 4 servings.

TERIYAKI CHICKEN

6 chicken breasts, boned and
   skinned
1¼ cups water
2 Tbsp. Kikkoman soy sauce
   (or other low-sodium product)
No-calorie sweetener to taste
1 clove garlic, minced or 1 tsp.
   garlic powder
½ tsp. powdered ginger

Put water, soy sauce, sweetener, garlic, and ginger in a large saucepan and bring to simmer. Add chicken breasts and simmer 30 minutes or until done. Do not overcook! Remove from heat and let cool, uncovered. Refrigerate for at least 4 hours or up to 2 days, tightly covered. Serve cold or reheat for a few minutes in the marinade just before serving.

Yield: 6 servings.

See also: Chicken Salad Supreme and Melon and Chicken Salad in the Salads and Salad Dressings section (page 326).

FISH AND SEAFOOD

CRAB CASSEROLE

4 oz. crab
2 Wasa Brod (Lite Rye),
   crushed
½ cup green pepper
1 Tbsp. onion, minced
1 tsp. lemon juice
Dash pepper

Toss all ingredients. Bake at 350° for 15 minutes or cook in microwave on high 4 to 5 minutes, turning once at half cooking time.

Yield: 1 serving.

HERB-BAKED HADDOCK

1½ lbs. haddock
4 tsp. lemon juice
1 tsp. powdered mustard
¼ tsp. oregano leaves
¼ tsp. marjoram
Dash pepper
Paprika
1 tsp. instant minced onion, re-
   hydrated in water and
   drained

Wipe fish with damp cloth and arrange in baking dish. Pour lemon juice over fish and add all remaining ingredients. Marinate at least 10 minutes. Bake at 375° for 20 minutes or until fish flakes easily with fork. Serve with lemon wedges (optional).

Yield: 6 servings.

LEMON TROUT

1 lb. trout fillets
4 slices lemon, cut in halves
¼ cup apple cider vinegar
4 Tbsp. minced onion
1 tsp. grated lemon peel
¼ tsp. pepper
1 tsp. parsley flakes
Diet Center "the good stuff
   seasoning"*

Arrange fillets in baking dish. Put 2 lemon slices on each. Combine remaining ingredients and pour over fish. Bake at 350° for 25 minutes or cover with wax paper and microwave on high 4 to 6 minutes, turning at half cooking time.

Yield: 4 servings.

RED SNAPPER

1 lb. red snapper
8 lime slices
¼ tsp. tarragon
½ tsp. onion powder
Dash pepper
Dillweed to taste

Divide snapper in four equal pieces. Place in baking dish. Combine seasonings and sprinkle on fish. Cover with wax paper. Bake at 350° for 30 minutes or microwave on high for 3 minutes. Turn dish and place 2 lime slices on each piece. Cover. Bake at 350° for 30 minutes or microwave for 3 to 4 more minutes.

Yield: 4 servings.

SHRIMP AND VEGETABLE KABOBS

26 fresh mushrooms or 1 8-oz.
   can whole mushrooms
1 green pepper, cut in large
   pieces
1 sweet onion, cut in wedges
1 lb. cooked, cleaned shrimp
½ cup apple cider vinegar
2 Tbsp. lemon juice
1 tsp. salt
1 tsp. pepper
½ tsp. garlic powder (optional)
4 large skewer sticks

Place mushrooms, green pepper, onion, and shrimp in bowl. In separate bowl, mix all remaining ingredients together; pour over vegetable-shrimp mixture. Cover and marinate overnight in refrigerator. Place drained vegetables and shrimp alternately on skewers and grill in oven or over outdoor grill until browned. Do not overcook.

Yield: 4 servings.

SHRIMP AND ZUCCHINI CASSEROLE

4 cups sliced zucchini
¼ cup onion, finely minced
2 eggs, beaten
10 oz. shrimp, precooked
4 Wasa Brod crackers (Lite
   Rye), crushed
2 tsp. celery flakes
4 tsp. parsley flakes
¼ tsp. garlic powder
¼ tsp. onion powder
¼ tsp. dry mustard
Dash of black pepper

Spray skillet and 2-quart casserole with Pam (or similar product). In skillet, stir-fry zucchini and onion until tender-crisp. In large bowl, combine eggs, shrimp, half of the crushed Wasa Brod, and seasonings. Pour into casserole. Sprinkle remaining Wasa Brod on top. Cook in preheated 350° oven for 30 minutes.

Yield: 4 servings.

TANGY SHRIMP

12 oz. shrimp
¼ cup apple cider vinegar
1 tsp. minced garlic
½ tsp. parsley flakes
⅛ tsp. tarragon
1 small bay leaf
Dash each of salt, pepper

Combine all ingredients in a 2-quart casserole dish. Cover with wax paper. Bake at 350° for 30 minutes or microwave on high for 3½ to 5 minutes, or until shrimp are opaque, stirring at half cooking time. When cooking time is up, leave in microwave for additional 3 or 4 minutes.

Yield: 3 servings.

OTHER PROTEIN DISHES

1½ lbs. ground beef heart
½ cup onions, chopped
½ cup green pepper, chopped
½ cup celery, chopped
½ cup Melba rounds, crushed
3 eggs
Dash each of:
 Salt
 Pepper
 Garlic powder

2 lbs. rabbit
Juice of 1 lemon
Diet Center "buttery flavor
 salt"*
Pepper
1 tsp. grated orange rind
1 cup orange juice with pulp
 (use 3 fresh oranges)
⅛ tsp. nutmeg
½ tsp. rosemary

1 lb. tofu
Dash onion powder
Dash garlic powder
Diet Center "nice 'n spicy"*
Diet Center "the good stuff sea-
 soning"* (or other seasonings
 as desired)

DIET CENTER MEAT LOAF

Mix all ingredients together. Place in casserole dish and bake at 350° for 1 hour.

Yield: 7 servings.

ORANGE RABBIT

Cut meat in pieces. Wash; pat dry. Rub with lemon juice. Sprinkle with pepper and "buttery flavor salt." Combine orange rind, orange juice, nutmeg, and rosemary. Pour over meat and cook at 350° for 1 hour.

Yield: 8 servings.

TOFU CROUTONS

Place tofu in freezer overnight. (Tofu changes consistency when frozen and becomes more like bread.) Take out of freezer and thaw. Pat as dry as possible without crumbling. Cut in small cubes and place on no-stick cookie sheet. Sprinkle with onion powder, garlic powder, and "the good stuff seasoning." Bake at 250° for 2 hours.

Yield: 2 servings.

TACO SALAD

3½ oz. ground beef heart
¼ cup water
Diet Center "buttery flavor
    salt"*
Dash of each of the following:
    black pepper, chili powder,
    cumin, garlic powder, onion
    powder
1 Tbsp. Diet Center Mayon-
    naise (page 312)
Shredded lettuce
2 Melba rounds (or any other
    cracker on Reducing Diet
    equivalent to 1 bread serving)
½ cup each of any of following
    vegetables: celery, chopped;
    cauliflower; cucumber, sliced;
    green pepper, chopped; mush-
    rooms, chopped; green beans
    (raw), chopped; spinach
    leaves; sprouts (alfalfa/mung
    bean); zucchini, sliced

Spray a small skillet with Pam (or similar product). Add ground beef heart and water. Cook, stirring, until beef heart is browned. Add seasonings and onion; mix well. Mix 1 Tbsp. Diet Center Mayonnaise with shredded lettuce and vegetables. Top with meat and crushed Melba rounds.

Yield: 1 serving.

BEVERAGES

3 cans lime diet soda
4 peach halves
4 large strawberries
4 lemon slices
8 mint leaves
Additional diet soda

DIET CENTER LIME-FIZZ FRUIT PUNCH

Pour diet soda into a ring mold and place in freezer. Put a strawberry in the center of each peach half. When ring is partially frozen, place fruit in mold by alternating strawberry peach halves with lemon slices and mint leaves. Freeze. Unmold and place upright in punch bowl filled with additional diet soda.

DIET CENTER MOCK COLD DUCK

6 cans red diet soda (black
    cherry, raspberry, punch)
3 cans lemon-lime diet soda
¼ cup apple cider vinegar
6 drops no-calorie sweetener

Combine all ingredients in sealed container. Flavor is best if refrigerated up to 24 hours before serving. Serve chilled.

SALADS AND SALAD DRESSINGS

1 medium head cabbage
1 green onion, chopped
1 cup chopped celery
1 green pepper, cut in strips
1 tsp. salt
1 tsp. celery seed
½ tsp. white mustard seed
1 cup apple cider vinegar
6 tsp. corn oil
No-calorie sweetener to taste
Paprika

DIET CENTER COLE SLAW

Mix together cabbage, onion, celery, and green pepper. In separate bowl, mix remaining ingredients. Pour over cabbage and mix well. Chill 6 hours. Before serving, add 2 tsp. oil and sprinkle with paprika.

Yield: 3 cups.

1 cooked chicken breast,
   chopped
½ cup celery, chopped
½ cup green pepper, chopped
2 Tbsp. onion, chopped
2 mushrooms, chopped
1 radish, chopped
1 Tbsp. Vinegar and Oil Dressing (page 330), with 2 tsp. oil
Dash each of garlic salt, poultry
   seasoning, pepper, paprika
Lettuce leaves

CHICKEN SALAD SUPREME

Combine chicken, celery, pepper, onion, mushrooms, and radish. Toss with Vinegar and Oil Dressing. Add garlic salt, poultry seasoning, pepper, and paprika to taste. Serve on bed of lettuce.

Yield: 1 serving.

1 cantaloupe
4 3½-oz. cooked chicken breasts
1 cup celery, diagonally sliced
½ cup radishes, sliced
4 Tbsp. Diet Center Mayonnaise
   (page 312)
¼ cup Egg Salad Dressing (page
   329)
Dash each of salt, pepper

MELON AND CHICKEN SALAD

Peel cantaloupe and cut in half. Remove seeds. Slice two large rings from each half of melon. In large bowl, combine reserved melon, chicken, celery, and radishes. Mix with dressing, using only as much as needed to moisten. Cover salad and chill several hours. To serve, place melon rings on salad plates and spoon chicken salad into middle of each ring.

Yield: 4 servings.

POTATO (TOFU) SALAD

2 cups cauliflower (raw)
1 cup celery, diced
4 green onions
6 hard-boiled eggs
3 Tbsp. Diet Center Mayonnaise
  (page 312)
½ cup Egg Salad Dressing (page
  329)
8 oz. tofu
Dash each of salt, pepper

Chop cauliflower, onion, celery and eggs. Mix together with Diet Center Mayonnaise, Egg Salad Dressing, and seasonings. Cut tofu in small chunks and fold in. Stir and refrigerate.

Yield: 3 servings.

RED-CABBAGE SALAD

1 cup shredded red cabbage
½ cup chopped green pepper
3 or 4 fresh spinach leaves
¼ cup grated heart of Chinese
  cabbage
¼ cup watercress

Combine all ingredients. Serve with dressing of your choice.

Yield: 1 serving.

RIBBON LAYER SALAD

1ST LAYER
2 cans diet soda (lemon-lime diet
  soda)
2 packages unflavored gelatin
3 drops green food coloring

Dissolve gelatin in soda over medium heat. Add green food coloring. Pour into mold and chill until set.

2ND LAYER
3 packages unflavored gelatin
¼ cup water
1 16-oz. can water-packed apricots
16 oz. tofu
3 drops almond flavoring
1 tsp. no-calorie sweetener

Over medium heat, dissolve gelatin in water and apricot liquid. Add remaining ingredients in blender and blend until smooth. Pour on top of first layer of gelatin. Chill until set.

3RD LAYER
2 cans orange diet soda
2 packages unflavored gelatin

Dissolve gelatin (see above instructions) in soda and pour over top of second layer. Chill until firm. Unmold onto a platter and serve.

Yield: 8 servings.

TASTY SPINACH SALAD

1 clove fresh garlic
2 tsp. corn oil
½ tsp. black pepper
1 Tbsp. apple cider vinegar
½ tsp. dry mustard
No-calorie sweetener
4 cups fresh spinach
1 hard-boiled egg, sliced

Rub the inside of the bowl, thoroughly, with garlic clove. Add next five ingredients as listed, stirring after each addition. Add spinach and toss thoroughly. Garnish with slice of hard-boiled egg.

Yield: 4 servings.

DIET CENTER SPINACH-TOSSED SALAD

2 cups raw spinach, washed and torn in bite-size pieces
2 hard-cooked eggs, sliced
2 Tbsp. Diet Center Crunchies*

Place spinach, eggs, and Crunchies on serving plate. Serve with Garlic-Vinaigrette Dressing (page 329).

Yield: Up to 3 cups equals daily salad allowance.

DIET CENTER FRESH-FRUIT SALAD

1 cup each of (frozen or fresh): blueberries, strawberries, apples, honeydew melon, peaches, blackberries, raspberries, oranges, cantaloupe

Thaw if frozen, then mix together. Serve 1 cup per person. Just before serving, pour a small amount of Diet 7-Up over it.

Yield: 9 1-cup servings.

SEAFOOD SALAD

1 recipe Tofu Dressing (page 330) or equivalent in mayonnaise (use only 2 tsp. per serving)
⅛ tsp. horseradish
2 Tbsp. lemon juice
½ cup celery, chopped
1 Tbsp. chives, minced, or green onion tops
3½ oz. cooked shrimp, diced
3½ oz. poached halibut, boned and flaked
3 hard-cooked eggs, chopped
Garnish: radish roses, fresh raw asparagus tips, tiny tender fresh raw green beans

In a large bowl, mix the Tofu Dressing, horseradish, and lemon juice. Add a bit of water if necessary. Stir dressing well. Add vegetables. Stir again. Add shrimp, halibut, and eggs. Stir well, but gently. Garnish each serving with radish roses, raw asparagus tips or fresh green beans.

Yield: 3 servings.

SHRIMP AND EGG SALAD

1 head lettuce, shredded
1 cucumber, diced
6 green onions, chopped
6 radishes, sliced
1 green pepper, chopped
2 stalks celery, chopped
¼ head cauliflower, cut in "flow-
   erettes"
Shrimp and Egg Salad Dressing
(see below)

Mix together all ingredients except last. Store in tightly sealed container in refrigerator up to 3 days. Add the Shrimp and Egg Salad Dressing before serving.

Yield: 4 servings.

DRESSINGS

SHRIMP AND EGG SALAD DRESSING

2 hard-boiled eggs
2 tsp. water
3 tsp. apple cider vinegar
2 tsp. lemon juice
Salt to taste
Pepper to taste
Garlic powder to taste
1 oz. water-packed shrimp

Put 2 hard-cooked eggs into blender; blend. Add water, vinegar, and lemon juice. Add salt, pepper, and garlic powder to taste. Blend until mixture becomes creamy. Add the shrimp to the egg mixture and serve on Shrimp and Egg Salad.

Yield: 1 serving.

EGG SALAD DRESSING

3 hard-cooked eggs
2 tsp. water
3 tsp. apple cider vinegar
2 tsp. lemon juice
Dash salt
Dash pepper
Dash garlic powder
Dash onion powder

Put 3 hard-cooked eggs in blender, blend. Add water, vinegar, and lemon juice. Add salt and pepper, and garlic powder to taste. Blend until mixture becomes creamy. Add the egg mixture to tossed salad.

Yield: 1 serving.

GARLIC-VINAIGRETTE DRESSING

2 large cloves garlic
1 cup apple cider vinegar
½ cup water
Dash coarsely ground black pepper (optional)
Dash salt
1 Tbsp. dry mustard
2 dashes no-calorie sweetener

Blend all ingredients together. Let stand one hour. You may use as much of this dressing as you wish on your salad. Add 2 tsp. oil for daily oil allowance. Refrigerate dressing in covered glass container up to 3 weeks.

Yield: 1½ cups.

VINEGAR AND OIL DRESSING

1 cup apple cider vinegar
Dash onion salt
1 Tbsp. no-calorie sweetener
Dash celery powder
Dash garlic powder
½ tsp. Diet Center "the good stuff seasoning"*
¼ tsp. black pepper
Lemon juice (optional)

Mix all ingredients together. Use as much of this dressing as desired, mixed with your 2 tsp. daily oil allowance.

Yield: 1 cup.

FRENCH DRESSING

½ cup apple cider vinegar
No-calorie sweetener to taste
1 tsp. parsley flakes
1 tsp. celery seed
1 tsp. dry mustard
Salt and pepper to taste
¼ tsp. onion powder

Mix all ingredients in a covered container and refrigerate. (A mason jar works nicely.) Shake well before using. Use 1 Tbsp. of oil (corn, safflower, or sunflower) per serving.

VARIATIONS: Any herbs or spices may be used in this recipe. Tarragon and basil are especially good.

TOFU DRESSING AND VEGETABLE DIP

8 oz. tofu, squeezed to remove excess moisture
½ cup cold water (more may be added if needed for proper consistency)
½ cup apple cider vinegar
1 cucumber, chopped, or 2 cups fresh spinach, washed and dried
6 green onions (including tops) cut in 1" pieces
3 stalks celery, chopped
No-calorie sweetener
Garlic powder
Diet Center "the good stuff seasoning"*
Dillweed
Pepper to taste

Place the first three ingredients in blender or food processor. Blend until smooth, adding more water if needed. Add remaining ingredients and blend until vegetables are mixed into the tofu mixture. It may be very smooth or chunky, depending upon your preference.

Yield: 4 servings.

VEGETABLES

3 cups "French-cut" frozen green
  beans
1 cups mushrooms, sliced
1 tsp. dehydrated onion
Diet Center "buttery flavor
  salt"*
Dash pepper, garlic powder

"FRENCH-STYLE" GREEN BEAN MEDLEY

Combine all ingredients in saucepan and simmer over low heat, steaming vegetables until tender.

Yield: 4 servings.

1 lb. fresh green beans, cut in
  1-inch pieces
1 cup mushrooms, sliced
⅓ cup onions, chopped
1 tsp. minced garlic
Dash pepper
¼ cup water
1 Tbsp. apple cider vinegar

FRESH BEANS AND MUSHROOMS

Combine all ingredients (except vinegar) in 2-quart casserole dish; cover. Bake at 375° for 45 minutes or microwave on high for 15 minutes, stirring every 3 or 4 minutes. Toss with vinegar and serve.

Yield: 3 servings.

¼ cup corn or safflower oil
1 cup whole mushrooms
1 cup frozen green beans,
  thawed
1 cup cauliflowerettes
1 green pepper, cut in strips
½ onion, cut in strips
⅔ cup apple cider vinegar
⅓ cup water
Dash each of salt, pepper
No-calorie sweetener
Hot pepper juice

MARINATED VEGETABLES

Mix oil, vinegar, water, sweetener, and seasonings. Pour over vegetables, cover and chill in the refrigerator at least 24 hours or up to 5 days. Stir occasionally.

Yield: 5 cups raw vegetables.

1 cup cabbage, finely chopped
2 Tbsp. onion, chopped
½ cup celery, finely chopped
½ cup green pepper, chopped
⅓ cup mushrooms, sliced
1 cup fresh bean sprouts
1 tsp. lemon juice
Dash garlic powder, Diet Center
  "buttery flavor salt"* (or other
  seasonings as desired), pepper

STIR-FRY VEGETABLES

Spray no-stick pan with Pam (or similar product). Combine vegetables and seasonings in pan. Cook until vegetables are clear (3 to 5 minutes). Stir in lemon juice. Serve.

Yield: 3 servings.

DIET CENTER MEN'S REDUCING AND WOMEN'S STABILIZATION RECIPES

DIET CENTER REDUCING RECIPES FOR MEN ONLY!

As noted in the chapter entitled "Dieting and Men," most men can tolerate larger quantities and varieties of foods than women and still lose optimum weight. The following recipes feature some of those foods (cottage cheese, tomatoes, tuna, turkey) which are allowed on Diet Center's Reducing Diet for Men, but are *NOT* allowed for women.

The key factor to success when using recipes is daily monitoring of your weight. Your metabolism, exercise, and stress levels may differ from the average dieter. If you fail to lose adequate weight (up to one pound per day), you may need to limit your intake to only those foods and portion sizes found on the Women's Reducing Diet.

Unlike women, men are allowed both cooked and raw vegetables at the same meal. Take advantage by enjoying a salad and cooked vegetable or soup. Men are also allowed tomatoes, which are featured in the following recipes.

ITALIAN TOMATO SAUCE

1 tomato, preferably fresh
½ cup water
½ tsp. Italian seasoning
⅛ tsp. basil
⅛ tsp. oregano
Pinch garlic powder
Pinch onion powder
Dash black pepper

Liquefy tomato in blender with water. Add seasonings. Simmer for 10 minutes or until thickened. Use as a sauce for meats or vegetables.

ITALIAN ZUCCHINI BAKE

1 zucchini, thinly sliced
½ cup low-fat cottage cheese
1 cup Italian Tomato Sauce
(page 332)

Line bottom of small casserole dish with zucchini. Spread a layer of cottage cheese. Repeat. Cover with Italian Tomato Sauce. Bake in preheated oven at 350° for 20 to 25 minutes, until sauce is bubbly and cottage cheese has started to melt.

RATATOUILLE (Tomato Vegetable Soup)

1 16-oz. can tomatoes, chopped,
or 4 fresh tomatoes, peeled
and diced
½ small onion, thinly sliced
1 cup zucchini, thinly sliced
½ green pepper, minced
Dash basil
Dash oregano
Dash black pepper
Dash salt (don't use salt if
canned tomatoes are used)

Place tomatoes in saucepan. If you are using fresh tomatoes, add a small amount of water if needed. Add onion and simmer for 2 minutes. Stir frequently. Add remaining vegetables and seasonings. Simmer, uncovered, until vegetables are tender-crisp. Delicious when made one day ahead. Serve hot or cold.

Yield: 3 servings.

TOMATO-AND-TUNA BOWL SALAD

1 fresh tomato
3½ oz. water-packed tuna,
drained
2 Tbsp. onion, minced
3 Tbsp. celery, minced
3 Tbsp. Diet Center Mayon-
naise (page 312)
¼ tsp. dillweed
Dash pepper

Cut fresh tomato in half. Remove pulp and dice. Add pulp to tuna, onion, celery, and mayonnaise. Gently mix. Add seasonings and mix. Stuff tomato halves with tuna mixture. Heat briefly under broiler or serve cold. Garnish with lettuce leaves.

Yield: 1 serving.

CHICKEN ITALIANA

2 chicken breasts, boned and
skinned
1 lb. fresh mushrooms, diced
1 onion, diced
1 clove garlic, minced
1 16-oz. can tomatoes, diced
1 green pepper, diced
1 cup water
1 tsp. Italian seasoning
½ tsp. garlic powder
¼ tsp. basil
¼ tsp. oregano
Dash pepper

Place chicken in the bottom of a large saucepan. Combine remaining ingredients and pour over chicken. Cover and simmer for 20 minutes or until chicken is done.

Yield: 2 servings.

ITALIAN-STYLE SEAFOOD STEW

2½ cups fresh tomatoes, chopped
    (include liquid)
1 clove garlic
1 bay leaf
Pinch cayenne pepper
⅛ tsp. fennel seed (optional)
½ tsp. each of thyme, basil,
    oregano
Dash black pepper
Dash salt (optional)
¼ lb. cod or other white-fleshed
    firm fish, cut in 1″ cubes
¼ lb. scallops, cut in 1″ pieces
¼ lb. raw shrimp, shelled and
    deveined

Combine tomatoes and seasonings in saucepan. Simmer for 10 minutes. Add cod and simmer gently for 2 minutes. Add scallops and simmer for another 2 minutes. Add shrimp and simmer 3 to 5 minutes, just until shrimp turns pink. Serve hot.

Yield: 3 servings.

PROTEINS

Men are allowed additional amounts and types of protein each day as compared to women including: lean beef, salmon, water-packed tuna, turkey and cottage cheese. The following recipes use these foods in dips, main dishes, soups and salads.

COTTAGE CHEESE DIP

8 oz. low-fat cottage cheese
2-5 Tbsp. apple cider vinegar
Dash onion powder
Dash chili powder
Dash garlic powder

Place cottage cheese in blender. Blend, adding apple cider vinegar to achieve dip consistency. Add seasonings to taste from the above list or of your own choosing. Blend 2 minutes or until seasonings are incorporated into the dip. Use raw vegetables for "dippers."

VARIATIONS: Add minced green pepper, green onions, celery or fresh spinach to the dip for texture, flavor and color. Parsley flakes or paprika may be added for color.

Yield: ½ cup.

VEGETABLE COTTAGE CHEESE

8 oz. low-fat cottage cheese
5 red radishes, minced
½ green pepper, chopped
½ cucumber, chopped

Combine all ingredients. Mix well. Add more vegetables if desired and your favorite seasonings.

Yield: 1 serving.

WHIPPED COTTAGE CHEESE

16 oz. low-fat cottage cheese
2 Tbsp. lemon juice

Place cottage cheese in blender or bowl (if using an electric mixer). Whip at high speed for 3 to 5 minutes or until smooth. Combine with chopped green onions, dillweed, or minced green chili for topping vegetables. Use in tuna, chicken or turkey salads or in Creamy Garlic Dressing.

CREAMY GARLIC DRESSING

2 Tbsp. whipped cottage cheese
2 tsp. oil (corn, cottonseed, saf-
    flower, sunflower, or soybean)
2 tsp. apple cider vinegar
1 tsp. lemon juice
¼ tsp. Italian seasoning
Dash garlic powder

Combine all ingredients. Blend vigorously. Serve over salad.

TUNA TREATS

3½ oz. water-packed tuna,
    drained
2 Tbsp. whipped cottage cheese
Dash onion powder
Dash Diet Center "good stuff
    seasoning"*
4 stalks celery, cleaned and cut
    into 6-inch pieces
Paprika

Combine tuna with whipped cottage cheese and seasonings. Fill celery stalks. Sprinkle with paprika.

MIDDLE-EASTERN TUNA SALAD

3½ oz. water-packed tuna,
    drained
1 Tbsp. onion, minced
2 Tbsp. celery, minced
2 Tbsp. sunflower or safflower
    oil
2 Tbsp. apple cider vinegar
Pinch dillweed
Pinch black pepepr
Pinch dried mint

Mix tuna with onion and celery. Add apple cider vinegar and oil to moisten. Add seasonings. Toss. Serve on a bed of lettuce or spinach leaves. Garnish with alfalfa or mung bean sprouts.

Yield: 1 serving.

TURKEY SOUP

3½ oz. cooked turkey, cubed
2½ cups broth
1½ cups vegetables:
    Cabbage
    Celery
    Green beans
    Onion
    Spinach
    Tomatoes
    Zucchini
All Natural Herbs — Soup Seasoning*
All Natural Herbs — Poultry Seasoning*
Dash garlic powder
Dash onion powder

Cook turkey (boil) in 2½ cups water; save broth. Combine broth and vegetables in 1-quart saucepan. Simmer on low heat until vegetables are tender. Season with soup and poultry seasonings. Add dash of garlic and onion powders. Add turkey and heat until hot.

Yield: 1 serving.

TURKEY BREAST BAKED IN MUSTARD SAUCE

4 oz. turkey breast
¼ cup prepared mustard (preferably no sugar added)
1 tsp. dehydrated parsley
¼ tsp. black pepper
¼ tsp. basil
Diet Center "the good stuff seasoning"*

Mix seasonings with mustard. Place skinned turkey breast on large piece heavy-duty foil. Spread mustard mixture over top of turkey breast. Seal foil tightly. Bake at 350° for 30 to 40 minutes. Serve hot or cold. (Handy to keep in refrigerator for a quick lunch or protein snack.)

Yield: 1 serving.

DIET CENTER WHOLE-GRAIN BREAD AND CEREAL RECIPES FOR MAINTENANCE DIETS

Nutrition-conscious homemakers should learn to use whole wheat. It has many uses: breads, cereals, rolls, or cookies. You can also substitute whole-wheat flour or other whole grains for white, sifted and unsifted flours in baking. Use 2 cups sifted whole-wheat flour when the recipe requires 2 cups unsifted flour; and use 1¾ cups of sifted whole-wheat flour when the recipe requires 2 cups sifted flour.

BRAN COOKIES

¾ cup tahini
1 cup unprocessed bran
½ cup oats
½ cup sunflower seeds
⅜ cup honey

Mix ingredients, adding honey last. Mix thoroughly. Using your hands, shape into 20 cookies. Bake on cookie sheet sprayed with Pam (or similar product) for 20 minutes at 350°.

Yield: 20 cookies.

BROWN-AND-SERVE WHOLE-WHEAT BREAD

6 cups whole-wheat flour
2 Tbsp. (2 packages) dry yeast
⅔ cup instant dry milk or scant
 ½ cup noninstant
⅓ cup brown sugar
2 Tbsp. salt
⅓ cup margarine
4 cups warm water (115° F)
3 cups enriched white flour (unbleached preferred)

In large mixer bowl, mix thoroughly: 4 cups whole-wheat flour, dry yeast, dry milk, brown sugar, and salt. Stir margarine into warm water until melted. Add to flour mixture. Beat at low speed of electric mixer ½ minute, scraping sides of bowl constantly. Beat 3 minutes at high speed.

By hand, stir in remaining 2 cups whole-wheat flour and enough white flour (approximately 1½ to 2 cups) to make a moderately stiff dough. Using remaining cup of white flour, knead dough for 10 to 12 minutes or until smooth and elastic. Place in greased bowl, turning once to grease surface. Cover and let rise in warm place until triple in bulk.

Punch down. Divide into loaves and let rest 10 minutes. Shape leaves and place in mini-loaf pans. (Mini-loaf pan size is 5x2½x2 — bottom measure.)

Shape remaining dough into 24 rolls. Let rise in warm place until double in bulk — 20 to 25 minutes.

Bake loaves at 325° for 20 to 25 minutes. Bake rolls in 325° oven for 12 to 15 minutes. *Do not brown.* Remove breads from oven and take out of pans. Cool loaves and rolls on racks. Wrap, label, and freeze loaves and rolls in plastic storage bags; secure at ends.

When ready to use, thaw to room temperature. Bake at 350° oven 10 to 12 minutes or until golden brown.

Yield: 5 mini-loaves and 2 dozen rolls.

CRACKED-WHEAT CEREAL

1 cup cracked wheat
4 cups water
1 tsp. salt

Bring cereal to a boil. Reduce heat to warm and let sit 20 to 30 minutes with lid on. (Reduce water to 3 cups if desired.) Stir frequently.

VARIATION: Cook cereal in fresh milk or reconstituted powdered milk instead of water.

Leftover cracked wheat cereal can be stored in the refrigerator in a straight-sided container. When ready to eat, slice and eat. Serve with butter and honey if desired.

Yield: 10 servings.

FRENCH TOAST

1 slice whole-wheat bread
1 egg
¼ cup milk
Dash cinnamon
No-calorie sweetener to taste

Combine milk, egg, sweetener and cinnamon. Beat to frothy foam. Dip bread in mixture and cook in no-stick pan until golden brown on both sides.

RAISIN WHOLE-WHEAT CEREAL

2 cups wheat, washed and drained (do not soak)
1 cup raisins
¼ cup brown sugar
¼ tsp. salt
2 Tbsp. honey
2 Tbsp. lemon juice
½ cup cornstarch
1 cup water

Cook wheat slowly for 2 hours in 4 cups water. Cook 1 cup raisins in enough water to cover for 15 minutes. Mix together remaining ingredients and add to raisins. Cook 2 to 5 minutes until thick, stirring often. Add to cooked wheat. Serve hot with milk. (The cereal should not need added sweetener.) May be kept in refrigerator for up to a week and warmed up as needed.

Yield: 20 servings.

SOURDOUGH STARTER

2 cups whole-wheat flour
2 cups warm water
1 package dry yeast

Make this starter only when you have forgotten to save a start or when you are making it for the first time. Combine ingredients and mix well. Place in a warm place or closed cupboard overnight. In the morning, put ½ cup of the starter in a scalded pint jar with a tight lid and store in the refrigerator or a cool place for future use. This is a sourdough starter. The remaining batter can be used immediately for pancakes, waffles, muffins, bread, or whatever you wish.

SOURDOUGH BRAN-AND-MOLASSES BREAD

2 cups sourdough starter
2 eggs
¾ cup safflower oil
¾ cup molasses
1½ cups buttermilk
3 cups bran
2 cups whole-wheat flour
1½ tsp. salt
2 tsp. baking powder
1 tsp. baking soda

Mix starter, eggs, oil, molasses, and buttermilk. Then stir in bran, whole-wheat flour, salt, baking powder and soda. Pour into a Pam-sprayed pan. Bake at 375° for 20 minutes or until done.

WHOLE-WHEAT CEREALS
Whole Wheat (Crockpot)

2 cups whole wheat, cleaned
4 cups water
1½ tsp. salt

Place all ingredients in 3½-quart crockpot. Cover and cook on low heat for 8 to 9 hours.

Yield: 20 servings.

Whole Wheat (Steamed)

1 cup whole wheat, cleaned
2 cups water
1 tsp. salt

Place ingredients in 2-quart casserole dish. Place, without lid, on a raised shelf or adapter ring of a steamer or deep kettle. Fill steamer with water within 1 inch of adapter ring. The steamer should have a tight-fitting lid, but the filled casserole should remain uncovered all the time. Bring water in bottom of pan to a full rolling boil and boil for about 15 minutes. Reduce heat to low. Steam for 10 to 12 hours or overnight.

Yield: 10 servings.

Whole Wheat (*Thermos*)

1 cup whole wheat, cleaned
2 cups boiling water
1 tsp. salt (optional)

Boil wheat for 3 minutes in water. Preheat thermos by rinsing with boiling water. Pour in boiling wheat mixture. Seal tightly and let stand overnight. It is then ready for morning cereal.

Yield: 10 servings.

NOTE: Any of the above cereals can be served with honey, milk, dates, raisins, sliced fresh fruits, etc. You can also use cooked wheat cereal from any of the above methods to make delicious pudding! (*See below.*)

WHOLE-WHEAT PUDDING

1½ cups cooked wheat
¼ cup honey
2 eggs
2 cups milk
3 drops vanilla
Cinnamon to taste

Mix sweetener, eggs, and milk in blender. Pour over cooked cereal; stir in vanilla and sprinkle with cinnamon. Bake at 325° for 30 minutes.

Yield: approximately 15 servings.

WHOLE-WHEAT FRENCH BREAD

2 Tbsp. (2 packages) yeast
½ cup warm water
2 cups hot water
3 Tbsp. sugar
1 Tbsp. salt
¼ cup melted shortening
3 cups whole-wheat flour
3 cups unbleached white flour

Dissolve yeast in ½ cup warm water. Mix hot water, sugar, salt, shortening and allow to stand until lukewarm. Add yeast and 3 cups whole-wheat flour. Beat well. Add rest of flour, beating in well. Let rest 10 minutes. Stir down. Let rest 20 minutes. Repeat 5 times. Divide into two portions. Roll each portion into 9″ x 12″ rectangle. Roll up jelly-roll style. Place in pans. Slash top three times. Brush with egg white and sprinkle sesame seed on top. Let rise 30 minutes. Bake at 400° for 35 minutes.

Yield: 2 loaves

100% WHOLE-WHEAT ROLLS (OVERNIGHT)

3 Tbsp. (3 packages) yeast
1 tsp. brown sugar
½ cup warm water (110° F)
½ cup noninstant dry milk or ¾ cup instant dry milk
½ cup vegetable oil
2 tsp. salt
½ cup brown sugar
2 cups water
2 eggs, beaten
6 cups whole-wheat flour in 2 additions

Sprinkle yeast and 1 tsp. brown sugar in ½ cup warm water. Set aside. In mixing bowl combine dry milk, vegetable oil, salt, and ½ cup brown sugar. Mix well. In a separate bowl, combine the yeast mixture, 2 cups water and eggs. Beat well for 2 minutes with electric hand mixer at medium speed. Add in dry milk, oil, etc. and mix well. Add whole-wheat flour, 3 cups at a time.

Knead slightly. Cover and refrigerate overnight. Take out of refrigerator 30 minutes before shaping into rolls. Let sit for 30 minutes and then shape into rolls. Let rise until double in bulk. Bake at 400° for 15 to 20 minutes on oiled baking sheet.

Yield: 4–5 dozen rolls.

APPENDIX

DIET CENTER'S FOOD COMPOSITION CHARTS

How to Use Diet Center's Food Composition Charts

Diet Center's Food Composition Charts can help you to become your own nutritionist! Hundred of food items have been divided into thirteen different categories:

Beverages
Breads, Flours, Cereals and Grains
Dairy Products
Desserts and Sweets
Fish, Seafood and Seaweed
Fruits
Meat and Poultry
Nut Products and Seeds
Oils, Fats and Shortening
Salad Dressings and Sauces
Soups
Spices and Herbs
Vegetables

Each food item appears in alphabetical order within its category. (For example, if you wanted to find, "roasted almonds," you would turn to page 365, "Nut Products and Seeds.")

Each food has been analyzed in terms of macronutrients (proteins, fats, carbohydrates), water, food energy (calories), and sodium. "Fats" have been subdivided into "saturated" and "unsaturated."

All foods on the Reducing Diet are indicated by bold type. Please consult footnotes for additional information.

WOMEN'S REDUCING DIET FIVE-DAY NUTRIENT SUMMARY

Dieters on the Diet Center Reducing Diet have a wide variety of foods from which to select. This versatility offers not only a nutritious, well-balanced diet, but one which dieters can enjoy.

This chart provides a complete nutrient analysis of foods consumed during a typical five-day period for women on the Reducing Diet. Daily summaries include standard fruit, vegetable and whole-grain consumption, coupled with interchanged protein selections.

Note: This analysis includes 1 egg each day. Dieters may replace egg as a protein source by increasing chicken breast portion to 4 oz. (raw weight). A maximum of 5 eggs is allowed per week.

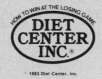

HOW TO WIN AT THE LOSING GAME

DIET CENTER INC.®

1983 Diet Center, Inc.

		Water	Food energy	Protein	Fat	(Total) Saturated	Unsaturated Oleic	Linoleic
		Per-cent	Calories	Grams	Grams	Grams	Grams	Grams
Diet Supplement	8		37	3.4	.69			
Hot lemonade	2 Tbsp.	91.6	6	0.2	T	--	--	--
Vitamin C	250 mg. (4)							
Cal-Mag Plus	700 mg.							
Tea	1 cup	--	4	0.1	T	--	--	--
Egg, hard cooked	1 large	73.7	82	6.5	5.8	1.8	2.5	0.4
Wasa Brod	4		120	4	0			
Chicken breast	3 oz. raw	74.8	94	19.7	1.02	.29	.218	.143
Safflower oil	2 tsp.	0	83	0	9.3	.73	1.3	6.5
Lettuce, Iceberg	1 cup	95.5	10	0.7	0.1	--	--	--
Dark leafy greens	1 cup		33	2.74	.491	--	--	--
Cabbage, sliced	½ cup	92.4	9	.45	.05	--	--	--
Cucumber, sliced	½ cup	95.1	8	.45	.05	--	--	--
Cauliflower, raw	½ cup	91	14	1.35	0.1	--	--	--
Mung bean sprouts	¼ cup	88.8	9	1	.05	--	--	--
Radishes, red	5 medium	94.5	4	.25	T	--	--	--
Mushrooms, raw	¼ cup	90.4	5	.475	.05	--	--	--
Green beans, cooked	1 cup	92.4	31	2	0.3	--	--	--
Vinegar	2 Tbsp.	93.8	4	T	0	--	--	--
Orange	1 large	86	100	2.02	.47	--	--	--
Apple	1 extra large	84.4	149	.467	1.56	--	--	--
Halibut	4 oz. raw	--	114	23.7	1.25	.228	.68	
Milk, skim	2 Tbsp.	90.5	11	1.1	.025	.036	.017	
Lemon, raw peeled	1 medium	90.1	20	0.8	0.2	--	--	--
Lime, raw	1 small	89.3	19	0.5	0.1	--	--	--
Bran, unprocessed	2 Tbsp.		20	*	0			
Gelatin	1 packet	13	23	6	T	--	--	--
Protein powder	2 Tbsp.		70	16	0			
Crunchies	2 Tbsp.		59	11.05	.215			

1st day		Total	1138	104.9	21.82	3.08		11.76

Summary of Days 2 Through 5 with Protein Replacements

2nd day Replace Halibut with Shrimp, canned	3½ oz.	Total	1137	105.93	21.64	2.9		11.08
3rd day Replace Halibut with Tofu	8 oz.	Total	1188	99.9	30.17	4.4		17.93
4th day Replace Halibut with Trout	4 oz.	Total	1245	105.6	33.52	5.7		14.4
5th day Replace Halibut with Sole	4 oz.	Total	1114	100.1	21.97	3.2		11.72
RDA (Women - Ages 23-50)			1600-2900	44	66			

Sodium can vary drastically depending upon how much salt is added to foods. One teaspoon of salt contains 2,132 mg. of sodium. * Contains less than 2% of U.S. RDA's. Dashes (--) denote lack of reliable data for a constitute believed to be present in a measurable amount.

Carbohydrates	Vitamin A	Vitamin B1	Vitamin B2	Vitamin B6	Vitamin B12	Biotin	Folic Acid	Niacin	Pantothenic Acid	Vitamin C	Vitamin E	Sodium	Phosphorus	Potassium	Calcium	Iron	Magnesium	Copper	Manganese	Selenium	Zinc	Fiber
Grams	International units	Milligrams	Milligrams	Milligrams	Micrograms	Micrograms	Milligrams	Milligrams	Milligrams	Milligrams	Milligrams	Milligrams	Milligrams	Milligrams	Milligrams	Milligrams	Milligrams	Milligrams	Milligrams	Milligrams	Milligrams	Grams
4.4	12	16	6	30				120	30													
2.4	T	T	T	.014	0	—	T	T	.03	12	—	T	4	42	2	T	.24	.024	.002	—	.004	T
										1000												
	4000												67		700	10	400				12	
0.9	0	0	.04	—	—	—	—	0.1	—	1	—	1.6	4	58	5	0.2	8	1.13	1.66	0.1	.04	T
0.5	590	.04	.14	.065	.749	—	.027	T	.985	0	—	61	103	65	27	1.2	6.84	—	—	—	.821	0
24	*	.06	.068					*		*			120	52	*	1.44						
0	18	.06	.077	.469	.325	—	.004	9.535	.698	1.02	—	56	167	218	10	.613	23.84	.04	.016	—	.68	—
0	T	T	T	—	—	—	—	T	—	T	7	0	0		T	T	—	—	—	—	.017	0
2.2	250	.05	.05	.028	0	.35	.02	0.2	0.1	5	—	7	17	131	15	0.4	5	.035	—	.675	0.3	.35
6.27	8629	.124	.229	.06	0	1.42	.045	.502	.148	66	.22	74	53	467	158	3.32	55.3	.169	.607	—	.083	1.26
1.9	45	.02	.02	.056	0	.035	.023	0.1	.55	17	0.1	7	10	82	17	.15	6.5	.046	—	.77	.15	0.4
1.8	130	.015	.02	.021	0	0.5	.008	0.1	.125	6	4.2	3	14	84	13	0.6	6	.045	.075	—	.11	0.3
2.6	30	.055	.05	.105	0	.75	.003	.35	0.5	39	.075	7	28	148	13	.55	12	.065	.085	.35	.185	0.5
1.7	5	.035	.035	—	—	—	.003	0.2	—	5	—	1.3	17	59	5	.35	—	—	—	—	.23	.18
0.8	T	.005	.005	.019	0	—	.006	.05	.046	6	—	4	7	73	7	.25	3.5	.04	.013	1.1	.065	.175
.78	T	.018	.08	.022	0	2.8	.004	.725	.385	0.5	.145	3	20	73	1	.15	1.93	.27	.014	2.14	.228	.14
6.8	680	.09	.11	.087	0	—	.05	0.6	.168	15	—	5	46	189	63	0.8	—	.125	—	—	0.4	1.2
1.8	—	—	—	T	0	—	—	—	—	—	—	T	2	30	2	0.2	0.4	.028	—	—	.03	0
24.9	404	.20	.08	.168	0	2.8	.129	.78	0.7	103	.67	1.6	40	409	84	.78	30.8	.17	.07	3.9	.404	1.4
37.3	233	.078	.047	.078	0	2.8	.022	.31	.296	10.8	2.069	3	26	283	19	.78	22.4	.249	.196	1.4	.14	2.8
0	500	.073	.08	.488	1.13	2.27	.0023	9.5	.313	T	—	61	239	509	15	0.8	—	.26	.0113	—	0.8	0
1.563	1	.011	.055	.012	.116	.63	.004	.03	.101	0.3	T	16	29	44	37	.013	3.5	.013	—	1.38	.123	0
6	10	.03	.01	.08	0	—	.012	0.1	.19	39	—	1	12	102	19	0.4	9	.15	.04	—	—	0.4
6.4	10	.02	.01	—	0	—	.003	0.1	.217	25	—	1	12	69	22	0.4	—	—	—	—	—	0.5
4	*	.03	*				.008	1.2		*		10	100		*	.72	40	.08				0.6
0	—	—	—	—	—	—	—	—	—	—	—	—	—	—	—	—	—	—	—	—	—	—
1	*	*	*					*		*						*	40					
6.69																						
146.7	15,535	13.0	17.21	7.8	32.32	14.36	.373	24.5	35.6	1352	14.48	324	1137	3187	1274	24.1	635.3	2.94	2.79	11.82	17.41	9.61
147.4	15,096	12.94	17.2	7.4	31.19	12.09	.373	16.8	35.5	1352	14.48	2517	1156	2797	1372	26.4	635.3	2.92	2.779	11.82	16.61	9.61
152.2	15,035	13.07	17.2	7.312	31.19	12.09	.371	15.3	35.29	1352	14.48	279	1184	2774	1550	27.6	889	2.7	2.779	11.82	16.61	9.84
146.7	15,035	13.01	17.4	8.1	36.9	12.09	.371	24.5	37.5	1352	14.48	307	898	3210	1281	24.4	635.3	3.06	2.813	11.82	16.61	9.61
146.7	15,035	12.99	17.2	7.5	32.6	12.09	.371	16.9	36.26	1352	14.48	352	1119	3066	1273	24.2	669.3	2.884	2.802	49.82	17.41	9.61
300	4000	1.0	1.2	2.0	3	100-200	0.4	13	4-7	60	8	1100-3300	800	1875-5625	800	18	300	2.0-3.0	2.5-5.0	.05-0.2	15	

FOOD PRODUCT[1]	AMOUNT	WEIGHT IN GRAMS	WATER (PERCENT)	FOOD ENERGY (CALORIES)	PROTEIN (GRAMS)	FAT (GRAMS)	(TOTAL) SATURATED (GRAMS)	UNSATURATED OLEIC (GRAMS)	UNSATURATED LINOLEIC (GRAMS)	CARBOHYDRATES (GRAMS)	SODIUM (MILLIGRAMS)
BEVERAGES											
Alcoholic											
Beer, 4.5% alcohol	8 oz.	240	—	101	.72	0	—	—	. —	9.1	17
Gin, rum, vodka, whiskey, 86 proof	1 oz.	28	—	70	0	0	—	—	—	T	T
Tom collins	10 oz.	300	—	180	0.3	—	—	—	—	9	—
Wines											
Sweet, 18.8% alcohol	1 cup	240	—	329	.24	0	—	—	—	18.4	10
Dry, 12.2% alcohol	1 cup	240	—	204	.24	0	—	—	—	9.6	12
Coffee, clear	1 cup	240	—	5	0.3	0.1	—	—	—	0.8	2.3
Cola drinks	1 cup	240	—	94	0	0	—	—	—	19	2
Diet drinks	1 cup	240	—	1	0	0	—	—	—	—	—
Fruit-flavored drinks	1 cup	240	—	110	0	0	—	—	—	29	18
Ginger ale	1 cup	240	—	74	0	0	—	—	—	19	18
Root beer	1 cup	240	—	98	0	0	—	—	—	25	18
Tea, clear	1 cup	240	—	4	.1	T	—	—	—	0.9	1.6
BREADS, FLOURS, CEREALS, AND GRAIN[2]											
Barley, pearled											
Light	1 cup	200	11.1	698	16.4	2	T	2	—	157.6	6
	½ cup	100	11.1	349	8.2	1	T	1	—	78.8	3
Pot or Scotch	1 cup	200	10.8	696	19.2	2.2	.48	1.52	—	154.4	—
	½ cup	100	10.8	348	9.6	1.1	.24	.76	—	77.2	—
Bran flakes, 40% fortified	1 cup	35	3.0	106	3.6	0.6	—	—	—	28.2	207[3]
	½ cup	18	3.0	53	1.8	0.3	—	—	—	14.1	104[3]
Bran, unprocessed[4]	2 Tbsp.	7	—	20	*	0	—	—	—	4	10
Bread											
Biscuit (2-in. diameter)	1 biscuit	28	27.4	103	2.1	4.8	1.8	2.2	.5	12.8	175
Cracked wheat, enriched											
Fresh	1 slice	23	34.9	60	2.0	.506	0.1	0.2	0.2	11.97	122
Toasted	1 slice	19	22.5	59	1.97	.49	0.1	0.2	0.2	11.77	120

Food	Measure	g									
French or Vienna, enriched	1 slice - - -	20	30.6	58	1.82	.599	0.1	0.3	0.2	11.07	116
Italian, enriched	1 slice - - -	20	31.8	55	1.82	.158	T	.17	—	11.26	117
Raisin, enriched	1 slice - - -	23	35.3	60	1.51	.64	0.1	0.3	0.2	12.32	84
Rye, American	1 slice - - -	23	35.3	56	2.09	.25	—	—	—	11.97	128
White, enriched											
Fresh	1 slice - - -	23	35.6	62	2.0	.734	0.2	0.3	0.2	11.60	117
Toasted	1 slice - - -	20	25.1	63	2.01	.726	0.2	0.3	0.2	11.74	118
Whole wheat											
Fresh	1 slice - - -	23	36.4	56	2.41	.69	0.1	0.3	0.2	10.96	121
Toasted	1 slice - - -	19	24.3	55	2.37	.68	0.1	0.3	0.2	10.76	119
Breadcrumbs, enriched, dry	1 cup - - -	100	6.5	392	12.6	4.6	1.1	2.1	1.2	73.4	736
Cornflakes, fortified	1 cup - - -	25	3.8	97	2.0	0.1	—	—	—	21.3	251
	½ cup - - -	13	3.8	49	1.0	.05	—	—	—	10.7	126
Corn grits (hominy), degermed, enriched											
Cooked	1 cup - - -	245	87.1	125	2.9	0.2	.03	.17	—	27	502[5]
	½ cup - - -	123	87.1	63	1.45	0.1	.015	.085	—	13.5	251
Crackers											
Ak-Mak (whole wheat)	1 cracker	7	—	29	1.16	.583	—	—	—	4.73	—
Finn Crisp	1 cracker	5	—	18	1.25	.25	—	—	—	3.5	—
Graham, plain	2, 2½ in. sq.	14	6.4	55	1.1	1.3	0.3	0.6	0.3	10.4	95
Melba rounds[4]											
Onion	2 rounds -	6	—	20	0.8	0.4	—	—	—	3.6	—
Sesame	2 rounds -	6	—	24	0.8	0.8	—	—	—	3.2	—
White	2 rounds -	6	—	20	0.8	0.4	—	—	—	3.6	—
Whole grain	2 rounds -	6	—	24	0.8	0.8	—	—	—	3.2	—
Melba toast[4]											
White	1 slice - - -	5	—	16.6	.667	0	—	—	—	3.33	—
Whole grain	1 slice - - -	5	—	16.6	.667	0	—	—	—	3.33	—
Norwegian flatbread[4]	1 wafer - -	20	4	20	0.5	.25	—	—	—	4	—
Soda	10 crackers	28	4	125	2.6	3.7	0.9	1.8	0.9	20.1	312
	1, 1⅛ in. sq.	3	4	13	.26	.37	.09	.18	.09	2.01	31
Soup or oyster	10 crackers	8	4	33	0.7	1	0.2	0.5	0.2	5.3	83
Wasa Brod (Lite Rye)[4]	2 wafers -	14	—	60	2	0	—	—	—	12	—
Farina, enriched											
Cooked	1 cup - - -	245	89.5	103	3.2	0.2	.074	.25	—	21.3	353
	½ cup - - -	123	89.5	52	1.6	0.1	.037	.125	—	10.7	177

FOOD PRODUCT[1]	AMOUNT	WEIGHT IN GRAMS	WATER (PERCENT)	FOOD ENERGY (CALORIES)	PROTEIN (GRAMS)	FAT (GRAMS)	(TOTAL) SATURATED (GRAMS)	UNSATURATED OLEIC (GRAMS)	UNSATURATED LINOLEIC (GRAMS)	CARBOHYDRATES (GRAMS)	SODIUM (MILLIGRAMS)
Flour											
Gluten	1 cup ---	140	8.5	529	58	2.7	—	—	—	66.1	3
White, all-purpose, unsifted	1 cup ---	125	12	455	13.1	1.3			—	95.1	3
Whole wheat	1 cup ---	120	12	400	16	2.4	T	2		85.2	4
Rye, dark	1 cup ---	128	11	419	20.9	3.3	.42	1		87.2	1
Muffins											
Plain	1 muffin -	40	38	118	3.1	4	1	2	0.8	16.9	176
Bran	1 muffin -	40	35.1	104	3.1	3.9	1.2	1.7	0.7	17.2	179
Bran, Diet Center recipe[6]	1 muffin -	72	—	69.2	3.62	1.69	.5		0.7	10.3	40
Cornmeal, whole ground	1 muffin -	45	3.4	130	3.2	4.6	1.7	1.9	0.6	19.1	223
Noodles, egg, enriched, cooked	1 cup ---	160	70.8	200	6.6	2.4	1	1	—	37.3	3[7]
Oatmeal, rolled oats, cooked	1 cup ---	240	86.5	132	4.8	2.4	0.5	0.8	1	23.3	523[8]
	½ cup ---	120	86.5	66	2.4	1.2	.25	0.4	5.0	11.7	262[8]
Pancakes											
Plain, enriched (4-in. diameter)	1 pancake	27	50.1	62	1.9	1.9	0.5	0.9	0.4	9.2	115
Buckwheat (4-in. diameter)	1 pancake	27	57.9	54	1.8	2.5	0.8	1.1	0.4	6.4	125
Pizza, cheese (14-in. diameter; ⅛ pizza)	1 piece --	65	48.3	153	7.8	5.4	2.1	2.3	0.5	18.4	456
Popcorn, plain	1 cup ---	6	4	23	0.8	0.3	T	0.1	0.2	4.6	T
Rice											
Brown, large grain, cooked w/salt	1 cup ---	195	70.3	232	4.9	1.2	.31	.94	—	49.7	550[8]
White, cooked w/salt	1 cup ---	205	72.6	223	4.1	0.2	0.1	.24	—	49.6	767[8]
Rice, puffed, fortified, w/o salt, sugar	1 cup ---	15	3.7	60	0.9	0.1	—	—	—	13.4	T
	½ cup ---	8	3.7	30	.45	.05	—	—	—	6.7	T
Rolls											
Danish, enriched	1 average	42	22	179	3	10	3	4.7	1.8	19.4	156
Hard, enriched	1 average	50	25.4	156	4.9	1.6	0.4	0.7	0.4	29.8	313
Whole wheat	1 average	35	0	90	3.5	1	—	—	—	18.3	197

Shredded wheat, biscuit	1 average	25	6.6	89	2.5	0.5	.09	.38	—	20	1
Spaghetti, enriched, cooked	1 cup	140	73	155	4.8	0.6	—	—	—	32.2	1[7]
Tapioca, dry	1 cup	152	12.6	535	0.9	0.3	—	—	—	131.3	5
Waffles (7-in. diameter)	1 waffle	75	41.4	209	7.0	7.4	2.4	3.3	1.1	28.1	356
Wheat germ, toasted	1 Tbsp.	6	4.2	23	1.8	0.7	0.1	0.2	0.3	3	T
Wheat, puffed	1 cup	15	3.4	54	2.3	0.2	—	—	—	11.8	1
	½ cup	8	3.4	27	1.2	0.1	—	—	—	5.9	0.5
Wheatmeal cereal, cooked	1 cup	245	87.7	110	4.4	0.7	—	—	—	23	519
	½ cup	123	87.7	55	2.2	.35	—	—	—	11.5	260

DAIRY PRODUCTS[2]

Cheese										
Natural cheeses										
Blue	1 oz.	28	40	104	6.1	8.6	4.8	2.9	0.3	0.6	396
Camembert (domestic)	1 oz.	28	52.2	85	5	7	3.8	2.3	0.2	0.5	239
Cheddar (domestic type)	1 oz.	28	37	113	7.1	9.1	5.0	3.0	0.3	0.6	198
shredded	1 cup	113	37	450	28.3	36.4	20.0	12.0	1.1	2.4	791
Cottage cheese										
2% fat (not packed)	1 cup	226	—	203	31	4.36	3.76	1.37		8.2	918
4.2% milk fat (not packed, small curd, with creaming mixture)	1 cup	210	78.3	223	28.6	8.8	4.9	2.9	0.3	6.1	481
0.3% milk fat (not packed, dry curd, without creaming mixture)	1 cup	145	79	125	24.7	0.4	.396	.182		3.9	421
Cream cheese	1 oz.	28	51	106	2.3	10.7	5.9	3.5	0.3	0.6	71
Mozzarella	1 oz.	28	—	80	5.51	6.12	3.73	2.08		.63	106
Parmesan, grated	1 Tbsp.	5	17	23	2.1	1.5	0.8	0.5	T	0.2	44
Swiss (domestic)	1 oz.	28	39	105	7.8	7.9	4.4	2.6	0.2	0.5	201
Pasteurized, processed cheese										
American	1 oz.	28	40	105	6.6	8.5	4.7	2.8	0.3	0.5	322[9]

FOOD PRODUCT[1]	AMOUNT	WEIGHT IN GRAMS	WATER (PERCENT)	FOOD ENERGY (CALORIES)	PROTEIN (GRAMS)	FAT (GRAMS)	(TOTAL) SATURATED (GRAMS)	UNSATURATED OLEIC (GRAMS)	UNSATURATED LINOLEIC (GRAMS)	CARBOHYDRATES (GRAMS)	SODIUM (MILLIGRAMS)
Cheese Spread (packed in glass jars and pressurized cans)	1 oz.	28	48.6	82	4.5	6.1	3.3	2.0	0.2	2.3	461[10]
Ricotta											
Whole milk	1 cup	246	—	428	27.7	31.9	20.4	9.87		7.48	207
Part skim	1 cup	246	—	340	28	19.5	12.1	6		12.6	307
Swiss (prepackaged slices)	1 slice or 1 oz.	28	40	101	7.5	7.6	4.2	2.5	0.2	0.5	331[11]
Cream											
Half-and-half	1 cup	242	79.7	324	7.7	28.3	15.6	9.3	0.8	11.1	111
Light, coffee or table	1 Tbsp.	15	71.5	32	0.5	3.1	1.7	1.0	0.1	0.6	6
Sour	1 cup	230	—	493	7.27	48.7	30	15.7		9.8	123
Whipping cream											
Light	1 cup	239	62.1	717	6	74.8	41.2	24.7	2.2	8.6	86
	1 Tbsp.	15	62.1	45	.38	4.68	2.58	1.544	.138	.538	5
Heavy	1 cup	238	56.6	838	5.2	89.5	49.2	29.5	2.7	7.4	76
	1 Tbsp.	15	56.6	52	.33	5.6	3.08	1.844	.169	.463	5
Eggnog[4]	1 cup	354	—	342	9.68	19	11.3	6.53		34.4	138
Eggs											
Hard-cooked	1 lg.	57	73.7	82	6.5	5.8	1.8	2.5	0.4	0.5	61
Poached	1 lg.	50	73.7	82	6.5	5.8	1.8	2.5	0.4	0.5	136
Raw											
Large	1 egg	57	73.7	82	6.5	5.8	1.8	2.5	0.4	0.5	61
Medium	1 egg	50	73.7	72	5.7	5.1	1.6	2.2	0.4	0.4	54
Scrambled[12]	1 egg	64	72.1	111	7.2	8.3	2.8	3.1	0.5	1.5	164
Scrambled, without fat	1 egg	57	73.7	82	6.5	5.8	1.8	2.5	0.4	0.5	61
Yolk, fresh, raw	1 lg. egg	17	51.1	59	2.7	5.2	1.7	2.3	0.4	0.1	9
Whites, fresh, raw	1 lg. egg	33	87.6	17	3.6	T	0	0		0.3	48
Ice cream	1 cup	133	63.2	257	6	14.1	7.8	4.7	0.4	27.7	84[13]
Ice milk	1 cup	131	66.7	199	6.3	6.7	3.7	2.2	0.2	29.3	89[13]
Milk											
Buttermilk	1 cup	245	90.5	88	8.8	0.2	1.34	0.7	0.4	12.5	319
Condensed, sweetened	1 cup	306	27.1	982	24.8	26.6	14.7	8.8	0.8	166.2	343

Food	Measure	Grams	Water %	Food energy	Protein	Fat	Sat.	Oleic	Linoleic	Carbohydrate	Calcium
Chocolate, whole	1 cup	250	81.5	213	8.5	8.5	4.7	2.8	0.3	27.5	118
Dry, nonfat, regular	1 cup	120	3.0	436	43.1	1.0	0.6	.28		62.8	638
Dry, nonfat, instant	1 cup	68	4.0	244	24.3	0.5	.32	.15		35.1	358
Evaporated, unsweetened, whole	1 cup	252	73.8	345	17.6	19.9	10.9	6.6	0.6	24.4	297
Skim, unsweetened	1 cup	256	—	198	19.3	.52	.31	.174		28.9	294
Goat	1 cup	244	87.5	163	7.8	9.8	6.1	2.4	0.5	11.2	83
Low-fat 2% nonfat, milk solids added	1 cup	246	87	145	10.3	4.9	2.7	1.6	0.1	14.8	150
Skim	1 cup	245	90.5	88	8.8	0.2	.287	.132		12.5	127
	2 Tbsp.	31	90.5	11	1.1	.025	.036	.017		1.563	16
Whey, dried	1 Tbsp.	7.5	.074	26	.97	.083	.05	.02		5.51	—
Whole	1 cup	244	87.4	159	8.5	8.5	4.7	2.8	0.2	12	122
	2 Tbsp.	31	87.4	20	1.063	1.063	.588	0.4	.03	1.5	15
Sherbet, orange	1 cup	193	67	259	1.7	2.3	—	—	—	59.4	19
Yogurt Whole mild	8 oz.	226	88	140	6.8	7.7	4.2	2.5	0.2	11.1	106
Partially skimmed	8 oz.	226	89	113	7.7	3.8	2.1	1.3	0.1	11.8	115

DESSERTS AND SWEETS[2]

Food	Measure	Grams	Water %	Food energy	Protein	Fat	Sat.	Oleic	Linoleic	Carbohydrate	Calcium
Boston cream pie (8-in. diameter)	1 piece	103	34.5	311	5.2	9.7	3	4.5	1.6	51.4	192
Brownie, with nuts (2×2×3/4)	1 brownie	30	14.7	146	1.95	9.45	2.1	4.9	1.7	15.3	75
Cake											
Angel Food (1/8 cake)	1 piece	45	31.5	121	3.2	0.1	—	—	—	27.1	127
Devils Food (3×3×2)											
Plain	1 piece	88	24.6	322	4.2	15.1	5.4	6.8	2.3	45.8	259
With chocolate icing	1 piece	120	22	443	5.4	19.7	7.8	8.5	2.4	67	282
With uncooked white icing	1 piece	118	21.3	435	4.5	17.2	6.5	7.5	2.4	69.9	270
Gingerbread (3×3×2)	1 piece	117	31.5	371	4.4	12.5	3.2	6.1	2.6	60.8	227
Pound, old-fashioned (3×3×1/2)	1 piece	30	17.2	142	1.7	8.9	2.3	4.4	1.8	14.1	33
Sponge (1/16 cake)	1 piece	49	31.8	146	3.7	2.8	0.9	1.2	0.1	26.5	82
White (2 layer, 9 in. diam, 3 in. high)											
Plain	1/12 cake	71	24.2	264	3.2	11.3	2.9	5.5	2.4	38.1	228
With uncooked white icing	1/12 cake	104	20	391	3.4	13.5	4.1	6.3	2.5	65.6	244

FOOD PRODUCT[1]	AMOUNT	WEIGHT IN GRAMS	WATER (PERCENT)	FOOD ENERGY (CALORIES)	PROTEIN (GRAMS)	FAT (GRAMS)	(TOTAL) SATU-RATED (GRAMS)	UNSATURATED OLEIC (GRAMS)	UNSATURATED LIN-OLEIC (GRAMS)	CARBO-HYDRATES (GRAMS)	SODIUM (MILLI-GRAMS)
Cake icing											
Chocolate	1 cup ---	275	14.3	1,034	8.8	38.2	21.3	13.6	0.9	185.4	168
	1 Tbsp. --	17	14.3	65	.55	2.39	1.3	0.9	.06	11.59	11
White, boiled	1 cup ---	94	17.9	297	1.3	0	.06	134			
	1 Tbsp. --	6	17.9	19	.08	0	—	—	—		3.7 8
Candy											
Chocolate chips, semisweet	1 oz. ----	28	1.1	144	1.2	10.1	5.7	3.7	1		
Chocolate fudge	1″ cube --	21	8.2	84	0.6	2.6	0.9	1.2	0.4	15.8	40
Peanut brittle	1 oz. ----	28	2	119	1.6	2.9	0.6	1.3	0.9	23	9
Cookies											
Chocolate chip (2⅓-in. diam.)	4 cookies	40	3	206	2.2	12	3.4	5.1	2.8	24	139
Fig bars (1½×1¾×¼)	4 cookies	56	13.6	200	2.2	3.1	0.9	1.5	0.6	42.2	141
Gingersnap (2-in. diam.)	10 cookies	70	3.1	294	3.9	6.2	1.6	3	1.3	55.9	400
Macaroon (2¾-in. diam.)	2 cookies	38	4.4	181	2	8.8	6.08	2.28		25.1	13
Oatmeal, with raisins (2⅝-in. diam.)	4 cookies	52	2.8	235	3.2	8	2.1	3.8	1.8	38.2	84
Custard, baked, regular	1 cup ---	265	77.2	305	14.3	14.6	6.8	5.4	0.7	29.4	209
Doughnut											
Cake, plain (3¼-in. diam.)	1 dough-nut	42	23.7	164	1.9	7.8	2	3.9	1.7	21.6	210
Raised, plain (3¾-in. diam.)	1 dough-nut	42	28.3	176	2.7	11.3	2.8	5.6	2.5	16	99
Eclair (5-in. diam.)	1 eclair --	100	56.2	239	6.2	13.6	4.4	6.2	2.1	23.2	82
Egg Custard, Diet Center recipe[6]	1 cup ---	224	—	170	14.2	91.4	2.92	4.50		6.94	155
	3 Tbsp. --	42	—	32	2.66	17.14	.548	.844		1.30	29
Honey, strained or extracted	1 Tbsp. --	21	17.2	64	0.1	0	—	—	—	17.3	1
Jams and Preserves	1 Tbsp. --	20	29	54	0.1	T	—	—	—	14	2
Jellies	1 Tbsp --	18	29	49	T	T	—	—	—	12.7	3
Pie											
Apple (⅙ of 9″)	1 piece --	160	8	410	3.52	17.8	4.6	8.7	3.8	60.95	482
Meringue, lemon (⅙ of 9″)	1 piece --	140	47.4	357	5.2	14.3	5.5	6.3	1.2	52.8	395
Pecan (⅙ of 9″)	1 piece --	160	3.78	669	8.16	36.7	5.1	21.1	7.3	82	354
Pumpkin (⅙ of 9″)	1 piece --	150	59.2	317	6.02	16.84	7.1	6.9	1.3	36.7	321

Food	Measure	g									
Piecrust, enriched, baked, 9", made with vegetable shortening											
	1 crust --	180	14.9	900	11	60.1	14.9	29.9	13.4	78.8	1,100
	½ crust --	30	14.9	150	1.8	10	2.5	4.9	2.2	13.1	183
Pudding											
Bread w/raisins, enriched	1 cup ---	265	58.6	496	14.8	16.2	7.7	5.9	1	75.3	533
Chocolate (cornstarch)	1 cup ---	260	65.8	385	8.1	12.2	6.7	4.6	0.3	66.8	146
Rice w/raisins	1 cup ---	265	65.8	387	9.5	8.2	4.5	2.7	0.3	70.8	188
Tapioca cream	1 cup ---	165	71.8	221	8.3	8.4	3.9	3.1	0.4	28.2	257
Sugar											
Beet or cane	1 cup ---	200	0.5	770	0	0	—	—	—	199	2
	1 Tbsp.--	12	0.5	46	0	0	—	—	—	11.9	.125
Brown, packed	1 cup ---	220	2.1	821	0	0	—	—	—	212.1	66
Powdered	1 cup ---	120	0.5	462	0	0	—	—	—	119.4	1
Syrup											
Corn	1 Tbsp --	20	—	57	0	0	—	—	—	14.8	—
Maple	1 Tbsp --	20	—	50	0	0	—	—	—	12.8	3
FISH, SEAFOOD, AND SEAWEED[2]											
Abalone, raw	1 lb. -----	454	—	445	84.8	2.3	—	—	—	15.4	—
	4 oz. -----	114[15]	—	111	21.2	.58	—	—	—	3.85	—
Bass, raw	1 lb. -----	454	—	472	85.7	9.5	2.04	5.8	—	0	308
	4 oz. -----	114[15]	—	118	21.4	2.4	.51	1.5	—	0	77
Bluefish, raw	1 lb. -----	454	—	531	93	15	—	—	—	0	336
	4 oz. -----	114[15]	—	133	23.3	3.8	—	—	—	0	84
Carp, raw	1 lb. -----	454	—	522	81.6	19.1	3.44	13.1	—	0	227
	4 oz. -----	114[15]	—	131	20.4	4.78	.86	3.28	—	0	57
Caviar, raw, sturgeon, granular	1 tsp. ---	10	—	26	2.7	1.5	—	—	—	3.3	220
Clams, raw, fresh	4 lg. or 9 sm.	100	—	82	14	1.9	—	—	—	1.3	36
canned[16]	1 cup ---	200	—	104	15.8	1.4	—	—	—	5.6	—
Cod, raw	1 lb. -----	454	—	354	79.8	3.3	.544	1.54	—	0	318
	4 oz. -----	114[15]	—	89	19.9	.83	.136	.39	—	0	80
Crab, steamed	1 lb. -----	454	—	422	78.5	8.6	—	—	—	2.3	—
	4 oz. -----	114[15]	—	106	19.6	2.2	—	—	—	.58	—

FOOD PRODUCT[1]	AMOUNT	WEIGHT IN GRAMS	WATER (PERCENT)	FOOD ENERGY (CALORIES)	PROTEIN (GRAMS)	FAT (GRAMS)	(TOTAL) SATURATED (GRAMS)	UNSATURATED OLEIC (GRAMS)	UNSATURATED LINOLEIC (GRAMS)	CARBOHYDRATES (GRAMS)	SODIUM (MILLIGRAMS)
Crab canned, drained[16]	1 cup	160	—	162	27.8	4	—	—	—	1.8	1,600
	3½ oz.	99	—	100	17.2	2.48	—	—	—	1.1	990
Flat fish, raw, flounder and sole	1 lb.	454	—	358	75.8	5.4	1.26	2.54	—	0	354
	4 oz.	114[15]	—	90	18.9	1.4	.32	.64	—	0	89
Haddock, raw	1 lb.	454	—	358	83	2.9	.498	1.22	—	0	277
	4 oz.	114[15]	—	90	21	.73	.125	.31	—	0	69
Halibut, raw	1 lb.	454	—	454	94.8	4.98	.91	2.72	—	0	245
	4 oz.	114[15]	—	114	23.7	1.25	.228	.68	—	0	61
Herring, raw, fresh	1 lb.	454	—	798	78.5	28.1	8.7	16.2	—	0	535
	4 oz.	114[15]	—	200	19.6	7.03	2.18	4.1	—	0	134
canned	1 cup	200	—	416	39.8	—	—	—	—	0	—
Kelp	1 Tbsp.	14	—	—	1.03	.157	—	—	—	5.5	429
Lobster, raw	1 lb.	454	—	413	76.7	8.6	—	—	—	2.3	1,359
	4 oz.	114[15]	—	103	19.2	2.2	—	—	—	.575	340
Mackerel, raw, fresh	1 lb.	454	—	866	86.2	44.4	11	27.5	—	0	652
	4 oz.	114[15]	—	217	21.6	11.1	2.8	6.88	—	0	163
canned, drained[16]	1 cup	210	—	384	40.4	12.4	—	—	—	0	—
Oysters, raw, fresh	1 lb.	454	—	299	38.1	8.2	—	—	—	15.4	331
	4 oz.	114[15]	—	75	9.53	2.05	—	—	—	3.85	83
canned[16]	1 cup	240	—	158	20.2	4.3	1.97	2.02	—	8.2	175
Perch											
Ocean, raw	1 lb.	454	—	431	86.2	11.3	1.86	7.57	—	0	286
	4 oz.	114[15]	—	108	21.6	2.83	.47	1.89	—	0	72
Yellow	1 lb.	454	—	413	88.5	4.1	—	—	—	0	308
	4 oz.	114[15]	—	103	22.1	1.03	—	—	—	0	77
Pike, walleye, raw	1 lb.	454	—	422	87.5	5.4	.725	2.08	—	0	231
	4 oz.	114[15]	—	105	21.9	1.35	.181	.52	—	0	58
Pollock, fillet, raw	1 lb.	454	—	431	92.5	4.1	.544	2.49	—	0	218
	4 oz.	114[15]	—	108	23.1	1.03	.136	.623	—	0	55
Salmon, raw, fresh	1 lb.	454	—	984	102	60.8	22	23	—	0	217
	4 oz.	114[15]	—	246	25.5	15.2	5.5	5.8	—	0	54

canned, pink[16]	1 cup	220	—	310	45.1	13	4	2	0	851
Scallops, raw	1 lb.	454	—	367	69.4	0.9	—	—	15	1,155[17]
	4 oz.	114[15]	—	92	17.4	.225	—	—	3.75	289[17]
Shrimp, raw, fresh	1 lb.	454	—	413	82.1	3.6	—	—	6.8	635
	4 oz.	114[15]	—	103	20.5	0.9	—	—	1.7	159
canned[16]	1 cup	128	—	148	31	1.4	—	—	0.9	2,944[18]
	3½ oz.	98	—	113	23.73	1.072	—	—	.69	2,254[18]
Snapper, raw	1 lb.	454	—	422	89.8	5.4	1.09	2.9	0	304
	4 oz.	114[15]	—	106	22.5	1.4	.273	.73	0	76
Trout, rainbow, raw	1 lb.	454	—	885	97.5	51.7	11	13	0	177
	4 oz.	114[15]	—	221	24.38	12.93	2.8	3.3	0	44
Tuna										
canned in water[16]	1 cup	200	—	254	56	1.6	—	—	0	824[19]
canned in oil[16]	1 cup	160	60.6	315	46.1	13.1	3.5	2.7	0	1,280[20]
Whitefish, raw	1 lb.	454	—	703	85.7	37.2	3.9	15.7	0	236
	4 oz.	114[15]	—	176	21.4	9.3	.98	3.93	0	59

FRUITS[2]

Apple, raw	1 med.	180	84.4	96	0.3	1	—	—	24	2
	1 extra lg.	270	84.4	149	.467	1.56	—	—	37.3	3
Applejuice, canned or bottled unsweetened	1 cup	248	87.8	117	0.2	T	—	—	29.5	2
Applesauce, canned, unsweetened	1 cup	244	88.5	100	0.5	0.5	—	—	26.4	5
Apricots										
Raw	3 avg.	114	85.3	55	1.1	0.2	—	—	13.7	1
Canned, solids and liquid Syrup packed, heavy	1 cup	258	76.9	222	1.5	0.3	—	—	56.8	3
Water packed	1 cup	246	89.1	93	1.7	0.2	—	—	23.6	2
	½ cup	123	44.6	47	0.9	0.1	—	—	11.8	1
Apricot nectar, canned or bottled	1 cup	251	84.6	143	0.8	0.3	—	—	36.6	T
Avocado, raw, pitted	1 avg.	200	—	334	4.2	32.8	—	—	12.6	8
Banana, raw	1 avg.	150	75.7	87	1.1	0.2	—	—	22.6	1
Blackberries										
Raw	1 cup	144	84.5	84	1.7	1.3	—	—	18.6	1

FOOD PRODUCT[1]	AMOUNT	WEIGHT IN GRAMS	WATER (PERCENT)	FOOD ENERGY (CALORIES)	PROTEIN (GRAMS)	FAT (GRAMS)	(TOTAL) SATURATED (GRAMS)	UNSATURATED OLEIC (GRAMS)	LINOLEIC (GRAMS)	CARBOHYDRATES (GRAMS)	SODIUM (MILLIGRAMS)
Blackberries, canned, solids and liquids											
Syrup packed, heavy	1 cup ---	256	76.1	233	2	1.5	—	—	—	56.8	3
Water packed[21]	**1 cup** ---	244	89.3	98	2	1.5	—	—	—	22	2
Blueberries											
Raw	**1 cup** ---	145	85.2	90	1	0.7	—	—	—	22.2	1
Frozen, not thawed											
Unsweetened	**1 cup** ---	165	85	91	1.2	0.8	—	—	—	22.4	2
Sweetened	1 cup ---	230	72.3	242	1.4	0.7	—	—	—	61	2
Boysenberries											
Frozen, not thawed											
Unsweetened	1 cup ---	126	86.8	60	1.5	0.4	—	—	—	14.4	1
Sweetened	1 cup ---	143	74.3	137	1.1	0.4	—	—	—	34.9	1
Canned, solids and liquids, water packed[21]	1 cup ---	244	89.8	88	1.7	0.2	—	—	—	22.2	2
Cantaloupe, raw	¼ avg. ---	100	91.2	30	0.7	.11	—	—	—	7.49	12
	½ avg. ---	200	91.2	60	1.4	.22	—	—	—	14.9	24
Casaba melon, raw	1/10 avg. ---	245	91.5	38	1.7	T	—	—	—	9.1	17
	¼ avg. ---	613	91.5	95	4.3	T	—	—	—	22.8	43
	½ avg. ---	1,225	91.5	190	8.5	T	—	—	—	45.6	86
Cherries											
Sour, red											
Raw, pitted	1 cup ---	155	83.7	90	1.9	0.5	—	—	—	22.2	3
Canned											
Syrup packed, heavy[21]	1 cup ---	270	—	119	2.2	0.5	—	—	—	29.6	2
Water packed[21]	1 cup ---	244	88	105	2	0.5	—	—	—	26.1	5
Sweet											
Raw, whole	1 cup ---	130	80.4	82	1.5	0.4	—	—	—	20.4	2
Canned, solids and liquid, light or dark cherries											
Syrup packed	1 cup ---	279	78	208	2.3	0.5	—	—	—	52.6	3
Water packed, solids and liquids[21]	1 cup ---	270	86.6	119	2.2	0.5	—	—	—	29.6	2

Food	Measure										
Cranberry juice cocktail, bottled and sweetened	1 cup	253	83.2	164	0.3	0.3	—	—	—	41.7	3
Cranberry sauce, canned, sweetened	1 cup	277	62.1	404	0.3	0.6	—	—	—	103.9	3
Dates, pitted	10 dates	80	22.5	219	1.8	0.4	—	—	—	58.3	1
Figs, raw	2 lg.	100	77.5	80	1.2	0.4	—	—	—	20.4	2
Fruit Cocktail, canned, solids and liquid											
Syrup packed, heavy	1 cup	255	79.6	194	1	0.3	—	—	—	50.2	13
Water packed[21]	1 cup	245	89.6	91	1	0.2	—	—	—	23.8	12
Gooseberries, raw	**1 cup**	150	88.9	59	1.2	0.3	—	—	—	14.6	2
Grapefruit											
Raw, pink, red, white	½ med.	184	88.4	40	0.5	0.1	—	—	—	10.3	1
Canned, solids and liquid											
Syrup packed	1 cup	254	81.1	178	1.5	0.3	—	—	—	45.2	3
Water packed[21]	1 cup	244	91.3	73	1.5	0.2	—	—	—	18.5	10
Grapefruit juice, canned											
Unsweetened	1 cup	247	89.2	101	1.2	0.2	—	—	—	24.2	2
Sweetened[22]	1 cup	250	86.2	133	1.3	0.3	—	—	—	32	3
Grapes											
Raw, whole											
American type, as Concord, Delaware, Niagara, Catawba, Scuppernong (slip skin)	1 cup	153	81.6	70	1.3	1	—	—	—	15.9	3
European type, as Thompson Seedless, Emperor, Flame Tokay, Ribier, Malaga, Muscat (adherent skin)	1 cup	160	81.4	107	1	0.5	—	—	—	27.7	5
Canned, solids and liquid, Thompson Seedless											
Syrup packed, heavy	1 cup	256	79.1	197	1.3	0.3	—	—	—	51.2	10
Water packed[21]	1 cup	245	85.5	125	1.2	0.2	—	—	—	33.3	10
Grape juice											
Canned or bottled, unsweetened	1 cup	253	82.9	167	0.5	T	—	—	—	42	5
Frozen concentrate, sweetened, diluted[22]	1 cup	250	86.4	133	0.5	T	—	—	—	33.3	3

FOOD PRODUCT[1]	AMOUNT	WEIGHT IN GRAMS	WATER (PERCENT)	FOOD ENERGY (CALORIES)	PROTEIN (GRAMS)	FAT (GRAMS)	(TOTAL) SATURATED (GRAMS)	UNSATURATED OLEIC (GRAMS)	LINOLEIC (GRAMS)	CARBOHYDRATES (GRAMS)	SODIUM (MILLIGRAMS)
Honeydew melon, raw	**2" wedge**	226	90.6	49	1.2	0.4	—	—	—	11.5	18
	½ melon	1,130	90.6	245	6	2	—	—	—	57.5	90
Kumquats, raw	1 med.	20	81.3	12	0.2	T	—	—	—	3.2	1
Lemon, raw, peeled	**1 med.**	110	90.1	20	0.8	0.2	—	—	—	6	1
Lemon juice											
Raw	**2 Tbsp.**	30	91	8	0.2	T	—	—	—	2.4	T
Canned, unsweetened	**2 Tbsp.**	30	91.6	6	0.2	T	—	—	—	2.4	T
Lemonade, Frozen concentrate, diluted	1 cup	248	88.5	107	0.1	T	—	—	—	28.3	1
Lime											
Raw	**1 sm.**	80	89.3	19	0.5	0.1	—	—	—	6.4	1
Lime juice											
Raw	2 Tbsp.	31	91	8	T	T	—	—	—	2.8	T
Canned, unsweetened	2 Tbsp.	31	91.6	8	T	T	—	—	—	2.8	T
Loganberries, raw	1 cup	144	83	89	1.4	0.9	—	—	—	21.5	1
Loquats, raw	10 fruits	160	86.5	59	0.5	0.2	—	—	—	15.3	—
Lychees, raw	10 fruits	150	81.9	58	0.8	0.3	—	—	—	14.8	3
Mangos, raw	1 fruit	300	81.7	152	1.6	0.9	—	—	—	38.8	16
Nectarines, raw	1 avg.	150	81.8	88	0.8	T	—	—	—	23.6	8
Olives											
Green, pitted	2 med.	13	78.2	15	.18	1.65	—	—	—	.169	312
Ripe, pitted	2 lg.	20	80	37	.24	4.02	—	—	—	.64	150
Greek, pitted	3 med.	20	43.8	68	.44	7.15	—	—	—	1.74	657
Orange, all commercial varieties, raw, used for peeled fruit	1 sm.	180	86	64	1.3	0.3	—	—	—	16	1
	1 med.	224	86	80	1.6	.37	—	—	—	19.9	1.2
	1 lg.	280	86	100	2.02	.47	—	—	—	24.9	1.6
Orange juice											
Raw	1 cup	248	88.3	112	1.7	0.5	—	—	—	25.8	2
Canned											
Unsweetened	1 cup	249	87.4	120	2	0.5	—	—	—	27.9	2
Sweetened[22]	1 cup	250	86.5	130	1.8	0.5	—	—	—	30.5	2

Food	Measure										
Frozen concentrate, unsweetened, diluted	1 cup - - -	249	87.2	122	1.7	—	—	0.2	—	28.9	2
Papaya, raw	**½ med.** - -	150	88.7	58	.89	—	—	.17	—	15	5
Peach											
Raw	**1 med.** - -	115	89.1	38	0.6	—	—	0.1	—	9.7	1
Canned, solids and liquid											
Syrup packed, heavy	1 cup - - -	256	79.1	200	1	—	—	0.3	—	51.5	5
Water packed[21]	**1 cup** - - -	244	91.9	76	1	—	—	0.2	—	19.8	5
Pear											
Raw	1 avg. - - -	200	83.2	122	1.4	—	—	.79	—	30.5	4
Canned, solids and liquid											
Syrup packed, heavy	1 cup - - -	255	79.8	194	0.5	—	—	0.5	—	50	3
Water packed[21]	1 cup - - -	244	91.1	78	0.5	—	—	0.5	—	20.3	2
Persimmon											
Japanese, raw	**1 med.** - -	100	—	77	0.7	—	—	0.4	—	19.7	6
Native, raw	**1 med.** - -	100	—	127	0.8	—	—	0.4	—	33.5	1
Pineapple											
Raw	1 cup - - -	155	85.3	81	0.6	—	—	0.3	—	21.2	2
Canned, solids and liquid											
Syrup packed, heavy	1 cup - - -	255	79.9	189	0.8	—	—	0.3	—	49.5	3
Water packed[21]	1 cup - - -	246	89.1	96	0.7	—	—	0.2	—	25.1	2
Pineapple juice, canned, unsweetened	1 cup - - -	250	85.6	138	1	—	—	0.3	—	33.8	3
Plums											
Damson, raw	2 med. - -	100	81.1	66	.53	—	—	T	—	17.8	2
Prune type, raw	3 med. - -	100	78.7	75	.79	—	—	.18	—	19.7	1
Canned, solids and liquid, purple (Italian prunes), whole											
Syrup packed, heavy	1 cup - - -	272	77.4	214	1	—	—	0.3	—	55.8	3
Water packed[21]	1 cup - - -	262	86.8	114	1	—	—	0.5	—	29.6	5
Pomegranate, raw	1 lg. - - - -	275	82.3	97	0.8	—	—	0.5	—	25.3	5
Raisins, natural pack	1 cup - - -	165	18	477	4.1	—	—	0.3	—	127.7	45
Raspberries											
Black, raw	**1 cup** - -	134	80.8	98	2	—	—	1.9	—	21	1
Red, raw	**1 cup** - -	123	84.2	70	1.5	—	—	0.6	—	16.7	1
Canned, solids and liquid, **water packed**[21]	1 cup - - -	243	90.1	85	1.7	—	—	0.2	—	21.4	2

FOOD PRODUCT[1]	AMOUNT	WEIGHT IN GRAMS	WATER (PERCENT)	FOOD ENERGY (CALORIES)	PROTEIN (GRAMS)	FAT (GRAMS)	(TOTAL) SATURATED (GRAMS)	UNSATURATED OLEIC (GRAMS)	UNSATURATED LINOLEIC (GRAMS)	CARBOHYDRATES (GRAMS)	SODIUM (MILLIGRAMS)
Raspberries frozen, sweetened, thawed[22]	1 cup	255	71.3	278	1.3	0.5	—	—	—	70.9	3
Rhubarb, raw, diced	1 cup	122	94.8	20	0.7	0.1	—	—	—	4.5	2
	½ cup	61	47.4	10	.35	.05	—	—	—	2.3	1
Strawberries											
Raw	1 cup	149	89.9	55	1	0.7	—	—	—	12.5	1
Canned, solids and liquid, water packed[21]	1 cup	242	93.7	53	1	0.2	—	—	—	13.6	2
Frozen, sweetened[22]	1 cup	255	71.3	278	1.3	0.5	—	—	—	70.9	3
Tangelo, raw	1 med.	170	89.4	39	0.5	0.1	—	—	—	9.2	—
Tangerine, raw	1 med.	116	87	39	0.7	0.2	—	—	—	10	2
Tangerine juice											
Raw	1 cup	247	88.9	106	1.2	0.5	—	—	—	24.9	2
Canned											
Unsweetened	1 cup	247	88.8	106	1.2	0.5	—	—	—	25.2	2
Sweetened[22]	1 cup	249	87	125	1.2	0.5	—	—	—	29.9	2
Watermelon (slice, 6"×1½")	1 slice	600	92.6	156	3.04	1.19	—	—	—	38.3	7

MEAT AND POULTRY[2]

FOOD PRODUCT[1]	AMOUNT	WEIGHT IN GRAMS	WATER (PERCENT)	FOOD ENERGY (CALORIES)	PROTEIN (GRAMS)	FAT (GRAMS)	(TOTAL) SATURATED (GRAMS)	UNSATURATED OLEIC (GRAMS)	UNSATURATED LINOLEIC (GRAMS)	CARBOHYDRATES (GRAMS)	SODIUM (MILLIGRAMS)
Crunchies	2 Tbsp.	9	—	59	11.05	.215	—	—	—	6.69	—
Beef											
Chuck roast, raw, lean with fat, with bone (77% lean, 12% fat)	1 lb.	454	64.2	905	78.8	62.9	30.2	27.7	1.3	0	276
	4 oz.	114	64.2	266	19.7	15.73	7.6	6.93	.33	0	69
Club steak, raw, lean with fat, with bone (57% lean, 30% fat)	1 lb.	454	49	1,443	58.9	132.1	63.4	58.1	2.6	0	206
	4 oz.	114	49	361	14.8	33.03	15.9	14.53	0.7	0	52
Flank steak, raw (100% lean)	1 lb.	454	71.7	653	98	25.9	12.4	11.4	0.5	0	343
	4 oz.	114	71.7	163	24.5	6.48	3.1	2.9	.13	0	86
Ground beef											
Raw, lean with 10% fat	1 lb.	454	68.3	812	93.9	45.4	21.8	20	0.9	0	329

Food	Measure										
	4 oz.	114	68.3	203	23.5	11.4	5.5	5	.23	0	82
Raw, lean with 21% fat	1 lb.	454	60.2	1,216	81.2	96.2	46.2	42.3	1.9	0	284
	4 oz.	114	60.2	304	20.3	24.1	11.6	10.58	.48	0	71
Heart, raw, lean	1 lb.	454	—	490	77.6	16.3	5	7.72	—	3.2	390
	4 oz.	114	—	123	19.4	4.1	1.25	1.93	—	.8	98
Kidney, raw	1 lb.	454	—	590	69.9	30.4	—	—	—	4.1	798
	4 oz.	114	—	148	17.5	7.6	—	—	—	1.03	200
Liver, raw, lean	1 lb.	454	—	635	90.3	17.2	6.8	5	—	24	617
	4 oz.	114	—	159	22.6	4.3	1.7	1.3	—	6	154
Porterhouse steak, raw, lean with fat and bone (54% lean, 33% fat)	1 lb.	454	48.3	1,603	60.8	148.8	71.4	65.5	3	0	213
	4 oz.	114	48.3	401	15.2	37.2	17.9	16.38	0.8	0	53
Rib roast, raw, lean with fat, with bone (54% lean, 33% fat)	1 lb.	454	47.2	1,673	61.8	156.1	74.9	68.7	3.1	0	216
	4 oz.	114	47.2	418	15.5	39.03	18.73	17.18	.78	0	54
Round steak, raw, lean with fat, with bone (86% lean, 11% fat)	1 lb.	454	66.6	863	88.5	53.9	25.9	23.7	1.1	0	310
	4 oz.	114	66.6	216	22.1	13.48	6.48	5.93	.28	0	78
Rump roast, raw, lean with fat, with bone (63% lean, 22% fat)	1 lb.	454	56.5	1,167	67	97.4	46.8	42.9	1.9	0	235
	4 oz.	114	56.5	292	16.8	24.4	11.7	10.73	.48	0	59
Sirloin steak, raw, lean with fat, with bone (68% lean, 25% fat)	1 lb.	454	55.7	1,316	71.1	112.3	53.9	49.4	2.2	0	249
	4 oz.	114	55.7	329	17.8	28.08	13.48	12.4	0.6	0	62
T-Bone steak, raw, lean with fat, with bone (55% lean, 34% fat)	1 lb.	454	47.5	1,596	59.1	149.1	71.6	65.6	3	0	207
	4 oz.	114	47.5	399	14.8	37.28	17.9	16.4	0.8	0	52
Tongue, raw	1 lb.	454	—	714	56.5	52	—	—	—	1.4	252
	4 oz.	114	—	179	14.13	13	—	—	—	.35	63
Beef, corned, raw, boneless	1 lb.	454	54.2	1,329	71.7	113.4	54.4	49.9	2.3	0	5,897
	4 oz.	114	54.2	332	17.9	28.4	13.6	12.48	.58	0	1,474
Beef, dried, chipped, raw	4 oz.	114	11.93	230	38.9	7.2	3.4	3.2	.15	0	4,876

FOOD PRODUCT[1]	AMOUNT	WEIGHT IN GRAMS	WATER (PERCENT)	FOOD ENERGY (CALORIES)	PROTEIN (GRAMS)	FAT (GRAMS)	(TOTAL) SATURATED (GRAMS)	UNSATURATED OLEIC (GRAMS)	LINOLEIC (GRAMS)	CARBOHYDRATES (GRAMS)	SODIUM (MILLIGRAMS)
Chicken,[23] raw, all classes without skin, cut-up parts[24]											
Back	1 lb.	454	75.3	622	88.53	26.79	6.90	6.95	5.13	0	372
	4 oz.	114	75.3	156	22.13	6.69	1.73	1.74	1.28	0	93
Breast	1 lb.	454	74.8	499	104.9	5.45	1.5	1.14	.77	0	295
	4 oz.	114	74.8	125	26.2	1.36	.38	.29	.19	0	74
Drumstick	1 lb.	454	76.4	540	93.5	5.44	3.9	3.9	2.9	0	400
	4 oz.	114	76.4	135	23.38	1.4	.98	.98	.73	0	100
Heart	1 lb.	454	73.6	695	70.4	42.2	12.08	8.99	8.7	3.22	336
	4 oz.	114	73.6	174	17.6	10.6	3.02	2.25	2.18	.805	84
Liver	1 lb.	454	73.6	568	81.58	17.5	5.9	3.77	1.82	15.53	359
	4 oz.	114	73.6	142	20.4	4.38	1.48	.94	.46	3.883	90
Neck	1 lb.	454	71.2	699	79.5	39.9	10.22	10.31	7.6	0	368
	4 oz.	114	71.2	175	19.88	9.98	2.56	2.58	1.9	0	92
Thigh	1 lb.	454	75.8	540	88.98	17.71	4.54	4.59	3.41	0	390
	4 oz.	114	75.8	135	22.25	4.43	1.14	1.15	.85	0	98
Wing	1 lb.	454	75	572	99.9	15.9	4.27	3.31	2.31	0	368
	4 oz.	114	75	143	24.98	3.98	1.07	.83	.53	0	92
Chicken, raw											
Light meat	1 lb.	454	74.9	518	105.3	7.5	1.99	1.54	.99	0	241
	4 oz.	114	74.9	130	26.33	1.88	.49	.39	.25	0	60
Dark meat	1 lb.	454	76	568	91.3	19.6	4.99	5.04	3.72	0	459
	4 oz.	114	76	142	22.83	4.9	1.25	1.26	.93	0	115
Chicken, canned	1 cup	205	—	406	44.5	24	7.7	9.1	4.8	0	—
Chili con carne	1 cup	255	72.4	339	19.1	15.6	7.5	6.8	0.3	31.1	1,354
Frankfurter	1 lb.	454	55.6	1,402	56.7	125.2	51	72		8.2	4,990
	4 oz.	114	55.6	351	14.18	31.3	12.8	18		2.1	1,248
	1 frankfurter	57	55.6	176	7.12	15.72	6.4	9.04		1.03	626
Gelatin	**1 envelope**	7	13	23	6	T	—	—	—	0	—
Lamb											
Leg, raw, lean with fat, with bone (70% lean, 14% fat)	1 lb.	454	64.8	845	67.7	61.7	34.6	22.2	1.9	0	237
	4 oz.	114	64.8	211	16.93	15.43	8.7	5.6	.48	0	59

Food	Measure	Grams									
Chops, loin, raw (62% lean, 24% fat)	1 lb.	454	57.7	1,146	63.7	97	54.3	34.9	2.9	0	223
	4 oz.	114	57.7	287	15.93	24.3	13.58	8.73	.73	0	56
Liver pâté	1 Tbsp.	13	—	60	1.5	5.7	—	—	—	0.6	—
Pork[23] Bacon — Raw, sliced	1 lb.	454	19.3	3,016	38.1	314.3	100.6	150.9	28.3	4.5	3,084
	4 oz.	114	19.3	754	9.53	78.58	25.2	37.73	7.08	1.13	771
Cooked, broiled, drained	1 slice	8	8.1	43	.95	3.9	1.8	2.66	.499	.25	77
Bacon, Canadian, unheated	1 lb.	454	61.7	980	90.7	65.3	23.5	27.4	5.9	1.4	8,578
	4 oz.	114	61.7	245	22.68	16.33	5.88	6.9	1.48	.35	2,145
Cooked, broiled, drained	1 slice	21	49.9	58	5.7	3.7	1.09	1.27	.273	0.1	537
Boston butt, raw, lean with fat, with bone and skin (74% lean, 20% fat)	1 lb.	454	59.3	1,220	65.9	104.1	37.5	43.7	9.4	0	231
	4 oz.	114	59.3	305	16.48	26.03	9.38	10.93	2.4	0	58
Chops, loin, raw, lean with fat, with bone (63% lean, 16% fat)	1 lb.	454	57.2	1,065	61.1	89	32	37.4	8	0	214
	4 oz.	114	57.2	266	15.28	22.3	8	9.4	2	0	54
Ham — Cured, raw, medium fatness, lean meat with fat, bone, skin	1 lb.	454	42	1,535	66.7	138	49.7	58	12.4	1.2	3,415
	4 oz.	114	42	384	16.68	34.5	12.43	14.5	3.1	0.3	854
Deviled, canned	1 cup	225	51.5	790	31.3	72.7	26.2	30.5	6.5	0	—
	2 Tbsp.	28	51.5	99	3.91	9.09	3.28	3.813	.81	0	—
Picnic, raw, lean with fat and bone and skin (61% lean, 22% fat)	1 lb.	454	58.9	1,083	59	92.2	33.2	38.7	8.3	0	207
	4 oz.	114	58.9	271	14.8	23.1	8.3	9.68	2.08	0	52
Spareribs, raw, lean with fat and bone	1 lb.	454	51.8	976	39.2	89.7	32.3	37.7	8.1	0	137
	4 oz.	114	51.8	244	9.8	22.43	8.08	9.43	2.03	0	34
Protein powder	2 Tbsp.	9	—	70	16	0	1	—	—	—	—
Rabbit[23] raw, ready to cook	1 lb.	454	—	581	75	28.7	11	13	—	0	154
	4 oz.	114	—	145	18.8	7.18	2.8	3.3	—	0	39

FOOD PRODUCT[1]	AMOUNT	WEIGHT IN GRAMS	WATER (PERCENT)	FOOD ENERGY (CALORIES)	PROTEIN (GRAMS)	FAT (GRAMS)	(TOTAL) SATURATED (GRAMS)	UNSATURATED OLEIC (GRAMS)	UNSATURATED LINOLEIC (GRAMS)	CARBOHYDRATES (GRAMS)	SODIUM (MILLIGRAMS)
Sausage[23]											
Blood											
Blood pudding and blood											
Tongue sausage	1 lb.	454	46.4	1,787	64	167.4	—	—	—	1.4	—
	4 oz.	114	46.4	447	16	41.9	—	—	—	.35	—
Bologna, packaged	1 lb.	454	56.2	1,379	54.9	124.7	54	69	—	5	5,897
	1 slice	22	56.2	67	2.7	6.04	2.62	3.34	—	.24	286
Country style	1 lb.	454	49.9	1,565	68.5	141.1	50.8	59.2	12.7	0	—
	4 oz.	114	49.9	391	17.13	35.28	12.7	14.8	3.18	0	—
Headcheese, prepackaged, square	1 lb.	454	58.8	1,261	70.3	99.8	35.9	41.9	9	4.5	785
	4 oz.	114	58.8	315	17.58	24.9	8.98	10.48	2.3	1.13	196
Knockwurst, prepackaged, link	1 lb.	454	57.6	1,261	64	105.2	45.5	70.5	—	10	699
	4 oz.	114	57.6	315	16	26.3	11.38	17.63	—	2.5	175
Liverwurst, fresh, not smoked	1 lb.	454	53.9	1,393	73.5	116.1	—	—	—	8.2	1,080
	4 oz.	114	53.9	348	18.38	29.03	—	—	—	2.1	270
Pork, link, prepackaged links	1 lb.	454	38.1	2,259	42.6	230.4	83	96.8	20.7	T	3,357
	4 oz.	114	38.1	565	10.7	57.6	20.8	24.2	5.18	T	839
Salami, prepackaged	1 lb.	454	29.8	2,041	108	172.8	53.5	89.5	—	5.4	—
	4 oz.	114	29.8	510	27	43.2	13.38	22.38	—	1.4	—
Vienna sausage, canned, drained	7 sausages	113	63	271	15.8	22.4	—	—	—	0.3	—
Turkey,[23] raw, all classes without skin[24]											
Light meat	1 lb.	454	73.6	527	93.5	7.54	2.41	1.09	1.32	0	286
	4 oz.	114	73.6	132	23.38	1.89	.60	.27	.33	0	72
Dark meat	1 lb.	454	74	590	91.3	22.25	7.45	4.18	5.36	0	88
	4 oz.	114	74	148	22.83	5.56	1.86	1.05	1.34	0	350
Turkey, canned, meat only, boned	1 cup	205	64.9	414	42.8	25.6	7.4	11.0	5.4	0	—

Food	Measure										
Tofu[23]	8 oz	227	84.8	164	17.7	9.6	1.5	1.9	4.95	5.45	16
Veal[23]											
Chuck, raw, lean with fat, with bone (69% lean, 11% fat)	1 lb.	454	70	628	70.4	36	17.3	15.8	0.7	0	246
	4 oz.	114	70	157	17.6	9	4.33	3.95	.18	0	62
Cutlet, lean with fat, with bone (71% lean, 12% fat)	1 lb.	454	69	681	72.3	41	19.7	18	0.8	0	253
	4 oz.	114	69	170	18.08	10.3	4.93	4.5	0.2	0	63
Plate, breast, raw, lean with fat, with bone (58% lean, 21% fat)	1 lb.	454	64	828	65.6	61	29.3	26.8	1.2	0	230
	4 oz.	114	64	207	16.4	15.3	7.33	6.7	0.3	0	58
Rib roast, raw, with bone (63% lean, 14% fat)	1 lb.	454	66	723	65.7	49	23.5	21.6	1	0	230
	4 oz.	114	66	181	16.43	12.3	5.88	5.4	.25	0	58
Rump roast, raw, lean with fat, with bone (67% lean, 10% fat)	1 lb.	454	70	573	68.1	31	14.9	13.6	0.6	0	238
	4 oz.	114	70	143	17.03	7.8	3.73	3.4	.15	0	60
Venison[23]											
Raw, lean meat only	1 lb.	454	74	571	95.47	18.13	11.2	4.27	.53	0	318
	4 oz.	114	74	143	23.87	4.53	2.8	1.07	.133	0	80

NUT PRODUCTS AND SEEDS[30]

Food	Measure										
Almonds[25]											
Dried, shelled, raw	1 cup	142	4.7	849	26.4	77.0	6.2	51.6	15.4	27.7	6
Roasted (in oil), salted	1 cup	157	4.7	984	29.2	90.6	7.3	60.7	18.1	30.6	311
Almond meal,[25] partially defatted	1 cup	28	7.2	116	11.2	5.2	0.4	3.5	1.0	8.2	2
Brazil nuts, raw, shelled[25]	1 cup	140	4.6	916	20.0	93.7	18.7	45.0	24.3	15.3	1
Cashew nuts, roasted (in oil)[25]	1 cup	140	5.2	785	24.1	64.0	10.9	44.8	4.5	41.0	21[29]
Chestnuts, fresh, shelled[25]	1 cup	160	52.5	310	4.6	2.4	.44	2.04		67.4	10
Coconut meat, fresh, shelled,[25] not packed	1 cup	80	50.9	277	2.8	28.2	24.3	2.0	T	7.5	18
Coconut milk[26]	1 cup	240	65.7	605	7.7	59.8	51.4	4.2	T	12.5	

FOOD PRODUCT[1]	AMOUNT	WEIGHT IN GRAMS	WATER (PERCENT)	FOOD ENERGY (CALORIES)	PROTEIN (GRAMS)	FAT (GRAMS)	(TOTAL) SATURATED (GRAMS)	UNSATURATED OLEIC (GRAMS)	LINOLEIC (GRAMS)	CARBOHYDRATES (GRAMS)	SODIUM (MILLIGRAMS)
Coconut water, liquid from coconuts	1 cup ---	240	94.2	53	0.7	0.5	—	—	—	11.3	60
Hazelnuts (filberts), raw, shelled	1 cup ---	135	5.8	856	17.0	84.2	4.2	45.5	13.5	22.5	3
Macadamia nuts, roasted	6 avg. ---	15		709	1.4	11.7	1.64	8.9		1.5	—
Peanuts, roasted,[25,27] shelled, chopped from	1 cup ---	144	1.8	838	37.7	70.1	15.4	30.2	20.3	29.7	7
Peanut butter[25]	1 Tbsp. ---	16	1.7	94	4.0	8.1	1.5	3.8	2.3	3.0	97
Pecans, shelled[25,27]	1 cup ---	108	3.4	742	9.9	76.9	5.4	48.4	15.4	15.8	T
Pine nuts, shelled[25]	1 oz. -----	28	3.1	180	3.7	17.2	1.7	11.7		5.8	—
Pistachio nuts, shelled[25]	30 avg. --	15	5.3	89	2.9	8.05	.81	5.23	1.5	2.85	—
Pumpkin and squash seeds, dried, hulled	1 cup ---	140	4.4	774	40.6	65.4	11.8	23.5	27.5	21.0	—
Sesame seeds, dried, hulled	1 cup ---	150	5.5	873	27.3	80.1	11.2	30.4	33.6	26.4	—
Sunflower seeds, dry, hulled[28]	1 cup ---	145	4.8	812	34.8	68.6	8.2	13.7	43.2	28.9	44
Walnuts, black,[25] shelled, chopped	1 cup ---	125	3.1	785	25.6	74.1	4.5	26.0	35.6	18.5	4
Walnuts, Persian or English, shelled, halves	1 cup ---	100	3.5	651	14.8	64.0	4.5	9.6	39.7	15.8	2

OILS, FATS AND SHORTENING[2]

FOOD PRODUCT	AMOUNT	WEIGHT IN GRAMS	WATER (PERCENT)	FOOD ENERGY (CALORIES)	PROTEIN (GRAMS)	FAT (GRAMS)	(TOTAL) SATURATED (GRAMS)	UNSATURATED OLEIC (GRAMS)	LINOLEIC (GRAMS)	CARBOHYDRATES (GRAMS)	SODIUM (MILLIGRAMS)
Corn	1 Tbsp. ---	14	0	120	0	13.6	1.4	3.8	7.2	0	0
	2 tsp. ---	9	0	80	0	9.1	.93	2.5	4.8	0	0
Cottonseed	1 Tbsp. ---	14	0	120	0	13.6	3.4	2.9	6.8	0	0
	2 tsp. ---	9	0	80	0	9.07	2.27	1.93	4.53	0.	0
Soybean	1 Tbsp. ---	14	0	120	0	13.6	2.0	2.7	7.1	0	0
	2 tsp. ---	9	0	80	0	9.1	1.3	1.8	4.73	0	0
Olive	1 Tbsp. ---	14	0	119	0	13.5	1.5	10.3	0.9	0	0
	2 tsp. ---	9	0	79	0	9	1.0	6.87	0.6	0	0
Peanut	1 Tbsp. ---	14	0	119	0	13.5	2.4	6.3	3.9	0	0
	2 tsp. ---	9	0	79	0	9	1.6	4.2	2.6	0	0

Safflower											
	1 Tbsp.	14	0	124	0	13.6	1.1	2.0	9.8	0	T
	2 tsp.	9	0	83	0	9.3	.73	1.3	6.5	0	T
Sunflower											
	1 Tbsp.	14	—	124	T	14	1.8	12		T	T
	2 tsp.	9	—	83	T	9.3	1.2	8		T	T
Butter	1 Tbsp.	14	15.5	102	0.1	11.5	6.3	3.8	0.3	0.1	140
Margarine											
Regular	1 Tbsp.	14	15.5	102	0.1	11.5	2.1	5.9	3.1	0.1	140
Whipped	1 Tbsp.	14	15.5	68	0.1	7.6	1.4	3.9	2.1	T	93
Vegetable fat (shortening)	1 Tbsp.	13	0	111	0	12.5	3.1	6.3	2.7	0	0

SALAD DRESSINGS AND SAUCES[2]

Barbecue sauce	1 cup	250	80.9	228	3.8	17.3	1.7	4.8	9.2	20	2,038
	1 Tbsp.	15	80.9	14	.24	1.08	.11	0.3	.58	1.3	127
Tomato catsup	1 Tbsp.	15	68.6	16	0.3	0.1	—	—	—	3.8	156[32]
Chili sauce	1 Tbsp.	15	68	16	0.4	T	—	—	—	3.7	201[32]
Horseradish, prepared	**1 Tbsp.**	15	87.1	6	0.2	T	—	—	—	1.4	14
Mayonnaise	1 Tbsp.	14	15.1	101	0.2	11.2	2	8		0.3	84
Mustard	**1 Tbsp.**	15	80.2	12	0.6	0.6	—	—	—	0.9	189
	1 tsp.	5	80.2	4	0.2	0.2	—	—	—	0.3	63
Salad Dressings											
Blue or Roquefort, regular	1 Tbsp.	15	32.3	76	0.7	7.8	1.6	1.7	3.8	1.1	164
Low calorie	1 Tbsp.	16	83.7	12	0.5	0.9	0.5	0.3	T	0.7	177
French, regular	1 Tbsp.	16	38.8	66	0.1	6.2	1.1	1.3	3.2	2.8	219
Low calorie	1 Tbsp.	16	77.3	15	0.1	0.7	0.1	0.1	0.4	2.5	126
Italian, regular	1 Tbsp.	15	17.5	83	T	9.0	1.6	1.9	4.7	1	314
Low calorie	1 Tbsp.	15	90.1	8	T	0.7	0.1	0.1	0.4	0.4	118
Russian, regular	1 Tbsp.	15	34.5	74	0.2	7.6	1.4	1.7	3.8	1.6	130
Thousand Island, regular	1 Tbsp.	16	32	80	0.1	8.0	1.4	1.7	4.0	2.5	112
Low calorie	1 Tbsp.	15	68.2	27	0.1	2.1	0.4	0.4	1.0	2.3	105
Soy sauce[31]	1 Tbsp.	18	62.8	12	1	0.2	—	—	—	1.1	1,319
Tartar sauce	1 Tbsp.	14	34.4	74	0.2	8.1	—	—	—	0.6	99
Vinegar, cider	**1 Tbsp.**	15	93.8	2	T	0	—	—	—	0.9	T
White sauce, medium	1 Tbsp.	16	5	25	0.6	1.96	1.03	.644	.063	1.4	59

SOUPS[33]

FOOD PRODUCT[1]	AMOUNT	WEIGHT IN GRAMS	WATER (PERCENT)	FOOD ENERGY (CALORIES)	PROTEIN (GRAMS)	FAT (GRAMS)	(TOTAL) SATURATED (GRAMS)	UNSATURATED OLEIC (GRAMS)	UNSATURATED LIN-OLEIC (GRAMS)	CARBO-HYDRATES (GRAMS)	SODIUM (MILLI-GRAMS)
Beans and pork, canned	1 cup	250	84.4	168	8	5.8	1.5	2.0	1.9	21.8	1,008
Beef, consommé or bouillon, canned	1 cup	240	95.8	31	5	0	—	—	—	2.6	782
Noodle, canned	1 cup	245	86.4	140	7.8	5.4	1.7	2.0	1.3	14.2	1,872
Celery, cream of, canned	1 cup	240	92.3	86	1.7	5.0	0.9	1.5	2.2	8.9	955
Chicken, cream of, canned	1 cup	240	91.9	94	2.9	5.8	0.9	1.7	2.6	7.9	970
Gumbo, canned	1 cup	240	93.8	55	3.1	1.4	—	—	—	7.4	950
Noodle, canned	1 cup	240	93.3	62	3.4	1.9	—	—	—	7.9	979
W/Rice, canned	1 cup	240	94.8	48	3.1	1.2	—	—	—	5.8	917
Clam chowder, Manhattan, canned	1 cup	245	91.9	81	2.2	2.5	—	—	—	12.3	938
Minestrone, canned	1 cup	245	89.5	105	4.9	3.4	—	—	—	14.2	955
Mushroom, cream of, canned	1 cup	240	89.6	134	2.4	9.6	1.3	2.7	4.6	10.1	955
Onion, canned	1 cup	240	93.4	65	5.3	2.4	—	—	—	5.3	1,051
Pea, split, canned	1 cup	245	85.4	145	8.6	3.2	1.0	1.5	0.3	20.6	941
Tomato, canned	1 cup	245	90.5	88	2	2.5	0.4	0.7	1.0	15.7	970
Turkey, noodle, canned	1 cup	240	92.3	79	4.3	2.9	0.8	1.2	0.6	8.4	998
Vegetable, beef, canned	1 cup	245	91.9	78	5.1	2.2	—	—	—	9.6	1,046
Vegetarian, canned	1 cup	245	91.8	78	2.2	2	—	—	—	13.2	838

SPICES AND HERBS[2]

FOOD PRODUCT[1]	AMOUNT	WEIGHT IN GRAMS	WATER (PERCENT)	FOOD ENERGY (CALORIES)	PROTEIN (GRAMS)	FAT (GRAMS)	(TOTAL) SATURATED (GRAMS)	UNSATURATED OLEIC (GRAMS)	UNSATURATED LIN-OLEIC (GRAMS)	CARBO-HYDRATES (GRAMS)	SODIUM (MILLI-GRAMS)
Allspice	1 tsp.	1.9		5	.12	.17	.05		.05	1.37	1
Anise seed	1 tsp.	2.1		7	.37	.33			.28	1.05	T
Basil, ground	1 tsp.	1.4		4	0.2	.06			—	.85	T
Bay leaf, crumbled	1 tsp.	0.6		2	.05	.05	.01		.02	.45	T
Caraway seed	1 tsp.	2.1		7	.42	.31	.01		.22	1.05	T
Cardamom, ground	1 tsp.	2		6	.21	.13	.01		.03	1.37	T
Celery seed	1 tsp.	2		8	.36	.5	.04		.39	.83	3
Chervill, dried	1 tsp.	0.6		1	.14	.02			—	0.3	T
Chili powder	1 tsp.	2.6		8	.32	.44			—	1.42	26

	Measure								
Cinnamon, ground	1 tsp.	2.3	6	.09	.07	.01	.02	1.84	1
Cloves, ground	1 tsp.	2.1	7	.13	.42	.09	—	1.29	5
Coriander leaf, dried	1 tsp.	0.6	2	.13	.03	—	—	.31	1
Coriander seed	1 tsp.	1.8	5	.22	.32	.02	.27	.99	1
Cumin seed	1 tsp.	2.1	8	.37	.47	—	—	.93	4
Curry powder	1 tsp.	2	6	.25	.28	—	—	1.16	1
Dill seed	1 tsp.	2.1	6	.34	.31	.02	.22	1.16	T
Dillweed, dried	1 tsp.	1	3	0.2	T	—	—	.56	2
Fennel seed	1 tsp.	2	7	.32	0.3	.01	.23	1.05	2
Fenugreek seed	1 tsp.	3.7	12	.85	.24	—	—	2.16	2
Garlic powder	1 tsp.	2.8	9	.47	.02	—	—	2.04	1
Ginger, ground	1 tsp.	1.8	6	.16	.11	.03	.04	1.27	1
Mace, ground	1 tsp.	1.7	8	.11	.55	.16	.26	.86	T
Marjoram, dried	1 tsp.	0.6	2	.08	.04	—	—	.36	T
Mustard seed, yellow	1 tsp.	3.3	15	.82	.95	.05	.83	1.15	T
Nutmeg, ground	1 tsp.	2.2	12	.13	0.8	.57	.08	1.08	1
Onion powder	1 tsp.	2.1	7	.21	.02	.04	—	1.69	T
Oregano, ground	1 tsp.	1.5	5	.17	.15	.04	.09	.97	1
Paprika	1 tsp.	2.1	6	.31	.27	—	0.2	1.17	1
Parsley, dried	1 tsp.	0.3	1	.07	.01	—	—	.15	1
Pepper									
Black	1 tsp.	2.1	5	.23	.07	.03	.03	1.36	1
Red or cayenne	1 tsp.	1.8	6	.22	.31	.06	0.2	1.02	1
White	1 tsp.	2.4	7	.25	.05	—	—	1.65	T
Poppy seed	1 tsp.	2.8	15	.5	1.25	.14	1.04	.66	1
Poultry seasoning	1 tsp.	1.5	5	.14	.11	—	—	.98	T
Pumpkin pie spice	1 tsp.	1.7	6	0.1	.21	—	—	1.17	1
Rosemary, dried	1 tsp.	1.2	4	.06	.18	—	—	.77	1
Saffron	1 tsp.	0.7	2	.08	.04	.05	.02	.46	1
Sage, ground	1 tsp.	0.7	2	.07	.09	—	—	.43	T
Salt	1 tsp.	5.5	0	0	0	—	—	0	2,132
Savory, ground	1 tsp.	1.4	4	.09	.08	—	—	.96	T
Tarragon, ground	1 tsp.	1.6	5	.36	.12	.04	.03	.8	1
Thyme, ground	1 tsp.	1.4	4	.13	.01	.04	—	.89	1
Turmeric, ground	1 tsp.	2.2	8	.17	22	—	—	1.43	1

VEGETABLES

FOOD PRODUCT[1]	AMOUNT	WEIGHT IN GRAMS	WATER (PERCENT)	FOOD ENERGY (CALORIES)	PROTEIN (GRAMS)	FAT (GRAMS)	SATURATED (TOTAL) (GRAMS)	UNSATURATED OLEIC (GRAMS)	UNSATURATED LINOLEIC (GRAMS)	CARBOHYDRATES (GRAMS)	SODIUM (MILLIGRAMS)
Asparagus											
Cooked spears, drained (spears, ½-in. diam. at base)	**4 spears** -	60	93.6	12	1.3	0.1	—	—	—	2.2	1[34]
Canned spears (drained solids) (spears, ½-in. diam. at base)	4 spears -	80	92.5	17	1.9	0.3	—	—	—	2.7	189[35]
Beans											
Lima, canned (drained solids)	1 cup - - -	170	74.7	163	9.2	0.5	—	—	—	31.1	401[35]
Snap											
Green											
Cooked, drained	**1 cup** - - -	125	92.4	31	2	0.3	—	—	—	6.8	5[34]
Canned (drained solids)	1 cup - - -	135	91.9	32	1.9	0.3	—	—	—	7	319[35]
Yellow or wax											
Cooked, drained	**1 cup** - - -	125	93.4	28	1.8	0.3	—	—	—	5.8	4[34]
Canned (drained solids)	1 cup - - -	135	92.2	32	1.9	0.4	—	—	—	7	319[35]
Beets, common, red											
Raw, peeled, diced	1 cup - - -	135	87.3	58	2.2	0.1	—	—	—	13.4	81
Cooked, drained, diced or sliced	1 cup - - -	170	90.9	54	1.9	0.2	—	—	—	12.2	73[34]
Canned (drained solids), diced or sliced	1 cup - - -	170	89.3	63	1.7	0.2	—	—	—	15	401[35]
Beet greens, common, edible leaves and stems											
Raw	**3.5 oz.**[38] -	100	90.9	24	2.2	0.3	—	—	—	4.5	129
Cooked, drained	**1 cup** - - -	145	93.6	26	2.5	0.3	—	—	—	4.8	110[34]
Broccoli, stalks											
Cooked, drained	1 cup - - -	155	91.3	40	4.8	0.5	—	—	—	7	16[34]
Brussels sprouts											
Cooked, drained	1 cup - - -	155	88.2	56	6.5	0.6	—	—	—	9.9	16[34]

Food	Measure										
Cabbage											
Common varieties											
Raw, shredded or sliced	1 cup ---	70	92.4	17	0.9	0.1	—	—	—	3.8	14
Cooked, drained	1 cup ---	145	93.9	29	1.6	0.3	—	—	—	6.2	20
Red, raw, shredded or sliced	1 cup ---	70	90.2	22	1.4	0.1	—	—	—	4.8	18
Savoy, raw, shredded or sliced	1 cup ---	70	92	17	1.7	0.1	—	—	—	3.2	15
Cabbage, Chinese (Cabbage Celery), raw	1 cup ---	75	95	11	0.9	0.1	—	—	—	2.3	17
Carrots											
Raw	1 carrot -	72	88.2	30	0.8	0.1	—	—	—	7	34
Grated or shredded	1 cup ---	110	88.2	46	1.2	0.2	—	—	—	10.7	52
Cooked, drained	1 cup ---	155	91.2	48	1.4	0.3	—	—	—	11	51[34]
Canned (drained solids)	1 cup ---	155	91.2	47	1.2	0.5	—	—	—	10.4	366[35]
Cauliflower flowerbuds (whole)											
Raw	1 cup ---	100	91	27	2.7	0.2	—	—	—	5.2	13
Cooked, drained	1 cup ---	125	93	28	2.9	0.3	—	—	—	5.1	11[34]
Celery											
Chopped or diced	1 cup ---	120	94.1	20	1.1	0.1	—	—	—	4.7	151
Cooked, diced pieces	1 cup ---	150	95.3	21	1.2	0.2	—	—	—	4.7	132
Stalk, small inner 5-in. long	1 stalk ---	17	94.1	3	.17	.03	—	—	—	.67	21
Chard, Swiss											
Raw	3.5 oz.[38] -	100	91.1	25	2.4	0.3	—	—	—	4.6	146
Cooked, drained	1 cup ---	145	93.7	26	2.6	0.3	—	—	—	4.8	25[34]
Chicory, raw, chopped	1 cup ---	90	95.1	14	0.9	0.1	—	—	—	2.9	6
Collards											
Raw, leaves including stems	3.5 oz.[38] -	100	86.9	40	3.6	0.7	—	—	—	7.2	43
Cooked, drained, leaves including stems	1 cup ---	145	90.8	42	3.9	0.9	—	—	—	7.1	36[34]
Corn, sweet											
Cooked, drained	1 cup ---	165	76.5	137	5.3	1.7	—	—	—	31	T[34]
Canned (drained solids)	1 cup ---	165	75.9	139	4.3	1.3	—	—	—	32.7	389[35]
Cream style	1 cup ---	256	76.3	210	5.4	1.5	—	—	—	51.2	604[35]
Cucumber, sliced ⅛-in. thick	1 cup ---	105	95.1	16	0.9	0.1	—	—	—	3.6	6

FOOD PRODUCT[1]	AMOUNT	WEIGHT IN GRAMS	WATER (PERCENT)	FOOD ENERGY (CALORIES)	PROTEIN (GRAMS)	FAT (GRAMS)	(TOTAL) SATURATED (GRAMS)	UNSATURATED OLEIC (GRAMS)	LINOLEIC (GRAMS)	CARBOHYDRATES (GRAMS)	SODIUM (MILLIGRAMS)
Dandelion greens											
Raw	3.5 oz.[38]	100	85.6	45	2.7	0.7	—	—	—	9.12	75
Cooked, drained	1 cup	105	89.8	35	2.1	0.6	—	—	—	6.7	46[34]
Dark leafy greens	1 cup	98	—	33	2.74	.491	—	—	—	6.27	74
Endive, curly (including escarole) raw, cut or broken, sm. pieces	1 cup	50	93.1	10	0.9	0.1	—	—	—	2.1	7
Fennel, common leaves, raw	3.5 oz.[38]	100	90	28	3	T	—	—	—	5	—
Kale											
Raw	3.5 oz.[38]	100	82.7	53	5.9	0.8	—	—	—	8.9	74
Cooked, drained	1 cup	110	87.8	43	5	0.8	—	—	—	6.7	47[34]
Lettuce, raw											
Butterhead varieties such as Boston types and Bib	1 head	220	95.1	23	2	0.3	—	—	—	4.1	15
Chopped or shredded	1 cup	55	95.1	8	0.7	0.1	—	—	—	1.4	5
Crisp head, as Iceberg	1 head	567	95.5	70	4.8	0.5	—	—	—	15.6	48
Sm. chunks	1 cup	75	95.5	10	0.7	0.1	—	—	—	2.2	7
Looseleaf (bunching varieties including Cos or Romaine)	1 cup	55	94	10	0.7	0.2	—	—	—	1.9	5
Mushrooms											
Agaricus campestris (commercial), raw, chopped or diced	1 cup	70	90.4	20	1.9	0.2	—	—	—	3.1	11
Mustard greens, raw	3.5 oz.[38]	100	89.5	31	2.9	0.5	—	—	—	5.6	32
Okra											
Raw, crosscut slices	1 cup	100	88.9	36	2.4	0.3	—	—	—	7.6	3
Cooked, drained	1 cup	160	91.1	46	3.2	0.5	—	—	—	9.6	3[34]
Onions											
Mature											
Raw, chopped	1 cup	170	89.1	65	2.6	0.2	—	—	—	14.8	17
	2 Tbsp.	21	89.1	8	0.3	.03	—	—	—	1.9	2
Cooked, drained, whole or sliced	1 cup	210	91.8	61	2.5	0.2	—	—	—	13.7	15[34]

Food	Measure	Weight (g)	Water	Calories	Protein	Fat	Carbohydrate				
Young green (bunching varieties), raw	1 cup	100	89.4	36	1.5	0.2	8.2	—	—	—	5
Parsley, raw, chopped	2 Tbsp.	12	89.4	5	.19	.03	1	—	—	—	.63
	1 cup	60	85.1	26	2.2	0.4	5.1	—	—	—	27
	1 Tbsp.	4	85.1	2	0.1	T	0.3	—	—	—	2
Parsnips, cooked, drained, diced or 2-in. lengths	1 cup	155	82.2	102	2.3	0.8	23.1	—	—	—	12[34]
Peas, green											
Raw	1 cup	145	78	122	9.1	0.6	20.9	—	—	—	3
Cooked, drained	1 cup	160	81.5	114	8.6	0.6	19.4	—	—	—	2[34]
Canned (drained solids)	1 cup	170	77	150	8	0.7	28.6	—	—	—	401[35]
Peppers, sweet											
Raw, sliced	1 cup	80	93.4	18	1	0.2	3.8	—	—	—	10
Cooked, drained	1 cup	135	94.7	24	1.4	0.3	5.1	—	—	—	12
Potato, cooked											
Baked, in skin	1 potato	202	75.1	145	4	0.2	32.8	—	—	—	6[34]
Boiled, in skin	1 potato	150	79.8	104	2.9	0.1	23.3	—	—	—	4[34]
Mashed, milk added	1 cup	210	82.8	137	4.4	1.5	27.3	—	—	—	632
Pumpkin, canned	1 cup	245	90.2	81	2.5	0.7	19.4	—	—	—	5[36]
Radishes, medium, raw	10 radishes	50	94.5	8	0.5	T	1.6	—	—	—	8
	5 radishes	25	94.5	4	.25	T	0.8	—	—	—	4
Sauerkraut, canned	1 cup	235	92.8	42	2.4	0.5	9.4	—	—	—	1,755[37]
Spinach											
Raw, chopped	1 cup	55	90.7	14	1.8	0.2	2.4	—	—	—	39
Cooked, drained	1 cup	180	92	41	5.4	0.5	6.5	—	—	—	90[34]
Canned (drained solids)	1 cup	205	91.4	49	5.5	1.2	7.4	—	—	—	484[35]
Sprouts											
Alfalfa, raw	1 cup	100	—	41	5.1	0.6	—	—	—	—	—
Mung bean	1 cup	105	88.8	37	4	0.2	6.9	—	—	—	5
Squash											
Summer varieties, cooked, drained, diced and drained	1 cup	180	85.5	25	1.6	0.2	5.6	—	—	—	2[34]
Winter varieties, cooked (baked), mashed	1 cup	205	81.4	129	3.7	0.8	31.6	—	—	—	2[34]
Sweet potato											
Baked, with skin	1 potato	146	63.7	161	2.4	0.6	.37	—	—	—	14

FOOD PRODUCT[1]	AMOUNT	WEIGHT IN GRAMS	WATER (PERCENT)	FOOD ENERGY (CALORIES)	PROTEIN (GRAMS)	FAT (GRAMS)	(TOTAL) SATURATED (GRAMS)	UNSATURATED OLEIC (GRAMS)	UNSATURATED LINOLEIC (GRAMS)	CARBOHYDRATES (GRAMS)	SODIUM (MILLIGRAMS)
Tomato, raw	1 tomato -	135	93.5	26	1.3	0.2	—	—	—	5.6	4
Canned, solids and liquids	1 cup ---	241	93.7	51	2.4	0.5	—	—	—	10.4	313
Tomato juice, cocktail											
Canned or bottled	1 cup ---	243	93	51	1.7	0.2	—	—	—	12.2	486
Turnips, raw	1 cup ---	130	91.5	39	1.3	0.3	—	—	—	8.6	64
Cooked, diced, drained	1 cup ---	155	93.6	36	1.2	0.3	—	—	—	7.6	53[34]
Turnip greens											
Raw	3.5 oz.[38] -	100	90.3	28	2.9	0.3	—	—	—	4.9	10
Cooked, drained	1 cup ---	145	93.2	29	3.2	0.3	—	—	—	5.2	—[34]
Watercress, raw, leaves including stems	1 cup ---	35	93.3	7	0.8	0.1	—	—	—	1.1	18

Footnotes

1. For each food product, the tabulated information includes the description of the item, the approximate measure or unit, the corresponding weight in grams, and the values for the edible parts of the food.
2. Boldface items allowed on Diet Center's Reducing Diet.

BREADS, FLOURS, CEREALS, AND GRAINS

3. Based on revised value per 100 gm. Value for Bran Flakes: sodium 590 mg.
4. Values taken from box panel and figured on percentage of U.S. RDA.
5. Based on value of 205 mg. per 100 gm. for product cooked with salt added as specified by manufacturers. If cooked without added salt, value is negligible.
6. Values based on ingredients of Diet Center recipe.
7. Value applies to product cooked in unsalted water.
8. Applies to product cooked in salt added as specified by manufacturers. If cooked without salt, value is negligible.

DAIRY PRODUCTS

9. Values for sodium are based on use of 1.5% anhydrous disodium phosphate as emulsifying agent. If emulsifying agent does not contain sodium, calculate content of this nutrient from these amounts per 100 gm.; sodium 650 mg.
10. Values for sodium are based on use of 1.5% anhydrous disodium phosphate as emulsifying agent. If emulsifying agent does not contain sodium, calculate content of this nutrient from these amounts per 100 gm.; sodium 1,139 mg.
11. Values for sodium are based on use of 1.5% anhydrous disodium phosphate as emulsifying agent. If emulsifying agent does not contain sodium, calculate content of this nutrient from these amounts per 100 gm.; sodium 682 mg.
12. Made with 1½ Tbsp. milk, ½ tsp. fat and dash of salt.
13. Value for product without added salt.
14. Made with 8 oz. whole milk, one egg, and 3 tsp. sugar.

FISH, SEAFOOD, AND SEAWEED

15. Four oz. raw is equivalent to 3½ oz. cooked.
16. Sodium content varies in canned products; check the label.
17. Based on frozen scallops, possibly brined.
18. Sodium content for shrimp taken from Salt Counter & Diet Book, by Lakewoods.
19. Sodium content taken from Ralston Purina Company, Pamphlet 1980.
20. Sodium content taken from Understanding Nutrition, by West.

FRUITS

21. Without artificial sweetener.
22. Sweetened with nutritive sweetener.

MEAT AND POULTRY

23. Values vary widely in meat (fat and lean) especially beef.
24. Values taken from the USDA Handbook #8–5.

NUT PRODUCTS AND SEEDS

25. Most of phosphorus in nuts, legumes, and outer layers of cereal grains is present.

26. Liquid from mixture of coconut meat and water.
27. Oxalic acid present may combine with calcium and magnesium to form insoluble compounds.
28. Data do not apply to product salted in shell.
29. Applies to unsalted nuts. For salted nuts, value for 1 cup of kernels is approx. 280 mg.; for 1 lb., 907 mg.; for 1 oz., 57 mg.
30. All nuts and seeds are unsalted, unless stated otherwise. For salted nuts, the sodium content is approx. 280 mg. per cup.

SALAD DRESSINGS AND SAUCES

31. Note: Soy sauce is high in sodium. Soy sauce allowed on Reducing Diet only in moderation, just a drop.
32. Applies to regular pack. For volume measures that apply to special dietary pack (low sodium), values for 12-oz. bottle range from 14 to 119 mg.; for No. 10 can from 163 to 1,141 mg.; for 1 cup, from 14 to 96 mg.; for 1 tsp. from 1 to 5 mg.; for 1 lb. 23 to 159 mg.

SOUPS

33. Note: High level of sodium (salt) in canned soups.

VEGETABLES

34. Value is for unsalted product. If salt is used, increase value by 236 mg. per 100 gm. of vegetable — an estimated figure based on typical amount of salt (0.6%) in canned vegetables.
35. Estimated value based on addition of salt in amount of 0.6% of finished product.
36. Applies to product without added salt. If salt is added, value for sodium estimated on basis of 236 mg. per 100 gm. is 1,070 mg. for 1-lb. can, 1,940 mg. for 29-oz. can, 7,092 for 16-oz. can, 578 mg. for 1 cup.
37. Values for sauerkraut are based on salt content of 1.9 and 2.0%, respectively, in finished products. Amounts in some samples may vary significantly from this estimate.
38. 3.5 oz. is for weight of product.

Index

Italics refer to recipes.